CORONARY ARTERY BYPASS GRAFTING

Collected Reprints (1972-2022)

By

William C. Roberts, MD

and

Colleagues

ISBN: 979-8-88680-078-4
Printed in the United States of America on acid-free paper.

Preface

This procedure revolutionized therapy for coronary heart disease. It was the first to successfully treat symptoms of coronary disease with an operative procedure, not a drug. The credit goes to Argentine Renè Favaloro, who at the time was working at the Cleveland Clinic. Initially, only one aortocoronary conduit was used, but rapidly the number of conduits and coronary anastomotic sites increased, providing more blood to the myocardium and better outcomes. A major innovation in the procedure came when it became apparent that the internal mammary artery was a much better conduit than the saphenous vein. Indeed, some believe the reason coronary bypass works so well is because of the use of an internal mammary artery as a conduit. What is it about the internal mammary artery that makes it such a magnificent conduit is unclear. The same cholesterol level presumably flows down the internal mammary conduit as the saphenous venous conduit, yet the latter narrows with time and the internal mammary artery does not.

Although coronary bypass is the most common cardiac operation performed, it is not the easiest cardiac operation. Some surgeons have a hard time with the procedure.

Despite its existence for >40 years, the amount of blood added to the myocardium by coronary bypass remains unclear. Coronary angioplasty with stent placement provides a splendid alternative to coronary bypass for many patients.

—William C. Roberts, MD

Table of Contents

*Articles are numbered based on WCR's CV.

The cause of luminal narrowing in internal mammary arteries implanted into canine myocardium

John W. Yarbrough, M.D.
William C. Roberts, M.D.
Ronald M. Abel, M.D.
Robert L. Reis, M.D.
Bethesda, Md.

Intimal proliferation has been implicated as a limiting factor in blood flow through internal mammary arteries implanted into myocardium. The cause of the proliferation is uncertain. This report summarizes observations from histologic examination of internal mammary arterial implants into canine myocardium, and provides evidence that thrombosis is the cause of the luminal narrowing.

Materials and methods

Bilateral internal mammary arterial implants were examined at necropsy in 6 mongrel dogs. In each animal one artery had been implanted deeply (average 8.9 ± 2.0 mm. [mean ± S.D.]) into the left ventricular myocardium, and the other one superficially (2.4 ± 0.7 mm.) into the subepicardial muscle (Figs. 1 and 2). Each mammary artery had been dissected from its origin from the subclavian artery to its epigastric bifurcation. No side holes had been made in it, and its distal branches were left patent. Each artery had been implanted over a length of 4 to 5 cm. in the left ventricular wall. The right internal mammary artery had been implanted

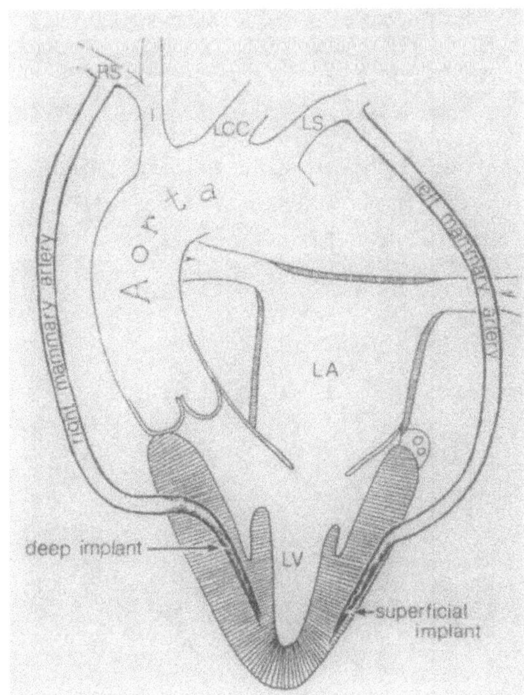

Fig. *1*. Diagram of left side of heart and ascending and transverse aorta illustrating the manner in which the internal mammary arteries were implanted into the left ventricular (*LV*) wall. *I* = innominate artery; *LA* = left atrium; *LCC* = left common carotid artery; *LS* = left subclavian artery; and *RS* = right subclavian artery.

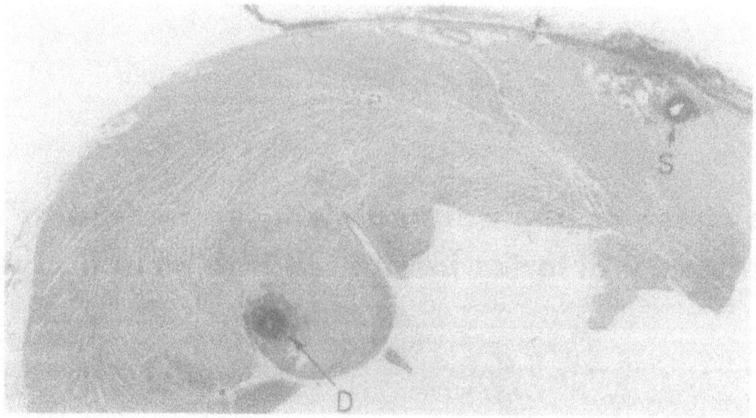

Fig. 2. Photomicrograph of transverse section of canine left ventricle showing location of the superficial (*S*) and deep (*D*) internal mammary implants. (Elastic tissue stain; ×3.)

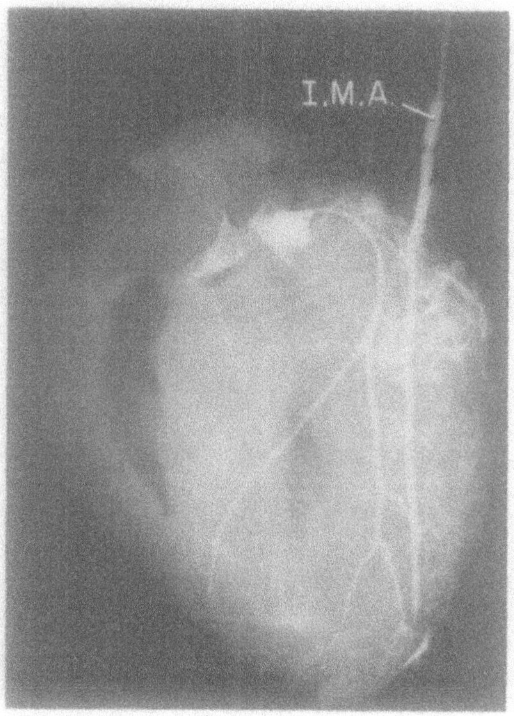

Fig. 3. Postmortem radiograph of heart taken after injection of contrast material into the internal mammary artery (*I.M.A.*) implanted into left ventricle. The lumen of the implanted artery is severely narrowed near the left ventricular apex. The left coronary artery is opacified by retrograde filling from the implanted internal mammary artery.

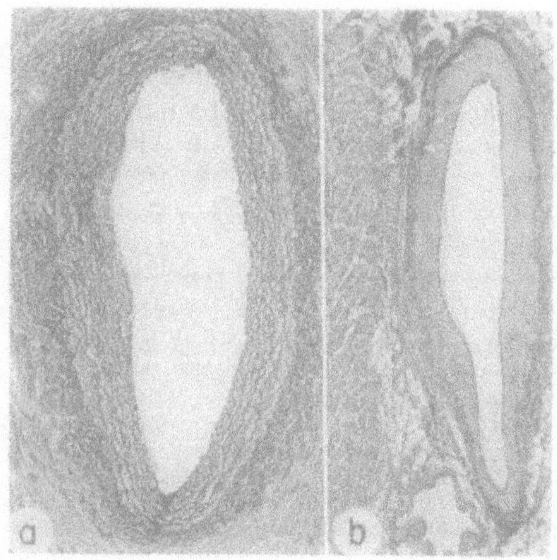

Fig. 4. Normal canine internal mammary artery (*a*) and normal coronary artery (*b*). The mammary is an elastic artery and the coronary, a muscular artery. (Elastic tissue stains; *a*, ×40; *b*, ×35.)

anterolaterally and the left, posterolaterally. The sequence of the depth of implantation of the arteries had been alternated for the right and left sides. Ameroid constrictors had been applied to the anterior descending and circumflex coronary arteries in one dog. The coronary arteries of the other 5 animals were not altered.

Seventeen months (506 ± 4 days) after mammary arterial implantation the dogs were studied hemodynamically.[1] Thereafter, each was put to death, and postmortem angiograms were performed after separate injection of contrast material into each of the implanted mammary arteries. The hearts and internal mammary arteries then were fixed in 10 per cent buffered formalin. After fixation each 4 to 5 cm. segment of implanted mammary artery into myocardium was cut, processed, em-

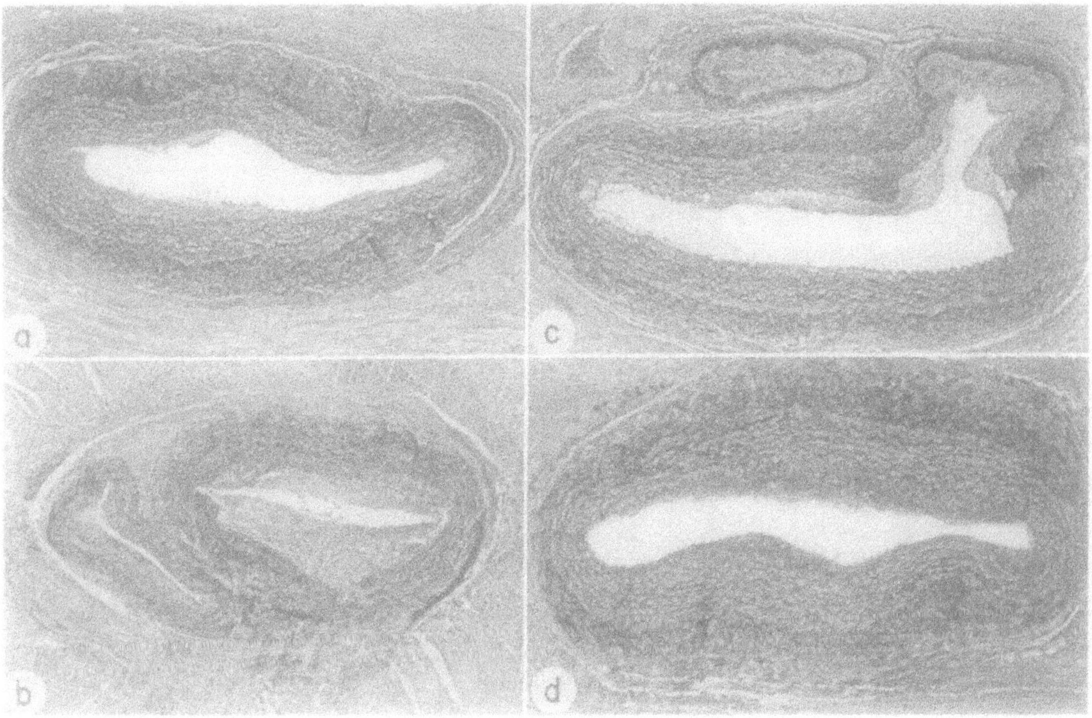

Fig. 5. Implanted internal mammary arteries in a dog in which the anterior descending and left circumflex coronary arteries had been narrowed by an Ameroid constrictor before implantation. *a*, Superficial implanted artery proximally. *b*, Superficial implanted artery distally. At this point the lumen is considerably narrowed by fibrous tissue devoid of elastic fibrils. *c*, Deep implanted artery proximally. A small branch, which shows mild intimal thickening, is arising at this point. *d*, Deep implanted artery distally. Only mild intimal proliferation is present. (Elastic tissue stains; *a*, ×50; *b* and *c*, ×45; and *d*, ×60.)

bedded, and sectioned at 6 micron intervals. Every even tenth section was stained by hematoxylin and eosin, and every odd tenth section by Verhoeff–van Gieson.

Results

Postmortem angiograms disclosed evidence of terminal narrowing in each of the 12 implanted mammary arteries. Nevertheless, retrograde filling of the coronary arteries occurred after injection of contrast material into each of the implanted mammary arteries (Fig. 3).

Both gross and histologic examination of each implanted mammary artery (elastic arteries in contrast to coronary arteries which are muscular arteries [Fig. 4]) showed varying degrees of luminal narrowing. The narrowing was least severe in the two internal mammary arteries implanted into the dog in which the left coronary arteries had previously been narrowed by Ameroid constrictors (Fig. 5). The luminal narrowing of the implanted internal mammary arteries consisted of fibrous tissue containing generally numerous elastic fibrils but no lipid deposits, cholesterol clefts, or calcific deposits (Figs. 6 to 9). Although some degree of intimal fibrous proliferation occurred along the entire length of the intramyocardial implants, the severest degrees of narrowing occurred at the most distal portions of the implants (Figs. 6 to 9). No fibrin or platelet aggregates were found in the lumens of any implanted mammary artery. In several implanted arteries, multiple luminal channels were present (Fig. 9). The media of all implanted arteries appeared normal, but usually the adventitia was obscured by dense fibrous tissue, which was devoid of elastic fibrils.

Comments

Intimal thickening develops within a short period in any internal mammary artery implanted into the myocardium.[2-7] When this artery is implanted into the ischemic myocardium, less intimal thicken-

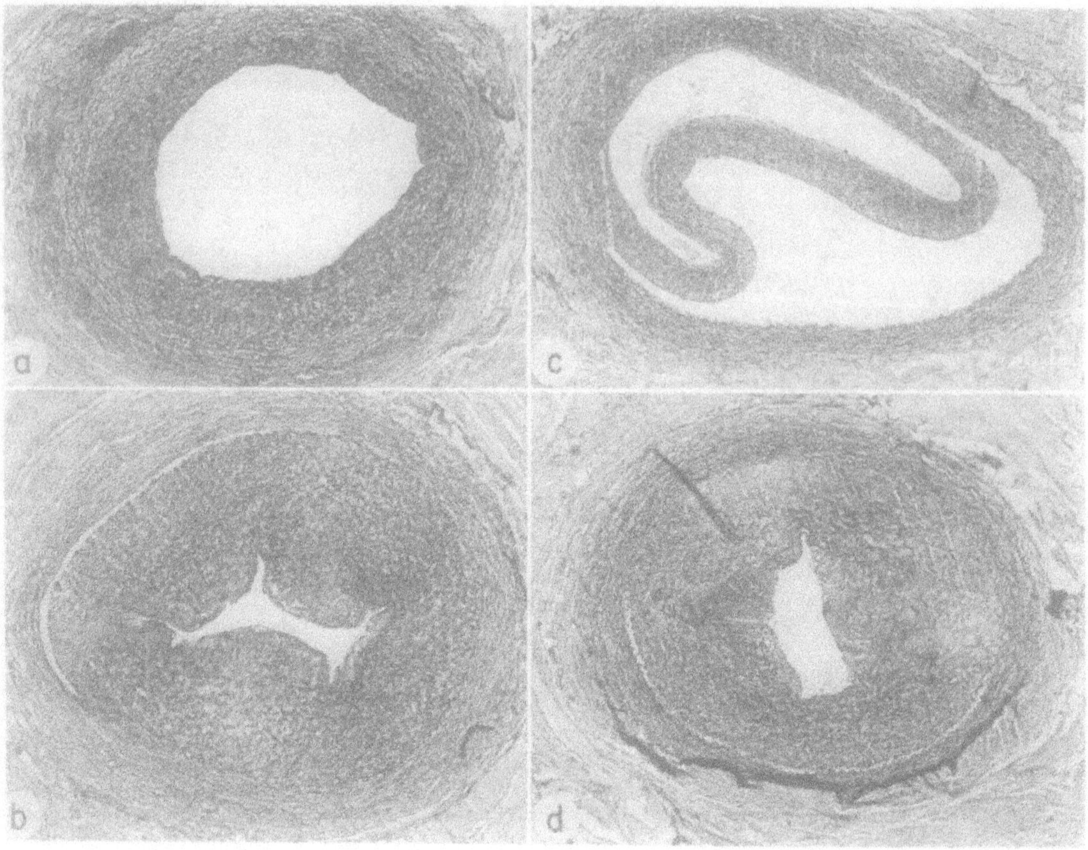

Fig. 6. Implanted internal mammary arteries in another dog. *a*, Proximal superficial implant showing only mild intimal thickening. *b*, Distal superficial implant showing severe intimal thickening by fibroelastic tissue. *c*, Proximal deep implant. The thin band of thickened intima partially dislodged. The disruption probably occurred at the time of arteriography. *d*, Distal deep implant showing severe intimal thickening by fibroelastic tissue. Generally, the degree of intimal thickening was similar in both superficial and deep implants. (Elastic tissue stains; each ×40.)

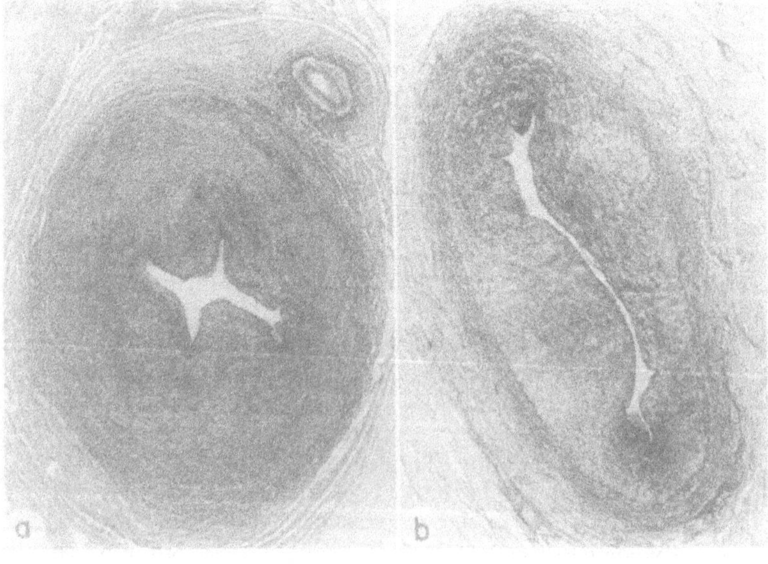

Fig. 7. Distal superficial (*a*) and deep (*b*) internal mammary implants in another dog. Each shows severe degrees of initimal thickening by fibrous tissue containing many elastic fibrils. (Elastic tissue stains; each ×40.)

ing occurs than when it is implanted into nonischemic myocardium.[7] The cause of the intimal thickening has been uncertain. Degeneration of the internal mammary artery itself due to lack of nutrition to its wall, trauma to the artery inflicted either at the time of implantation or by effects of ventricular contraction or dilatation, and thrombosis have been suggested as possible causes.

The present study provides evidence that the cause of the intimal proliferation in the implanted arteries is in situ thrombosis. The major evidence supporting organization of thrombi as the cause is the finding of multiple vascular channels within the intimal connective tissue (Fig. 9). Multiple luminal channels in arteries have long been recognized as the hallmark of organization of thrombi[8] (Fig. 10). The connective tissue in the lumens of the implanted internal mammary arteries with multiple luminal channels is similar to that in the vessels containing only one vascular channel, which suggests that the cause of each is similar. No fibrin or platelet aggregates, known components of thrombi, were observed in the implanted internal mammary arteries, but the 17 month interval between implantation and death of the animals provided more than enough time for organization into fibrous tissue. Actually, it would be surprising if thrombus did not form in the distal portions of the tunnelled internal mammary arteries since flow of blood at these sites at least initially is considerably slowed. Also, after induced myocardial infarction in the dog, marked reduction of flow in the anatomically patent coronary artery supplying the area of infarction occurs and this relative stasis may be responsible for thrombus formation in this vessel.[9] Injection of either fibrin or whole blood clots into systemic veins of rabbits also produces fibrous tissue within the pulmonary arteries similar to that observed in the internal mammary arteries implanted into the canine myocardium.[10]

Nachlas and associates[11] demonstrated that carotid arteries of dogs remained patent if implanted into the left ventricular myocardium and allowed to drain into the right ventricular cavity. Arteries implanted into the left ventricular myocardium, however, without distal egress or ones that had

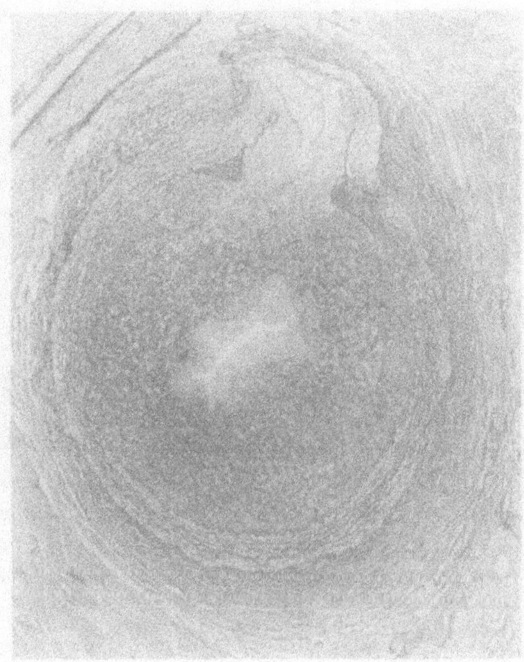

Fig. 8. Distal deep internal mammary implant in another dog. The lumen is severely narrowed, peripherally by fibroelastic tissue, but centrally by fibrous tissue devoid of elastic fibrils. The lumen of the small branch also is narrowed by fibrous tissue containing few elastic fibrils. (Elastic tissue stain; ×40.)

the distal lumen obstructed became occluded and developed intimal thickening. These authors concluded that intimal thickening did not develop from trauma by the contracting myocardium but from a lack of continuous blood flow through the vessel. From these reported findings plus the recanalization in the implanted arteries in the present experiments and others,[6] it would appear that stasis of blood in the implanted artery proceeds to thrombosis with later organization.

Summary

Attention is called to the cause of intimal thickening observed in the internal mammary arteries implanted in the myocardiums of 6 dogs. Each of the 12 implanted arteries showed varying degrees of fibrous intimal thickening, and several contained numerous channels. The multiple luminal channels strongly suggest that the intimal thickening was the result of organization of thrombi. The intimal thickening was less in the one animal in which the left coronary artery had been constricted before internal mammary artery implantation.

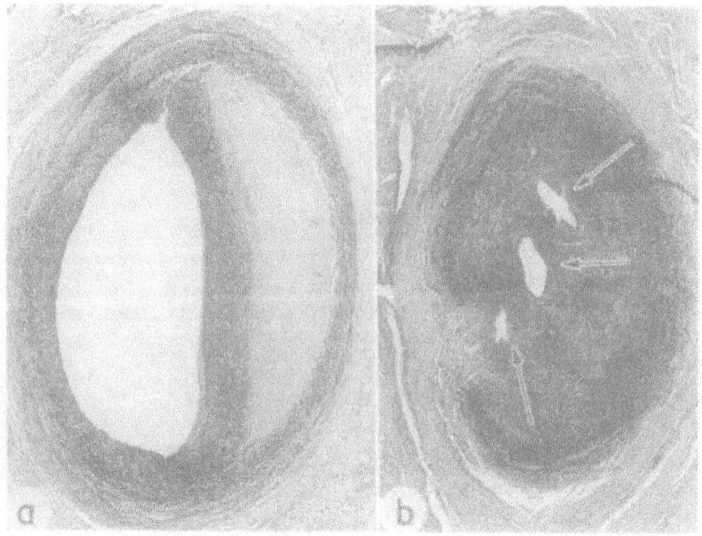

Fig. *9*. Intimal fibrous thickening in a deeply implanted internal mammary artery in another dog. *a*, Proximally. Here the luminal narrowing is caused primarily by fibrous tissue containing no elastic fibrils, although the "cap" over this fibrous tissue contains numerous elastic fibrils. *b*, Distally. The lumen at this point is occluded except for channels (arrows). The presence of the multiple channels strongly suggests that the intimal thickening resulted from organization of a thrombus. (Elastic tissue stains; *a*, ×42; *b*, ×40.)

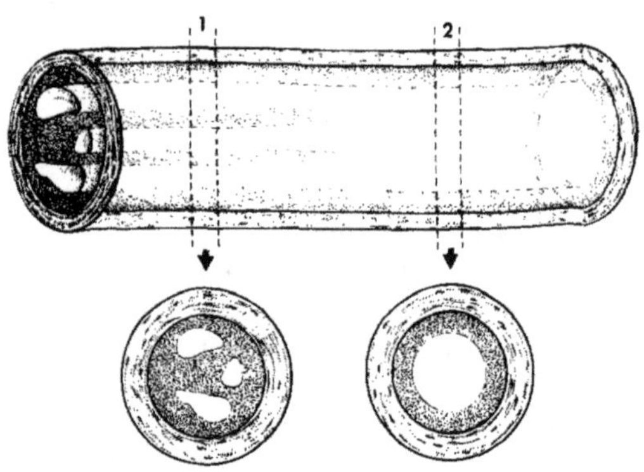

Fig. *10*. The multi- and unichanneled artery. Duguid,[12] when studying coronary arterial serial sections of an "organized thrombus," noted that the tissue present between channels was similar to that found in arteries with only one channel. Since the multichannel artery had been recognized as the hallmark of an organized thrombus, and since the tissue in both multi- and unichanneled arteries was similar, he reasoned that the causative process also was similar.

REFERENCES

1. Abel, R. M., Reis, R. L., Yarbrough, J. W., Staroscik, R. N., and Rodgers, B. M.: Determinants of flow through internal mammary artery implants, Submitted to Ann. Surg.
2. Provan, J. L.: Mammary-coronary anastomosis. A short histological study, Br. J. Surg. **49:**199, 1961.
3. Maruyama, Y., Warren, R., McCombs, H. L., Vickery, C. M., and Brener, B. J.: Morphologic observations of internal mammary artery-myocardial implantation, Surg. Gynecol. Obstet. **125:**799, 1966.
4. Patt, H. H., Golberg, M., Clift, J. V., and Lourvantij, B.: An evaluation of implantation of the internal mammary artery into the myocardium of pigs and dogs, J. Thorac. Surg. **35:**699, 1958.
5. Spencer, F. C.: A critique of implantation of a systemic artery for myocardial revascularization, Progr. Cardiovasc. Dis. **11:**351, 1969.
6. Criollos, R. L., Al-Shamma, A. M., and Roe, B. B.: Quantitative studies of extracoronary blood flow after double internal mammary artery implantation, Circulation **37** and **38** (Suppl. II):27 and 32, 1968.
7. Piccone, V. A., LeVeen, H. H., Potter, R. T., Falk, G., Manoli, A., and Oran, E.: Multiparameter evaluation of internal mammary artery implant function. An experimental study, Ann. Thorac. Surg. **8:**327, 1969.
8. Geiringer, E.: Intimal vascularization and atherosclerosis, J. Pathol. **63:**201, 1951.
9. Hellstrom, H. R.: Coronary artery stasis after induced myocardial infarction in the dog, Cardiovasc. Res. **5:**371, 1971.
10. Harrison, C. V.: Experimental pulmonary arteriosclerosis, J. Pathol. **60:**289, 1948.
11. Nachlas, M. M., Myers, M. J., Solomon, R. D., Kelly, A. B., and Seligman, A. M.: Maintenance of patency of carotid arteries implanted into the myocardium, J. Thorac. Surg. **35:**706, 1959.
12. Duguid, J. B.: Thrombosis as a factor in the pathogenesis of coronary atherosclerosis, J. Pathol. **58:**207, 1946.

Lesions Observed in Arterial Autogenous Vein Grafts

Light and Electron Microscopic Evaluation

By Michael Jones, M.D., David M. Conkle, M.D.,
Victor J. Ferrans, M.D., Ph.D., William C. Roberts, M.D., Frederick H. Levine, M.D.,
David B. Melvin, M.D., and Edward B. Stinson, M.D.

SUMMARY

Autogenous vein grafts used for canine femoral and aortocoronary arterial bypasses were evaluated from 2 to 365 days postoperatively. Femoral grafts showed focal endothelial disruption, mural fibrin deposition, and medial edema with inflammatory infiltrates during the first week; loss of medial smooth muscle cells and focal subendothelial lesions with intact endothelium by 2 weeks; and diffuse subendothelial lesions by 12 weeks, Coronary grafts studied at 6, 9, and 12 months had medial fibrosis and extensive intimal proliferation causing up to 90% luminal narrowing. Extension of the intimal process into the coronary artery distal to the bypass graft also compromised the arterial lumen. Coronary grafts obtained from humans dying 17 and 57 days after graft insertion revealed a similar subendothelial proliferation.

Electron microscopy showed that the subendothelial lesions were composed of mature smooth muscle cells and collagen primarily oriented parallel to the axis of blood flow. Recurrent endothelial cell damage, followed by mural fibrin deposition and organization, appears to be the cause of the subendothelial proliferative lesions.

Additional Indexing Words:

Subendothelial proliferation · Coronary arterial bypass graft · Mural thrombi · Luminal narrowing · Femoral arterial bypass graft · Fibrin deposition · Smooth muscle cells · Intimal thickening · Elastin · Collagen · Inflammatory infiltrates · Medial edema

STIMULATED BY the apparent success of femoral arterial bypass grafts using autologous saphenous veins, the aortocoronary bypass operation came into use and is now a common procedure. Partial or complete obstruction of the graft is a recognized and much too frequent complication of this operation. Because the etiology of the luminal narrowing in the bypass grafts has been debated, a detailed morphological evaluation of the lesions occurring in the walls of the transplanted veins was undertaken. Light and electron microscopic observations in the bypassing conduits (28 canine and 4 human) are described in the report which follows.

Materials and Methods

Autogenous grafts were obtained from saphenous or external jugular veins of 22 foxhounds weighing 15 to 22 kg. All vein grafts were reversed. Coronary arterial bypass grafts were anastomosed to the anterior descending coronary artery just distal to the first diagonal branch, using hypothermic anoxic cardiac arrest and cardiopulmonary bypass; the coronary artery proximal to the bypass was ligated. For peripheral arterial bypasses, a 3-cm segment of saphenous vein was substituted for a similar portion of the superficial femoral artery in the femoral triangle.

Canine tissues studied histologically consisted of control saphenous and external jugular veins (16); patent femoral arterial bypasses (16) obtained after 2 days and after 1, 2, 4, 8, and 12 weeks; patent coronary arterial bypass grafts (3) obtained at 6, 9, and 12 months; and occluded coronary arterial bypass grafts (9) obtained 1 to 9 months postoperatively. In addition, patent coronary arterial bypass grafts (4) were examined from 2 patients who died 17 and 57 days after operation. The patients had been anticoagulated with warfarin sodium beginning on the second postoperative day. The dogs in both the coronary and the femoral series received a single heparin dose of 200 units per kg at operation.

For light microscopy, all specimens were fixed in buffered 10% formalin, processed in alcohols and xylene, embedded in paraffin, and subserially sectioned. Selected 1- to 2-mm portions from each specimen were also processed for electron microscopy.

Results

The intima in control saphenous and external jugular veins consisted of an attenuated single layer

From the Clinic of Surgery and the Section of Pathology, National Heart and Lung Institute, National Institutes of Health, Bethesda, Maryland 20014.

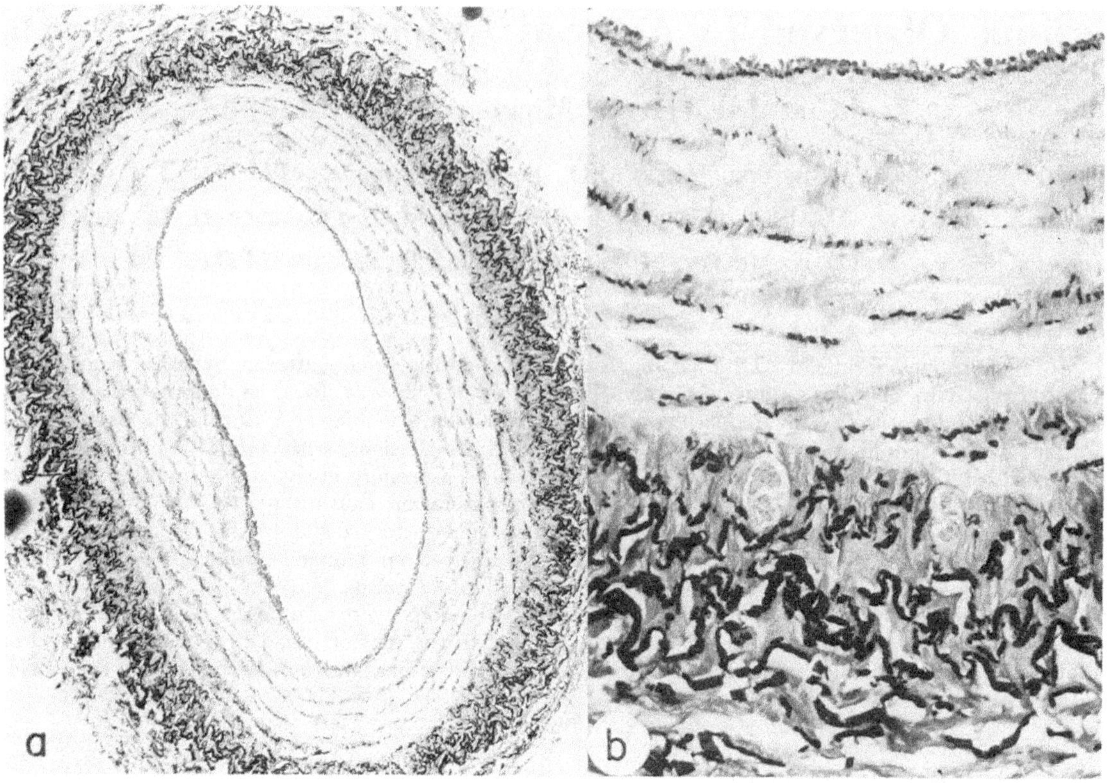

Figure 1

Normal canine saphenous vein, showing its single-cell–layered endothelium, rudimentary internal elastic membrane, concentric layers of smooth muscle, alternating with lamellae containing collagen and scant elastic fibers. Note vasa vasorum in the adventitia of **b**. *Elastic–Van Gieson stain,* × *52* (**a**), × *208* (**b**).

of endothelial cells separated from the media by a rudimentary internal elastic membrane. The media of the external jugular vein consisted of 6 to 10 concentric layers of smooth muscle cells alternating with lamellae of collagen and ground substance; these lamellae, characteristic of veins, contained only scant elastic fibers. Elastic fibers were more prominent in the adventitial layer, interlacing loosely with bands of collagen and occasional capillaries of the vasa vasorum. The saphenous vein, similarly composed but somewhat thicker, had 10 to 15 rows of smooth muscle cells. No control veins showed intimal thickening or medial fibrosis.

All vein bypasses were thicker than control veins, but much of the increased thickness was due to perivascular fibrosis and scarring. Aneurysmal dilatations were not found in any graft. During the first 2 weeks, medial edema, necrotic smooth muscle cells, and inflammatory infiltrates were apparent. Fibroblasts were rarely present in the media of control veins; however, concurrent with the loss of many smooth muscle cells, the media became infiltrated by spindle-shaped cells. Many of these cells had ultrastructural features typical of active fibroblasts. Other cells, however, resembled smooth muscle cells in that they contained thin myofilaments, 60 to 80 Å in diameter, but they also contained more organelles than did normal smooth muscle cells. Medial hypertrophy, as manifested by an increased size or number of smooth muscle cells or increased medial width, was never observed. Soon after transplantation some myocytes did show a transient increase in the dense bodies associated with the myofilaments, which suggests a hypertrophic change. In femoral bypass grafts examined after 3 months, and in the coronary arterial bypass grafts examined after 6 to 12 months, the media was reduced in thickness and the intercellular lamellae were widened and contained more collagen. The media had become focally sclerosed, especially near suture lines.

By 2 weeks, proliferative lesions were identified in the subendothelial space above the rudimentary internal elastic membrane. Most cells of these subendothelial thickenings were mature smooth muscle cells, identified by their blue cytoplasm with

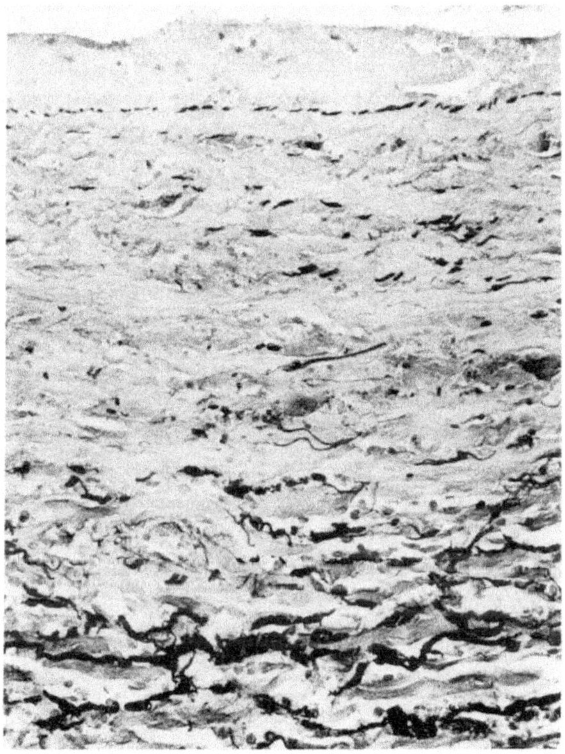

Figure 2

Canine saphenous vein femoral arterial bypass after one week's implantation. Endothelium has sloughed, and the internal elastic membrane is covered by a layer of fibrin; medial disorganization is apparent, reflecting edema and smooth muscle necrosis. Elastic–Van Gieson stain, × 224.

phosphotungstic acid–hematoxylin staining and by their ultrastructural morphology: myofilaments, dense bodies along the cytoplasmic membrane, basal laminae, pinocytotic vesicles, and perinuclear localization of mitochondria, endoplasmic reticulum, and ribosomes. The smooth muscle cells and their myofilaments were oriented parallel to the axis of blood flow. The extracellular space of the subendothelial proliferative lesions consisted of ground substance, collagen, microfibrils measuring approximately 100 Å in diameter, and, rarely, elastin; like the smooth muscle cells, the collagen was primarily oriented in the direction of blood flow.

During the first 2 weeks postoperatively, vein graft endothelium was focally disrupted and often covered by mural fibrin deposition. The intimal thickenings in vein grafts at all intervals had fibrin deposits on the luminal surfaces, beneath the endothelium, and within the proliferative lesions. In several-month-old coronary arterial bypass grafts, serial sections showed that the subendothelial thickening had become generalized, and in some areas significantly[1] compromised the bypass lumen (greater than 90% determined by planimetry). The subendothelial lesions in the late grafts took on an eccentric, laminated appearance suggesting intermittent deposition and organization. The most peripheral portions of the intimal lesions often contained capillaries, hemosiderin, and even calcium. Significantly, the lesions extended across the distal anastomoses into the adjacent arteries; in at least one coronary artery a subendothelial lesion narrowed the lumen at least 70%. Venous valves were noted in the bypasses, but they were not related either to graft occlusion or to proliferative lesions.

All occluded grafts contained elements of organizing thrombi, including fibrin, hemosiderin, and calcific deposits; recanalized channels; and smooth muscle cells. Only one dog with an occluded graft died naturally. The other dogs which had total occlusion of the grafts and of the coronary artery proximal to the grafts were killed 1 to 9 months later. The prolonged survival of these animals suggests that the graft occlusions were gradual.

Patent coronary arterial bypass grafts from 2 patients dying 17 and 57 days postoperatively had subendothelial lesions similar to those in canine vein grafts. In the 57-day-old grafts, the most severely affected portion was 50% narrowed.

Discussion

Johnson, Auer, and Tector[2] first observed in 3 patients a lesion which they called "massive subintimal fibroblastic hyperplasia," and Grondin et al.[3] described marked fibrosis of the vein wall, especially of the intima, in a patient dying 114 days after operation. Several patients have been reoperated because of graft stenosis.[4–6] Vlodaver and Edwards[7] described a fibrous subintimal proliferation characterized by avascular mucoid connective tissue containing "fibroblastic" cells in 29 grafts examined. Marti et al.,[8] studying 8 grafts, observed a similar intimal hyperplasia as well as medial atrophy.

Dedomenico et al.[9] evaluated external jugular coronary grafts in dogs for 4 to 5.5 years and found partial thrombotic occlusion of 1 graft and a threefold increase of medial fibromuscular tissue in 4 other grafts. In canine coronary arterial bypasses, Brody et al.[10] described focal intimal cushions of myointimal cells and early inflammatory and necrotic changes followed by fibrous replacement of the media.

Seven changes have been described in veins implanted as arteries: endothelial damage and disruption, intimal thickening, medial hypertrophy, medial necrosis, graft wall fibrosis, lipid deposition, and aneurysmal dilatation. Nunn et al.[11] studied graft endothelium *en face* and found endothelial cells to be slightly altered and enlarged, but viable, one week after transplantation. Brody et al.,[10] however, noted endothelial vacuolation and swelling, subendothelial edema, focal cell loss, and fibrin deposition.

Carrel and Guthrie[12] described intimal thickening in their first vein grafts performed in 1906, ascribing it to an attempt of the vein to assume the character of an artery. The matrix of the intimal lesion does contain elastic and fibrous tissue, and ground substance exhibiting the metachromasia of arterial mucopolysaccharides.[13, 14] Cells in these intimal lesions have been called fibroblasts by some authors, and smooth muscle cells by others.[15–17] The inference that these changes represent an "arterialization"[18] would appear inappropriate because of (1) the longitudinal orientation of the constituent cells; (2) the failure of the new growth to form circularly oriented layers, but rather longitudinal ones; and (3) diminution of elastic fibers.[19, 20] Extension of intimal lesions into the coronary artery in our study also argues against this process' being an arterialization. The thickened intimal tissue has been present as early as 10 to 20 days after grafting and progressed almost to luminal obliteration by 6 months in some peripheral vein grafts.[21]

Part of the vein graft's wall thickening has been attributed to medial muscular hypertrophy.[12, 22] Later studies would seem to indicate that medial thickening is first caused by edema and inflammatory infiltration and later by fibroblastic infiltration in areas of myocyte necrosis.[10, 23, 24] Late findings include further fibrous transformation of the media.[17, 25] In fact, Sako and Varco[26] reported a vena cava graft which, 10 years after aortic placement, consisted essentially of a fibrous tube. Carrel[25] noted a similar change after only 14 months, and Pena[27] after 6 weeks. Lipid deposition in vein grafts has not been common, and Penn et al.[17] stated that calcification and lipid accumula-

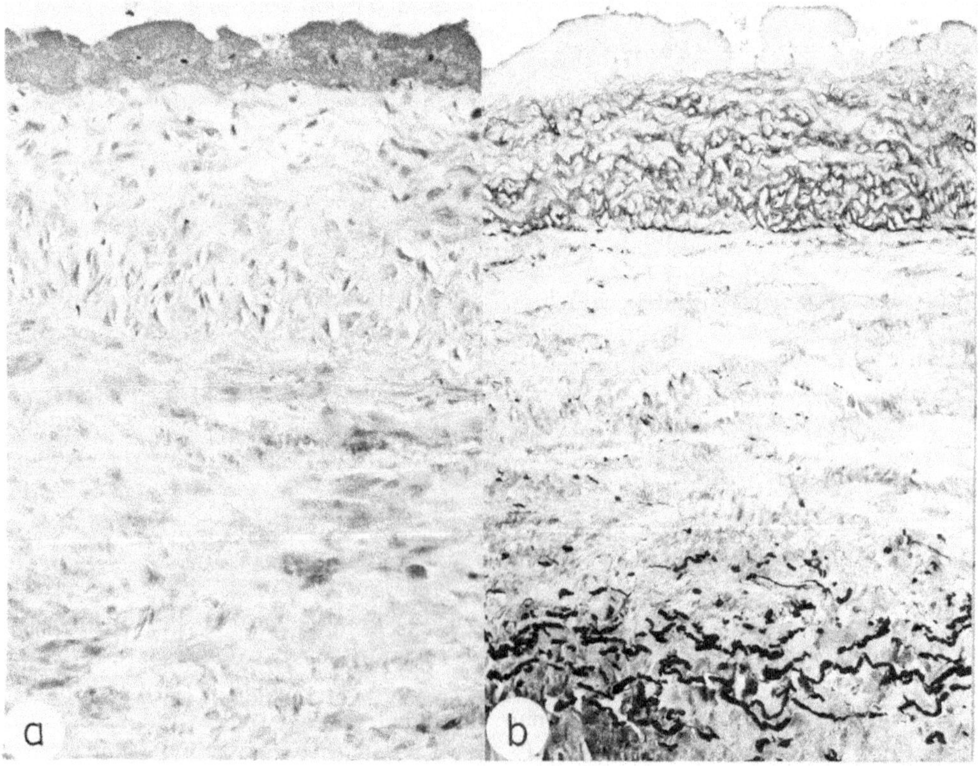

Figure 3

Canine saphenous vein femoral arterial graft at two weeks, with early subendothelial proliferation covered by secondary fibrin deposition. Hematoxylin and eosin stain, × 224 (a); *elastic–Van Gieson stain, × 140* (b).

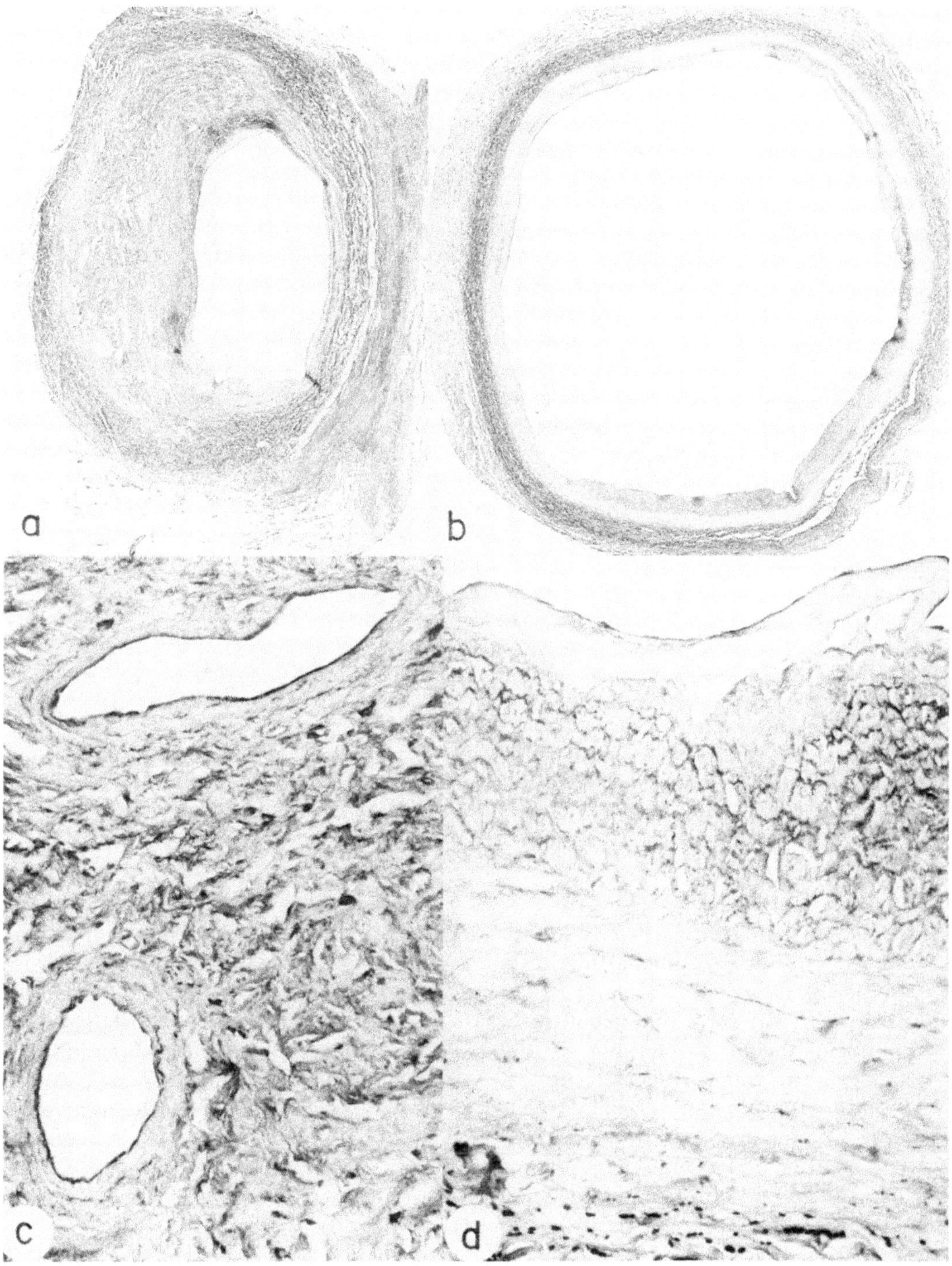

Figure 4

Patent canine external jugular vein coronary arterial bypass graft after 12 months. All sections are stained with elastic–Van Gieson stain. **(a)** *Eccentric, laminated area of about 50% luminal narrowing, with recanalization apparent in the more peripheral area of the subendothelial proliferative lesion at the left (× 108).* **(b)** *Portion of the graft at another site with minimal subendothelial proliferation (× 11).* **(c)** *Higher magnification of recanalized vessels seen in* a *(× 224).* **(d)** *Area of subendothelial proliferation from* b *with endothelialized fibrin (× 224).*

tion did not occur in vein grafts of atherosclerotic dogs. In contrast, Ejrup et al.,[28] McNamara et al.,[29] and Beebe et al.[30] all found intimal or subintimal lipid in human femoral bypass grafts examined several years after operation. Vein graft dilatations have been reported to involve external jugular

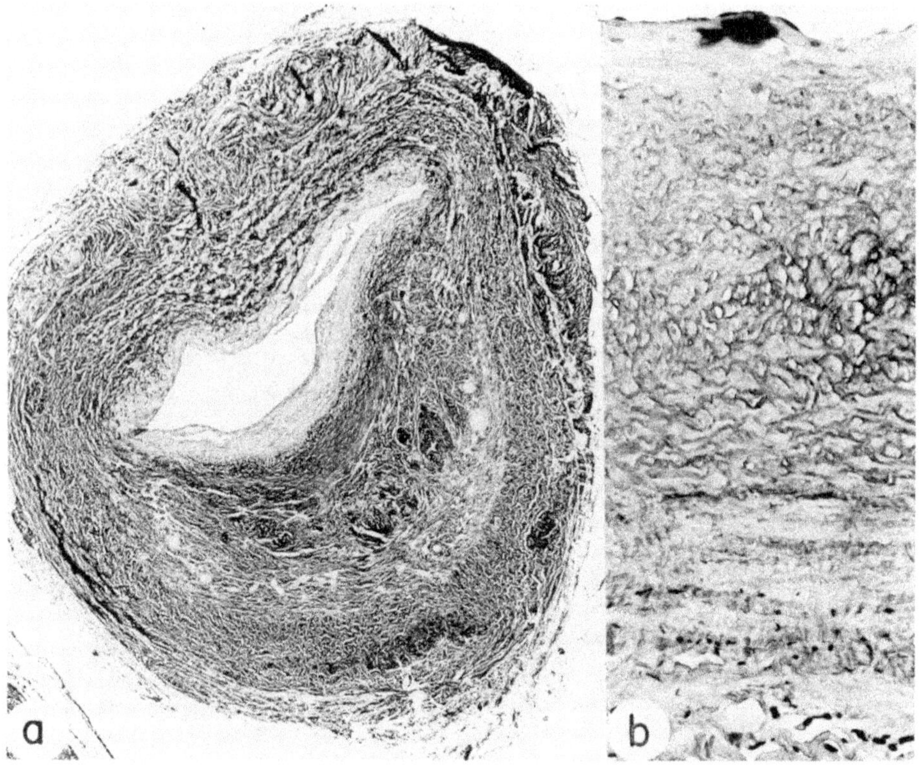

Figure 5

Canine external jugular vein coronary arterial bypasss graft (a) *after nine months, showing significant compromise of the lumen. Phosphotungstic acid–hematoxylin stain,* × *20. Another area* (b) *from the same graft with a threefold increase in the thickness of the vein wall, produced by subendothelial proliferation. A small accumulation of fibrin is apparent beneath the endothelium.*

grafts[9, 31, 32] and inferior vena caval grafts.[33–35] Subsequent clinical experience, particularly with saphenous vein grafts, has not found aneurysm formation to be of significance.[36]

Of the morphological changes in autogenous vein bypass grafts, subendothelial proliferation is the one which may lead to serious clinical complications. In the early stages, the intimal lesions consisted of fibrin, platelets, and necrotic endothelial cells. Later, smooth muscle cells were present along with collagen, ground substance, and occasional accumulations of elastin. Although after 6 to 12 months the smooth muscle cells appeared mature morphologically, a relative immaturity of the lesion was suggested by the appearance of extracellular spaces which contained a large proportion of ground substance, collagen fibrils of small diameter, and a large number of microfibrils. Microfibrils have been implicated as precursors of both collagen and elastin.[37, 38] Smooth muscle cell synthesis of collagen, mucopolysaccharides, basement membrane, and elastin has been demonstrated.[39–43]

Subendothelial proliferation, as we prefer to call the progressive intimal thickening and consequent luminal narrowing of vein graft walls, is characteristic of a number of vascular abnormalities. Veins subjected to increased hydrostatic pressure, such as the saphenous veins, often show intimal thickenings which may progress to the phlebosclerotic lesions of peripheral venous disease and varicosities.[44, 45] Phlebosclerotic lesions should be differentiated from subendothelial proliferation by examining control veins before bypass grafting.[20] Proliferation of intimal smooth muscle cells has been demonstrated experimentally and clinically in small pulmonary arteries in pulmonary hypertension.[46, 47] Because they contain fibrin, the lesions of pulmonary hypertension have been considered to represent the end stage of recurrent organizing thrombi.[48–50] Kapanci[51] and Wagenvoort et al.[48] have suggested that intimal fibrosis in pulmonary vascular disease may be related to thrombus organization. The vessels of chronic systemic hypertension[52] and of

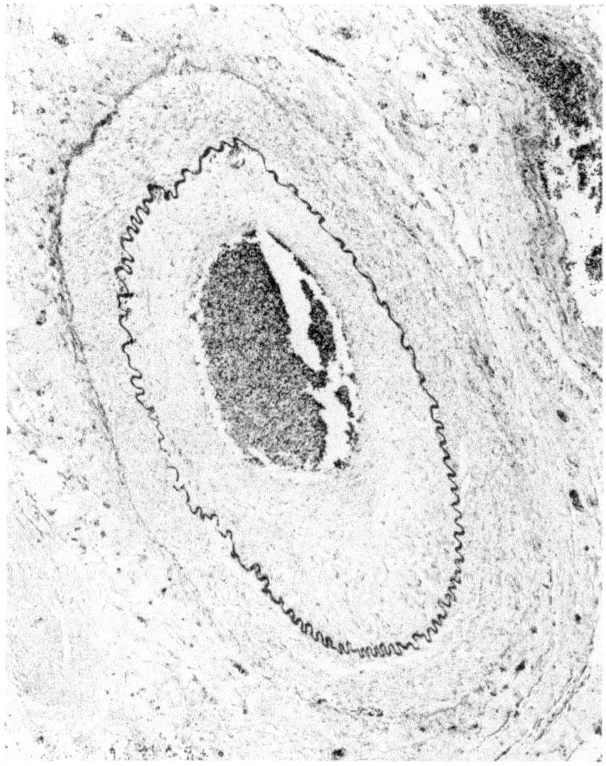

Figure 6

Canine coronary artery distal to the bypass seven months after grafting, with extension of the subendothelial lesion into the coronary artery above its internal elastic membrane. Lumen is 50% narrowed. Note the cellularity of the lesion. Movat stain, × 52.

cardiac homografts[53, 54] may show similar medial and intimal changes.

The lesions in bypass grafts are also similar to the atherosclerotic lesions for which the operation is performed. Foci of fibrous or musculoelastic intimal plaques occur in the arteries of children and progress with age.[55–58] The fibrous plaques resemble intimal thickenings of vein grafts in that both types of lesions contain ground substance of mucopolysaccharides, collagen, elastin (present but in decreased amounts), and smooth muscle cells with a longitudinal orientation.[59–62] Although the relationship of the fibromuscular intimal plaque to atherosclerosis, as defined by lipid accumulation, is not completely clear, it has been well established that smooth muscle cells both in experimental animals and in humans do accumulate lipid and may become foam cells.[63–66]

A variety of vascular injuries may result in thickened subintimal layers.[67] Surgical trauma such as occurs with anastomoses, or even with single sutures, will cause endothelial damage and mural thrombi; medial fibrous transformation follows vessel constriction.[68–70] Endothelial trauma, including flushes and transient preservation of the vein with heparinized saline, produces endothelial changes, including areas of slough.[10, 71] We observed, however, no difference in frequency or degree of subendothelial proliferation in veins left in heparinized saline for two hours and those transplanted immediately. Severing the vein's vasa vasorum, thus making the vein dependent on transmural diffusion from the lumen, has been implicated as the precipitating factor leading to medial necrosis and to endothelial slough,[10] but the vascular wall may be somewhat resistant to hypoxic damage since its oxygen consumption is low[72] and it is revascularized early.[73]

Following vascular endothelial trauma, fibrin and platelet microthrombi adhere to exposed fibrils of endothelial basement membranes,[74] elastin, and collagen.[10] Intimal tissue encircles and invades the original thrombus.[75] Fibrin lying beneath the regenerated endothelium may be identified by routine histological techniques[76–78] and by electron microscopy.[79] Incorporation of mural thrombi into intimal plaques, as shown by Duguid,[77, 80] is further evidenced by finding vascularization or recanalization in the subendothelial proliferative lesions.[81] Thus, the role that organization of mural thrombi may play in the genesis of the atherosclerotic plaque[82] directs attention to its significance in venous bypass graft changes.

Following the microthrombi produced by the initial endothelial insult, recurrent mural thrombi become superimposed on the subendothelial proliferative lesions. Their recurrence is suggested further by the eccentric, laminated appearance of lesions in some grafts. Mechanical stresses placed upon the vein graft endothelium would produce recurrent endothelial insult. Atherosclerotic plaques become located[83] and intravascular particulate matter is deposited[84] in response to local hemodynamic forces. These same forces may also disrupt vascular permeability barriers. Besides pressure, endothelial cells are subjected to shear forces in the direction of blood flow.[85] Such shear stresses may cause endothelial erosion and alter fluxes of blood substances without cytologically demonstrable change.[86] These shear forces may be responsible for the longitudinal orientation of smooth muscle cells and collagen in the subendothelial lesions. In addition to the hemodynamic forces occurring in a linear conduit, local irregularities—such as those produced by valves, discrepancies between vein

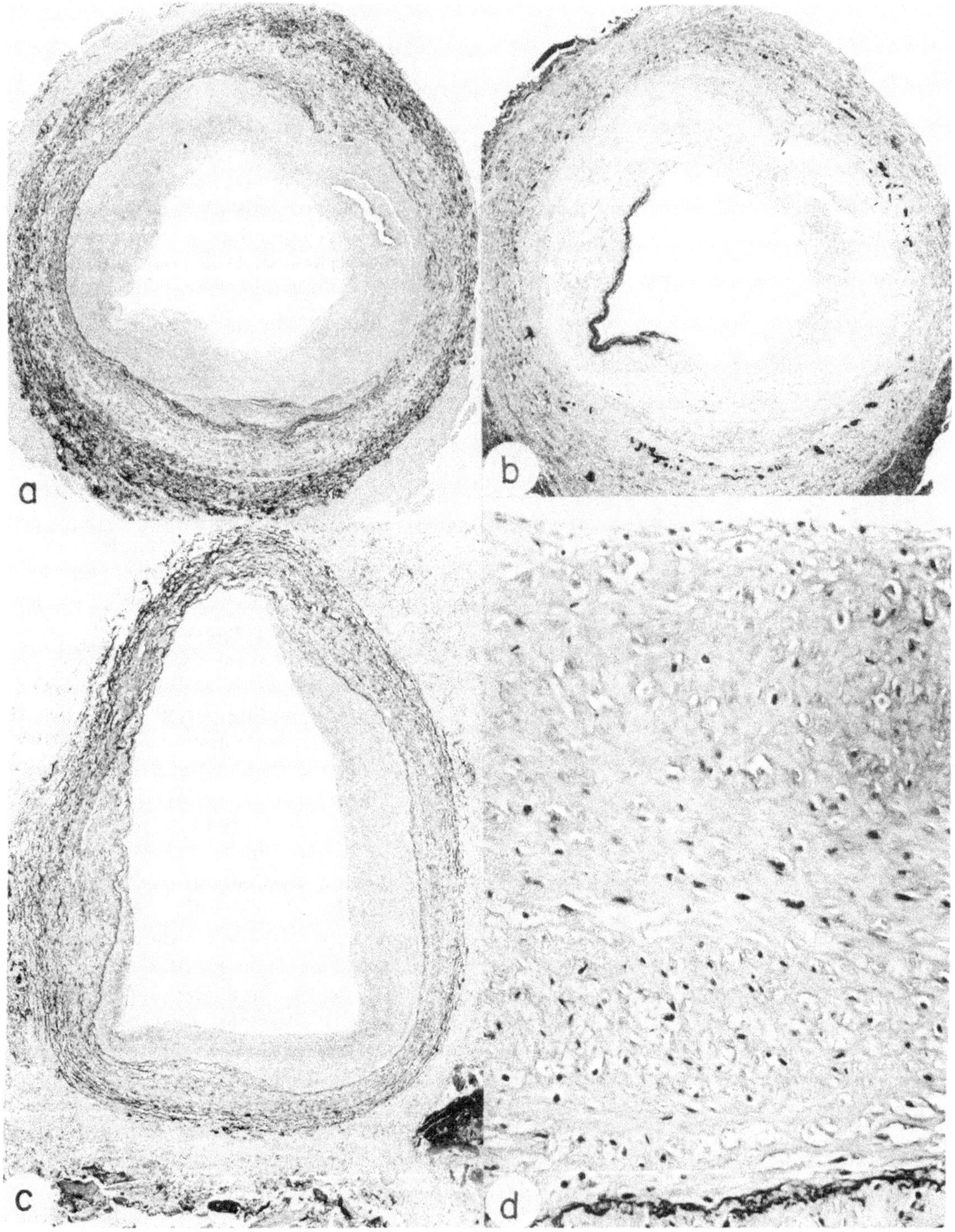

Figure 7

Human saphenous vein coronary arterial bypass grafts after 57 days. Subendothelial proliferation narrows the lumen of the right coronary arterial bypass by about 50% **(a)**; *elastic–Van Gieson stain,* × *20. Adjacent section* **(b)** *with subendothelial fibrin* (dark area); *hematoxylin and eosin stain,* × *20. Eccentric subendothelial proliferation in the left coronary artery bypass from the same patient* **(c)**; *Movat stain,* × *20.* **(d)** *A higher magnification of* c, *showing the lesion's cellularity and paucity of elastic fibers; Movat stain,* × *224.*

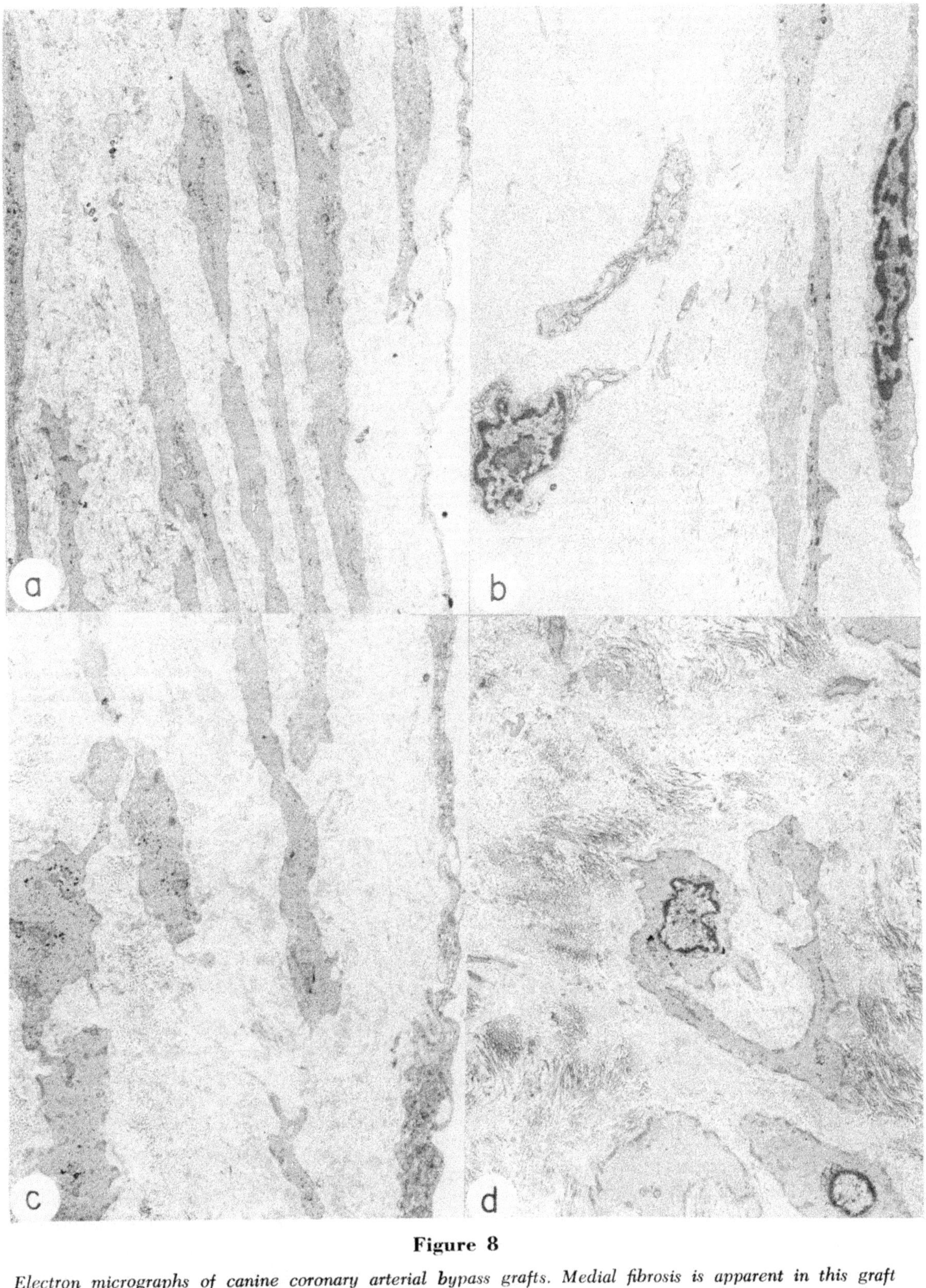

Figure 8

Electron micrographs of canine coronary arterial bypass grafts. Medial fibrosis is apparent in this graft 9 months postoperatively **(a)**, *and is more severe in another canine coronary arterial bypass at 12 months* **(b)**. c *and* **d** *show an area of subendothelial proliferation at 12 months, containing collagen and smooth muscle cells primarily oriented in the direction of blood flow. The only cells present in the lesion were such smooth muscle cells. The endothelium and lumen are at the right of* a, b, *and* c. *All four micrographs are* × *4,100.*

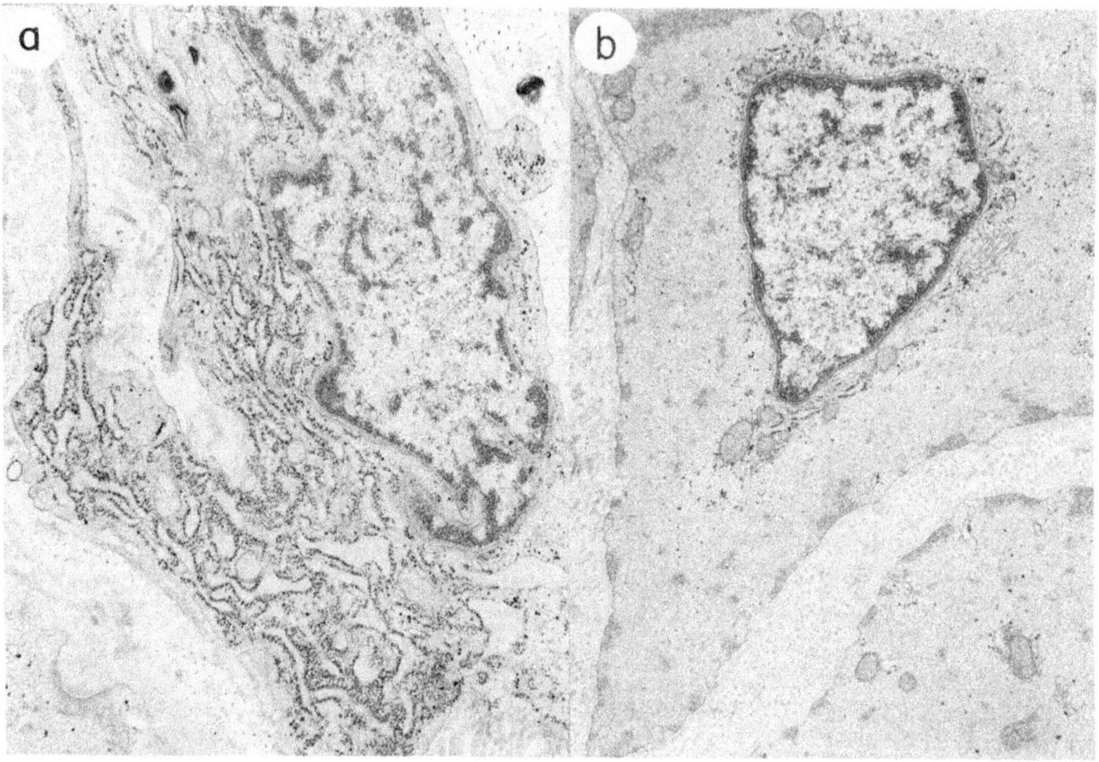

Figure 9

Electron micrograph of a fibroblast with its cytoplasm laden with endoplasmic reticulum and ribosomes, infiltrating the media of a 4-week canine femoral bypass graft (a). *A smooth muscle cell is at the lower right;* × *21,280. Mature smooth muscle cells* (b) *with perinuclear organelles, dense bodies, and myofilaments, from an area of subendothelial proliferation in a 12-month-old canine coronary arterial bypass graft. This cross section of the graft shows that the cells, their myofilaments, and the collagen fibers are oriented in the axis of blood flow. Electron micrograph,* × *21,280.*

graft caliber and the artery at both the proximal and distal anastomoses, and traction and torsion of the graft with the cardiac cycle—may all act to produce continuing endothelial damage.[4, 87] The possibility of a jet lesion where the vein graft enters the artery is borne out by the coronary arterial lesions in our study. Continued vascular insult may thus continue to produce conditions favorable for the development of proliferative subendothelial lesions, which lead to hemodynamically significant and progressive luminal compromise.

References

1. Brice JG, Dowsett DJ, Lowe RD: Effect of constriction on carotid blood flow and pressure gradient. Lancet **1**: 84, 1964
2. Johnson WD, Auer JE, Tector AJ: Late changes in coronary vein grafts (abstr). Amer J Cardiol **26**: 640, 1970
3. Grondin CM, Meere C, Castonguay Y, Lepage G, Grondin P: Progressive and late obstruction of an aorto-coronary venous bypass graft. Circulation **43**: 698, 1971
4. Bourassa MG, Lespérance J, Campeau L, Simard P: Factors influencing patency of aortocoronary vein grafts. *In* Cardiovascular Surgery 1971, edited by EB Mahoney. American Heart Assn Monograph 35. Supplements to Circulation **45** and **46** (suppl I): I-79, 1972
5. Grondin CM, Castonguay YR, Lepage G, Meere C, Grondin P: Aortocoronary bypass grafts: Early postoperative angiographic evaluation and reexploration for stenosis or thrombosis of the vein graft. Arch Surg (Chicago) **103**: 535, 1971
6. Hamaker WR, Doyle WF, O'Connell TJ, Gomez AC: Subintimal obliterative proliferation in saphenous vein grafts. Ann Thorac Surg **13**: 488, 1972
7. Vlodaver Z, Edwards JE: Pathologic changes in aortic-coronary arterial saphenous vein grafts. Circulation **44**: 719, 1971
8. Marti MC, Bouchardy B, Cox JN: Aorto-coronary bypass with autogenous saphenous vein grafts: Histopathological aspects. Virchow Arch [Path Anat] **352**: 255, 1971

9. Dedomenico M, Sameh AA, Berger K, Wood SJ, Sauvage LR: Experimental coronary artery surgery: Long-term follow-up, bypass venous autografts, longitudinal arteriotomies, and end-to-end anastomoses. J Thorac Cardiovasc Surg **56**: 617, 1968
10. Brody WR, Angell WW, Kosek JC: Histologic fate of the venous coronary artery bypass in dogs. Amer J Path **66**: 111, 1972
11. Nunn DB, Chun B, Whelan TJ Jr, Martins AN: Autogenous veins as arterial substitutes: A study of their histological fate with special attention to their endothelium. Ann Surg **160**: 14, 1964
12. Carrel A, Guthrie CC: Results of biterminal transplantation of veins. Amer J Med Sci **132**: 415, 1906
13. McCabe M, Cunningham GJ: Histological and histochemical examination of autogenous vein grafts. Brit J Surg **54**: 147, 1967
14. McCabe M, Wyatt AP, Cunningham GJ: Study on the ground substance of arteries, veins and grafted veins in dogs. Exp Molec Path **5**: 531, 1966
15. Fischer B, Schmeiden V: Experimentelle Untersuchungen über die funktionelle Anpassung der Gefässwand: Histologie transplantierter Gefässe. Frankfurt Z Path **3**: 8, 1909
16. Yamanouchi H: Über die zirkulären Gefässnahte und Arterienvenanastomosen, sowie über die Gefässtransplantationen. Deutsch Z Chir **112**: 1, 1911
17. Penn I, Schenk E, Rob C, DeWeese J, Schwartz SI: Evaluation of the development of athero-arteriosclerosis in autogenous venous grafts inserted into the peripheral arterial system. *In* Cardiovascular Surgery 1964, edited by FA Simeone. American Heart Assn Monograph 11. Supplements to Circulation **31** and **32** (suppl I): I-192, 1965
18. Jesseph JE, Jones TW, Sauvage LR, Kanar EA, Nyhus LM, Harkins HN: Five year observations on unsupported fresh venous grafts of the aorta in dogs. Surg Gynec Obstet **107**: 623, 1958
19. Chatterjee KN, Warren R, Gore I: Long term functional and histologic fate of arteriotomy patches of autogenous arterial and venous tissue: Observations on "arterialization." J Surg Res **4**: 106, 1964
20. Vlodaver Z, Edwards JE: The pathologist approaches clinical coronary disease. Hum Path **3**: 3, 1972
21. Kautzky R, Brussatis FR: Venentransplantation und Thromboendarteriektomien als Behandlung der Claudicatio intermittens. Langenbecks Arch Klin Chir **283**: 375, 1956
22. Allen P: Feasibility of autogenous vein grafts in the replacement of aortic aneurysms. Canad Med Ass J **76**: 922, 1957
23. Shumacker HB, Schloss G, Freeman LW, Wayson EE, Stahl NH: Studies in vascular repair: V. Experiments with the use of free venous transplants for bridging aortal defects. Yale J Biol Med **23**: 81, 1950
24. DeWeese JA, Terry R, Barner HB, Rob CG: Autogenous venous femoropopliteal bypass grafts. Surgery **59**: 28, 1966
25. Carrel A: Graft of the vena cava on the abdominal aorta. Ann Surg **52**: 462, 1910
26. Sako Y, Varco RL: Ten-year observations on autologous pericardial and venous grafts in the thoracic aorta: An experimental study. Surgery **51**: 465, 1962
27. Pena LI, Husni EA: Comparative study of autogenous vein and Dacron patch grafts in the dog. Arch Surg (Chicago) **96**: 370, 1968
28. Ejrup B, Hiertonn T, Moberg A: Atheromatous changes in autogenous venous grafts. Acta Chir Scand **121**: 211, 1961
29. McNamara JJ, Darling RC, Linton RR: Segmental stenosis of saphenous vein autografts. New Eng J Med **277**: 290, 1967
30. Beebe HG, Clark WF, DeWeese JA: Atherosclerotic change occurring in an autogenous venous arterial graft. Arch Surg (Chicago) **101**: 85, 1970
31. Carrel A, Guthrie CC: Uniterminal and biterminal venous transplantations. Surg Gynec Obstet **2**: 266, 1906
32. Carrel A: Results of transplantation of blood vessels, organs, and limbs. JAMA **51**: 1662, 1908
33. Nyhus LM, Kanar EA, Moore HG, Schmitz EJ, Sauvage LR, Zech RK, Harkins HN: Experimental vascular grafts: V. Unsupported venous autografts of the thoracic aorta. Northwest Med **54**: 359, 1955
34. Sauvage LR, Wesolowski SA: Healing and fate of arterial grafts. Surgery **38**: 1090, 1955
35. Nabatoff RA, Touroff ASW, Cross M: Four year studies concerning the fate of experimental vena cava autografts used to bridge aortic defects. Surg Gynec Obstet **101**: 20, 1955
36. Glenn WWL: Some reflections on the coronary bypass operation. Circulation **45**: 869, 1972
37. Haust MD: Fine fibrils of the extracellular space (microfibrils): Their structure and role in connective tissue organization. Amer J Path **47**: 1113, 1965
38. Oakes BW, North I, Rosen P, O'Brien B: Study of the development of arterial elastin in the dog and rabbit, following vascular surgery, and in the neonatal rat. J Anat **110**: 503, 1971
39. Wissler RW: The arterial medial cell, smooth muscle, or multifunctional mesenchyme? Circulation **36**: 1, 1967
40. Karrer HE, Cox J: Electron microscope study of the aorta in young and in aging mice. J Ultrastruct Res **5**: 1, 1961
41. Kadar A, Veress B, Jellinek H: Ultrastructural elements in experimental intimal thickening: II Study of the development of elastic elements in intimal proliferation. Exp Molec Path **11**: 212, 1969
42. Ross R, Klebanoff SJ: The smooth muscle cell: In vivo synthesis of connective tissue proteins. J Cell Biol **50**: 159, 1971
43. Ross R: The smooth muscle cell: II. Growth of smooth muscle in culture and formation of elastic fibers. J Cell Biol **50**: 172, 1971
44. Stein AA, Rosenblum J, Leather R: Intimal sclerosis in human veins. Arch Path (Chicago) **81**: 548, 1966
45. Zwillenberg LO, Laszt L, Zwillenberg H: Die Feinstruktur der Venenwand bei Varikose. Angiologica (Basel) **8**: 318, 1971

46. Esterly JA, Glagov S, Ferguson DJ: Morphogenesis of intimal obliterative hyperplasia of small arteries in experimental pulmonary hypertension. Amer J Path **52**: 325, 1968

47. Heath D, Edwards JE: Pathology of hypertensive pulmonary vascular disease: Description of six grades of structural changes in the pulmonary artery with special reference to congenital cardiac septal defects. Circulation **18**: 533, 1958

48. Wagenvoort CA, Nauta J, van der Schaar PJ, Weeda HWH, Wagenvoort N: Vascular changes in pulmonic stenosis and tetralogy of Fallot studied in lung biopsies. Circulation **36**: 924, 1967

49. Harrison CV: Experimental pulmonary arteriosclerosis. J Path Bact **60**: 289, 1948

50. Singh I, Khanna PK, Lal M, Hoon RS, Rao BDP: High altitude pulmonary hypertension. Lancet **2**: 146, 1965

51. Kapanci Y: Hypertensive pulmonary vascular disease. Amer J Path **47**: 665, 1965

52. McGee WG, Ashworth GF: Fine structure of chronic hypertensive arteriopathy in the human kidney. Amer J Path **43**: 273, 1963

53. Kosek JC, Chartrand C, Hurley EJ, Lower RR: Arteries in canine cardiac homografts. Lab Invest **21**: 328, 1969

54. Milam JD, Shipkey FH Jr, Lind CJ Jr, Nora JJ, Leachman RD, Rochelle DG, Bloodwell RD, Hallman GL, Cooley DA: Morphologic findings in human cardiac allografts. Circulation **41**: 519, 1970

55. Vlodaver Z, Neufeld HN: The musculo-elastic layer in the coronary arteries: A histological and hemodynamic concept. Vasc Dis **4**: 136, 1967

56. Vlodaver Z, Edwards JE: Pathology of coronary atherosclerosis. Progr Cardiovasc Dis **14**: 256, 1971

57. Movat HZ, More RH, Haust MD: Diffuse intimal thickening of human aorta with aging. Amer J Path **34**: 1023, 1958

58. Gresham GA, Howard AN, King AJ: Comparative histopathological study of the early atherosclerotic lesion. Brit J Exp Path **43**: 21, 1962

59. Haust MD, More RH, Movat HZ: Role of smooth muscle cells in the fibrogenesis of arteriosclerosis. Amer J Path **37**: 377, 1960

60. Geer JC: Fine structure of human aortic intimal thickening and fatty streaks. Lab Invest **14**: 1764, 1965

61. McCombs HL, Zook BC, McGandy RB: Fine structure of spontaneous atherosclerosis of the aorta in the squirrel monkey. Amer J Path **55**: 235, 1969

62. Moss NS, Benditt EP: Ultrastructure of spontaneous and experimentally induced arterial lesions: II. The spontaneous plaque in the chicken. Lab Invest **23**: 231, 1970

63. Geer JC, McGill NC Jr, Strong JP: Fine structure of the human atherosclerotic lesions. Amer J Path **38**: 263, 1961

64. Balis JU, Haust MD, More RH: Electron-microscopic studies in human atherosclerosis: Cellular elements in aortic fatty streaks. Exp Molec Path **3**: 511, 1964

65. Parker F, Odland GF: Correlative histochemical, biochemical and electron microscopic study of experimental atherosclerosis in the rabbit aorta with special reference to the myointimal cell. Amer J Path **48**: 197, 1966

66. Parker F, Odland GF: Light microscopic, histochemical and electron microscopic study of experimental atherosclerosis in rabbit coronary artery and a comparison with rabbit aorta atherosclerosis. Amer J Path **48**: 451, 1966

67. Schaper J, Schaper W: Ultrastructure of developing collaterals. *In* The Collateral Circulation of the Heart, by W Schaper. New York, American Elsevier Publishing Co, 1971

68. Poole JCF, Cromwell SR, Benditt EP: Behavior of smooth muscle cells and formation of extracellular structures in the reaction of arterial walls to injury. Amer J Path **62**: 391, 1971

69. Berry CL, Stark J, Aberdeen E: Histopathological change after aortic anastomosis. J Path **102**: 213, 1970

70. Ts'ao C: Myointimal cells as a possible source of replacement for endothelial cells in the rabbit. Circulation Research **23**: 671, 1968

71. Wyatt AP, Taylor GW: Vein grafts: Changes in the endothelium of autogenous free vein grafts used as arterial replacements. Brit J Surg **53**: 943, 1966

72. Kosan RL, Burton AC: Oxygen consumption of arterial smooth muscle as a function of active tone and passive stretch. Circulation Research **18**: 79, 1966

73. Wyatt AP, Rothnie NG, Griffiths IP: Experimental study of the histology, revascularization patterns and physiological activity of muscle in autogenous vein transplants (abstr). Brit J Surg **50**: 768, 1963

74. Ts'ao CH, Glagov S: Platelet adhesion to subendothelial components in experimental aortic injury: Role of fine fibrils and basement membrane. Brit J Exp Path **51**: 423, 1970

75. Byers SO, Friedman M: Experimental venous and arterial thromboatherosclerosis: A comparative study. Brit J Exp Path **43**: 198, 1962

76. Haust MD, More RH, Movat HZ: Mechanism of fibrosis in arteriosclerosis. Amer J Path **35**: 265, 1959

77. Duguid JB: Thrombosis as a factor in the pathogenesis of aortic atherosclerosis. J Path Bact **60**: 57, 1948

78. Crawford T, Levene CI: Incorporation of fibrin in the aortic intima. J Path Bact **64**: 523, 1952

79. Marshall JR, Adams JG, O'Neal RM, DeBakey ME: Ultrastructure of uncomplicated human atheroma in surgically resected aortas. J Atheroscler Res **6**: 120, 1966

80. Duguid JB: Thrombosis as a factor in the pathogenesis of coronary atherosclerosis. J Path Bact **58**: 207, 1946

81. Gerringer E: Intimal vascularization and atherosclerosis. J Path Bact **63**: 201, 1951

82. Roberts WC, Buja LM: Frequency and significance of coronary arterial thrombi and other observations in

fatal acute myocardial infarction: A study of 107 necropsy patients. Amer J Med **52:** 425, 1972

83. Santerre RF, Wight TN, Smith SC, Brannigan D: Spontaneous atherosclerosis in pigeons: A model system for studying metabolic parameters associated with atherogenesis. Amer J Path **67:** 1, 1972

84. Caro CG, Fitz-Gerald JM, Schroter RC: Arterial wall shear and distribution of early atheroma in man. Nature (London) **223:** 1159, 1969

85. Flaherty JT, Pierce JE, Ferrans VJ, Patel DJ, Tucker WK, Fry DL: Endothelial nuclear patterns in the canine arterial tree with particular reference to hemodynamic events. Circulation Research **30:** 23, 1972

86. Fry DL: Certain chemorheologic considerations regarding the blood vascular interface with particular reference to coronary artery disease. *In* Research on Acute Myocardial Infarction, edited by S Bondurant. American Heart Assn Monograph 27. Supplements to Circulation **39** and **40** (suppl IV): IV-38, 1969

87. Barner HB, Judd DR, Kaiser GC, Willman VL, Hanlon CR: Late failure of arterialized in situ saphenous vein. Arch Surg (Chicago) **99:** 781, 1969

Discussion

Dr. John H. Kennedy, Houston, Texas: Dr. Conkle and his co-workers are to be commended for their careful morphological study of fibrous subintimal hyperplasia in autogenous veins following aorto-coronary bypass graft. My colleagues, Dr. N. H. C. Hwang and Dr. David W. Wieting, and I have reported the results of an hydraulic study in computer analogy; to date these results suggest that the relative flows in the aorta and the vein bypass graft are influenced by the angle (θ) subtended by the vein and the aorta. Optimal flow occurs when angle (θ) approaches 90°. When (θ) was measured in postoperative angiograms in patients with proven subintimal hyperplasia, in each case (θ) fittted the theoretical curve in the computer analogy.

Isolated coronary arterial dissection

A complication of cardiac operations

Dissecting aneurysm limited to the coronary artery is described in 4 patients in whom cardiac operations had been performed. A tear into the dissected artery was identified in the 1 patient in whom coronary bypass grafting was performed. In the other 3, each of whom had undergone aortic valve replacement, no tear into the dissected coronary artery was observed. However, in 2 of them, the caged-ball aortic prosthesis was stenotic. It is speculated that the presumed sudden development of systolic hypertension in the coronary arteries of these 2 patients was an important factor underlying the dissection.

Bernadine H. Bulkley, M.D., and William C. Roberts, M.D., *Bethesda, Md.*

Dissecting aneurysm limited to the coronary artery is an infrequent and poorly recognized complication of cardiac operations. This lesion was observed, however, in four necropsy subjects who are described in the report which follows.

Patients studied

Aortic valve replacement had been carried out in 3 patients and coronary arterial bypass grafting in 1 (Table I). Two patients with valve replacement died from low cardiac output secondary to prosthetic aortic stenosis (Fig. 1). In Patient 1, severe atherosclerosis was present and the medial dissection caused minimal luminal narrowing. In Patient 2, atherosclerosis was minimal and the lumen of one coronary artery was nearly completely occluded by a medial hematoma (Fig. 2). Patient 3, who had had aortic valve replacement 4 years earlier, died of congestive cardiac failure secondary to an obstructing prosthetic thrombus. At necropsy, one coronary artery was severely narrowed by an organized medial hematoma (Fig. 3). A healed myocardial infarction was present in the anterior wall of the left ventricle. Patient 4, who had intractable angina, died immediately after aorto-coronary bypass grafting with the saphenous vein. A medial hematoma was present in one coronary artery proximal and distal to the anastomoses (Fig. 4).

In each case the medial hematoma developed in the outer media and separated the adventitia from the media. The extravasated blood was always contained within the external elastic membrane.

Comments

Acute dissection of a coronary artery is a potentially lethal complication of certain cardiac operations. The mural hematoma, which may be diagnosed by gross inspection, discolors and distorts the coronary artery, and the adjacent adipose tissue may contain extravasated blood. If this condition is suspected, a catheter passed via the aorta into the coronary artery might demonstrate an obstructed lumen, and appropriate operative correction could then be attempted.

The causes of iatrogenic primary coronary arterial dissection include blunt

From the Section of Pathology, National Heart and Lung Institute, National Institutes of Health, Bethesda, Md. 20014.

Received for publication July 30, 1973.

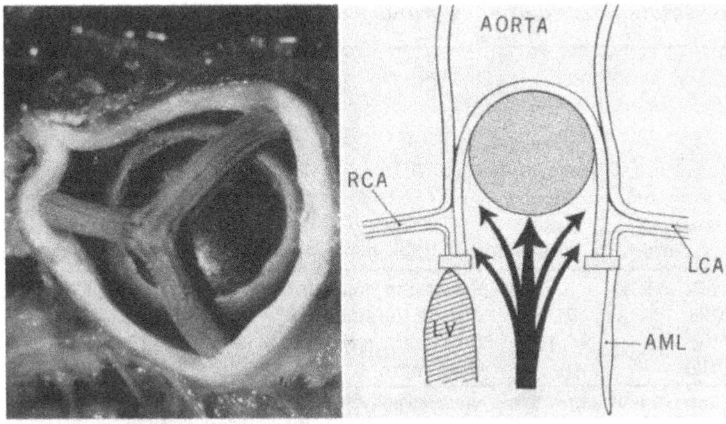

Fig. 1. Prosthetic aortic valvular stenosis and coronary dissection in Patient 1. The Starr-Edwards prosthesis from above *(left)*. She died 24 hours after replacement from low cardiac output. All three struts of the prosthesis contact the wall of the aorta, and movement of the poppet appears to have been severely impaired. Histologic examination of the entire coronary arterial tree disclosed medial dissections of the left circumflex, left anterior descending and left main coronary arteries. No medial or adventitial tears were identified. The dissections may have resulted from trauma by the coronary perfusion cannula. However, coronary arterial hypertension resulting from prosthetic valvular stenosis may have been another factor. The systolic pressure gradient across a stenotic, rigid-framed prosthesis may occur above the level of the coronary ostia and transmit elevated systolic pressures to the coronary arteries which normally receive only diastolic pressures *(right)*. *RCA,* Right coronary artery. *LV,* Left ventricle. *LCA,* Left circumflex coronary artery. *AML,* Anterior mitral leaflet.

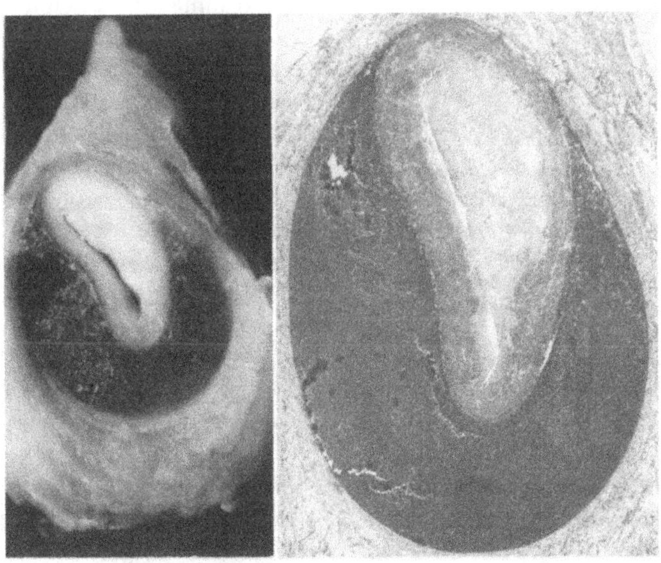

Fig. 2. Isolated coronary arterial dissection in Patient 2. The gross photograph *(left)* and histologic section *(right)* show a dissection in the right coronary artery of a woman who died unexpectedly 5 days after aortic valve replacement. The dissecting hematoma has separated the media from the adventitia. The hematoma has compressed the flexible portion of the arterial wall (i.e., the part not involved by atherosclerotic plaque), causing severe luminal narrowing. Severe stenosis of the prosthetic aortic valve also was present and may have been an important etiologic factor. (*Right,* Hematoxylin-eosin stain; ×23.)

Table I. *Iatrogenic isolated dissection of coronary artery: Data in 4 patients*

Patient No.	*Age/sex*	*Type of cardiac operation*	*Interval from operation to death (days)*	*Cause of death*	*Heart weight (Gm.)*	*CA dissected*	*Maximal luminal narrowing by old plaque (per cent)*	*Maximal luminal narrowing by medial hematoma (per cent)*
1	45/F	MVR, AVR	1	Prosthetic stenosis	310	LAD, LC	>75	<25
2	54/F	AVR	5	Prosthetic stenosis	700	R	25-50	>75
3	48/F	AVR	1,460	Prosthetic stenosis	600	LC	<25	>75
4	54/M	SVBG	0	Operation	385	LC	>75	<25

Legend: CA, Coronary artery. MVR, Mitral valve replacement. AVR, Aortic valve replacement. SVBG, Saphenous vein bypass graft. LAD, Left anterior descending. LC, Left circumflex. R, Right coronary artery.

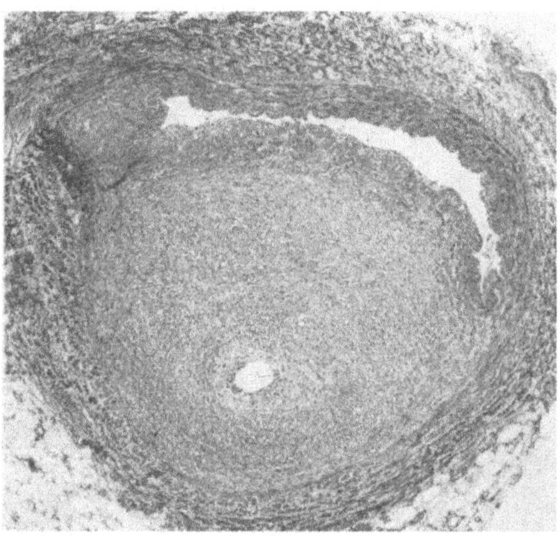

Fig. 3. Healed or chronic coronary arterial dissection in Patient 3, who survived an acute myocardial infarction after aortic valve replacement. At necropsy, 4 years after operation, she had a healed dissection of the left circumflex coronary artery, shown here, and a healed myocardial infarction. The hematoma within the media had organized and recanalized. (Hematoxylin-eosin stain; original magnification ×45.)

trauma, dissection at the site of operative incision into the artery (as for anastomosis for conduit bypassing), and direct intraluminal damage from a cannula. Isolated coronary arterial dissection after injection of contrast material into a coronary artery has been suspected during life in several patients[1-3] and confirmed by anatomic studies in 1.[4] Operative trauma from an intraluminal cannula has been described in 1 patient; a tear produced an intimal flap which caused fatal arterial occlusion.[5]

The mechanism of medial hematoma formation is uncertain. A partial tear originating in the intima or adventitia may lead to medial damage, hemorrhage, and dissection. Disruption of intima or adventitia, however, is not necessary for traumatic formation of a hematoma in media; in fact, a hematoma may develop spontaneously without trauma or associated abnormalities.[6] In 3 of our patients no intimal or adventitial tear was observed despite subserial sections, suggesting that blunt trauma led to medial bleeding with subsequent dissection.

Prosthetic stenosis may cause pressure trauma to the coronary arteries. Prosthetic "supravalvular" obstruction caused by the poppet's sticking in the cage above the ostia of the coronary arteries may produce isolated coronary arterial systolic hypertension, which might contribute to coronary dissection as systemic hypertension contributes to aortic dissection.

Medial dissection appears to cause more luminal narrowing in near normal coronary arteries than in severely atherosclerotic ones. The nonpliable rigid atherosclerotic plaque may protect the vessel against extraluminal compression and limit dissection. Similarly, aortic dissections of consequence rarely occur in heavily atherosclerotic vessels. Hence, the patient undergoing valve replacement may be more susceptible to this

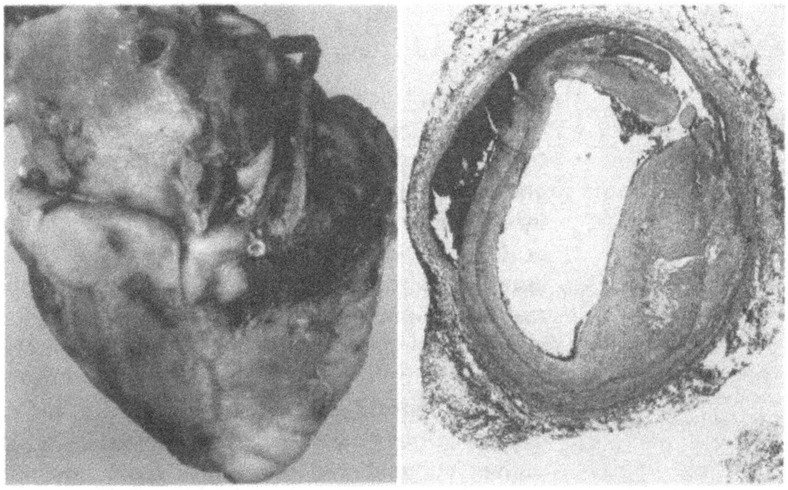

Fig. 4. Iatrogenic coronary arterial dissection in Patient 4, who underwent triple aorto-coronary bypass grafting with the saphenous vein and died in the operating room. Extensive hemorrhage into the atrioventricular sulcus occurred during the procedure *(left)*, and at necropsy a medial dissection of left circumflex coronary artery was identified *(right)*. Although the dissection did not cause significant luminal narrowing, the coronary arteries were not subjected to normal perfusion pressures. (Movat stain; original magnification ×27.)

complication than the patient undergoing coronary bypass grafting, in whom atherosclerosis is severe, even though the latter procedure involves direct operative trauma to the coronary artery.

The patient may survive after coronary dissection if, as suggested above, the narrowing of the true lumen by the medial hematoma is mild or if, as occurred in Patient 2, the subsequent myocardial infarction heals and the hematoma organizes and recanalizes. However, the latter is most unusual, as isolated coronary arterial dissection has heretofore been considered a universally fatal event.[6]

REFERENCES

1 Tsitouris, G., and Lekas, D.: Right Coronary Artery Occlusion During Retrograde Left Heart Catheterization Complicated by Rare Arrhythmias, Angiography **16:** 747, 1965.

2 Ross, R. S., and Gordon, R.: Coronary Arteriography, Circulation **27, 38:** 67, 1968 (Suppl. III).

3 Braunwald, E.: Deaths Related to Cardiac Catheterization, Circulation **37, 38:** 17, 1968 (Suppl. III).

4 Kitamura, K., Gobel, F. L., and Wang, Y.: Dissection of the Left Coronary Artery Complicating Retrograde Left Heart Catheterization, Chest **57:** 587, 1970.

5 Heilbrunn, A., and Zimmerman, J. M.: Coronary Artery Dissection: A Complication of Cannulation, J. Thorac. Cardiovasc. Surg. **49:** 767, 1965.

6 Claudon, D. G., Caludon, D. B., and Edwards, J. E.: Primary Dissecting Aneurysm of Coronary Artery: A Cause of Acute Myocardial Infarction, Circulation **45:** 259, 1972.

Heterografts as Aortocoronary Bypass Conduits in Human Beings

BERNADINE H. BULKLEY, MD
WILLIAM C. ROBERTS, MD, FACC

Bethesda, Maryland

Clinical and necropsy observations are described in a man in whom two sheep carotid arterial heterografts were inserted as aortocoronary bypass conduits 30 months before death, and in whom a canine saphenous vein heterograft was inserted several hours before death. All three grafts failed. The lumens of the sheep carotid arterial heterografts had closed by the time of catheterization 6 months after operation; at necropsy both grafts were totally occluded at their coronary and aortic ends and their media and adventitia were infiltrated by granulomatous inflammatory cells. Little information is available regarding the use of heterografts as coronary bypass conduits. Examination of previous reports describing heterografts for vascular reconstruction or bypass in both man and experimental animals and observations in our patient suggest that heterografts are unsatisfactory as aortocoronary bypass conduits.

Insertion of a conduit between the ascending aorta or one of its branches and a coronary artery is now a common form of treatment in patients with severe symptomatic coronary atherosclerosis. The vessel most commonly utilized for the conduit is an autogenous saphenous vein and the next most frequent, an autogenous mammary artery. A suitable substitute for these autogenous vessels in the aortocoronary position would be useful. Synthetic grafts small enough to anastomose to the coronary artery have been unsatisfactory because of clotting problems. Attention recently has been refocused on vascular heterografts as possible conduits between the aorta and the coronary artery. Stimulated by study at necropsy of a patient given two types of heterografts as aortocoronary conduits, we reviewed previous utilization of heterografts in man. Study of these previous reports and observations in our patient are summarized in this report.

Case Report

A 45 year old man with labile hypertension had angina pectoris at age 40 and a subendocardial myocardial infarction a year later. Coronary arteriography at age 42 disclosed severe (more than 90 percent) narrowing of the left main coronary artery, 26 to 50 percent narrowing of the right coronary artery and numerous irregularities of the left circumflex coronary artery. The left anterior descending coronary artery was not visualized. The left ventriculogram revealed apical akinesia. Because of bilateral strippings of the saphenous veins for varicosities several years earlier, and because the cephalic veins were small, sheep carotid arteries were used as aortocoronary conduits: one to the left anterior descending and a second to the left circumflex coronary artery.

The angina, rather than being relieved by the operation, gradually progressed. Coronary angiograms 6 months after operation demonstrated total occlusion of both grafts. In addition, the lumens of the left main, left circumflex and proximal left anterior descending coronary arteries were each more than 90 percent narrowed. Thirty months after the first operation, repeat coronary angiograms disclosed 100 percent occlusion of the left main, left an-

From the Section of Pathology, National Heart and Lung Institute, National Institutes of Health, Bethesda, Md. Manuscript accepted July 12, 1974.

Address for reprints: William C. Roberts, MD, Bldg. 10A, Rm 3E-30, National Institutes of Health, Bethesda, Md. 20014.

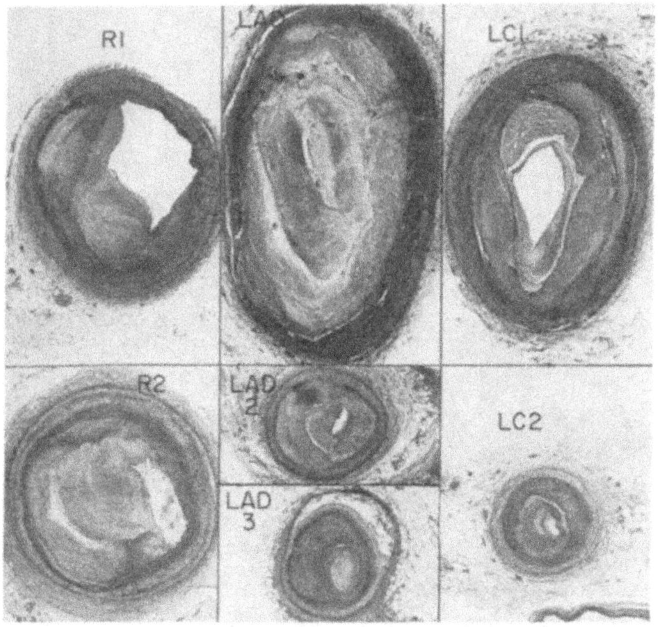

FIGURE 1. Native coronary arteries. Shown are histologic sections of proximal right (R1), left anterior descending (LAD) and left circumflex (LC1); of distal right (R2), and the left anterior descending (LAD2, LAD3); and left circumflex (LC2) immediately distal to the site of anastomosis of the bypass graft. The distal vessels are severely narrowed by atherosclerotic plaques. The distal left anterior descending and left circumflex coronary arteries are much smaller than their respective proximal vessels, and also much smaller than the heterografts anastomosed to them. (Movat stains, ×13.5, reduced by 24 percent.)

terior descending and left circumflex coronary arteries. The latter two arteries filled in retrograde manner from the right coronary artery. The heterografts never opacified. A bypass procedure between the aorta and the distal left anterior descending coronary artery was again performed: A canine glutaraldehyde-fixed saphenous vein was utilized. The patient died several hours after operation.

Pathologic findings: Portions of the native coronary arteries are illustrated in Figure 1 and the implanted heterografts in Figures 2 through 5. Both sheep heterografts were encased in fibrous tissue, densely adhering the heterografts to the underlying epicardium (Fig. 2). The lumens of the proximal and distal portions of each aortocoronary sheep carotid bypass artery were completely occluded by fibrous tissue (Fig. 3). The canine saphenous vein bypass heterograft from the aorta to the distal left anterior descending coronary artery, inserted hours before death, was open but the lumen of the artery into which it was inserted contained fresh thrombus (Fig. 5).

The caliber of the native coronary arteries was much smaller than that of the implanted grafts. In addition, the lumens of the native coronary arteries were diffusely and severely (more than 90 percent) narrowed by old atherosclerotic plaques. Atherosclerotic narrowing was severe proximal and distal to the inserted bypass grafts. Furthermore, at the sites of anastomosis between the heterografts and both coronary arteries the lumens of the natural vessels were severely (more than 75 percent) narrowed by old plaques.

The walls of the sheep heterografts were extensively infiltrated by granulomas containing numerous giant cells. These were present throughout the entire extent of the grafts and were unassociated with suture material. At several proximal and distal sites, the entire wall was obscured and replaced by granulomatous inflammation that also obliterated the lumen so that no remnants of the original graft wall remained.

Discussion

Autologous saphenous veins and internal mammary arteries are used routinely for coronary arterial bypass, but if these vessels are not usable, an alternative bypass conduit is not readily available. Synthetic knit (Dacron®) tubes have become the vessel of choice for aortic and iliofemoral repair and are suitable alternatives for femoral-popliteal or carotid arterial bypass if an autologous saphenous vein cannot be used (Table I). However, synthetic vessels with luminal diameters of less than 8 mm[1-4] are unsatisfactory because they clot and consequently cannot be used for coronary arterial bypass. Are vascular heterografts the next choice after autologous vessels for such procedures? Although their use is currently being investigated,[5] there is little or no information on the use of heterologous vessels as aortocoronary

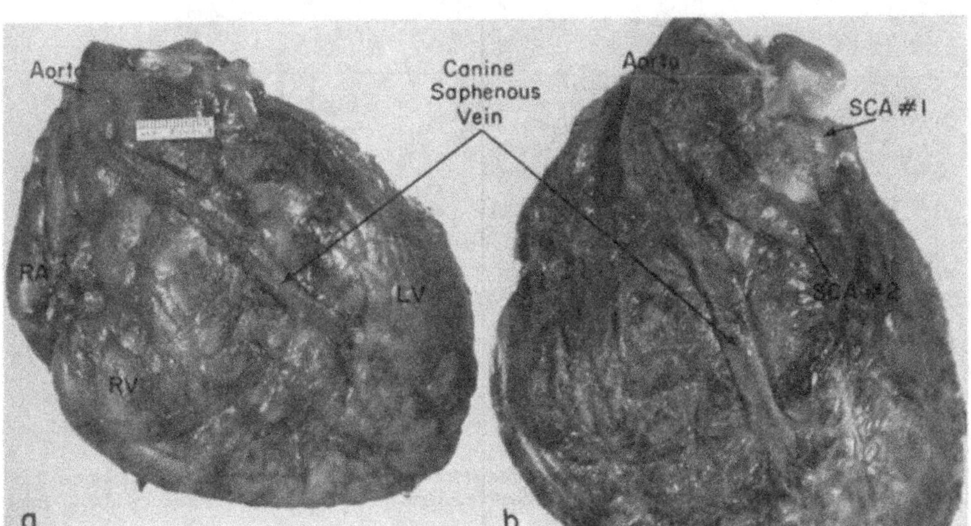

FIGURE 2. External surface of the heart showing the canine saphenous vein that was inserted between the aorta and the left anterior descending coronary artery hours before death. a, dense fibrous tissue, which had virtually concealed the two arterial heterografts implanted 30 months before death, was removed (**b**) to show the sheep carotid arterial bypass conduits between the aorta and left circumflex (SCA #1) and between the aorta and the left anterior descending coronary arteries (SCA #2). LV = left ventricle; RA = right atrium; RV = right ventricle.

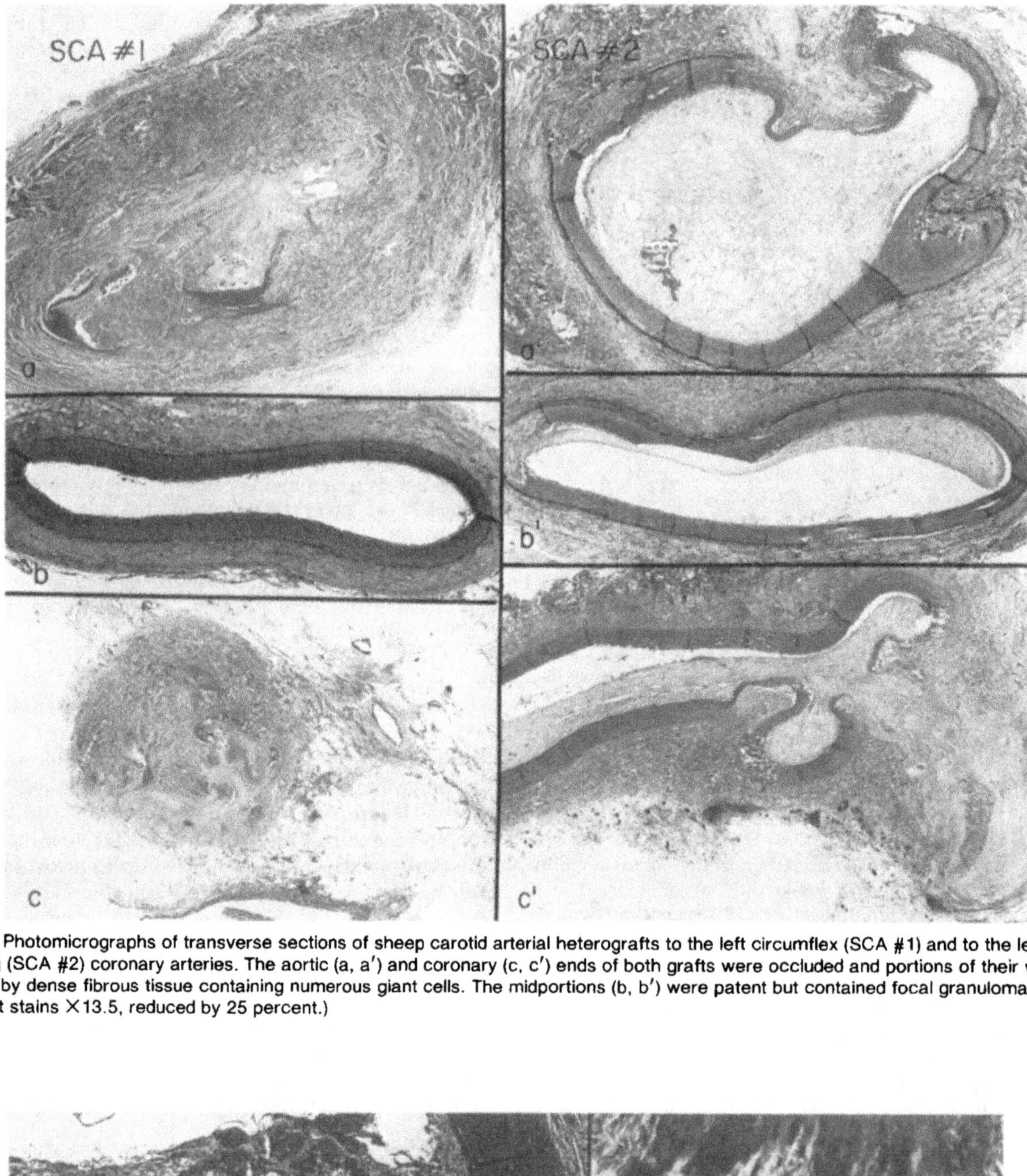

FIGURE 3. Photomicrographs of transverse sections of sheep carotid arterial heterografts to the left circumflex (SCA #1) and to the left anterior descending (SCA #2) coronary arteries. The aortic (a, a′) and coronary (c, c′) ends of both grafts were occluded and portions of their walls were obliterated by dense fibrous tissue containing numerous giant cells. The midportions (b, b′) were patent but contained focal granulomatous reaction. (Movat stains ×13.5, reduced by 25 percent.)

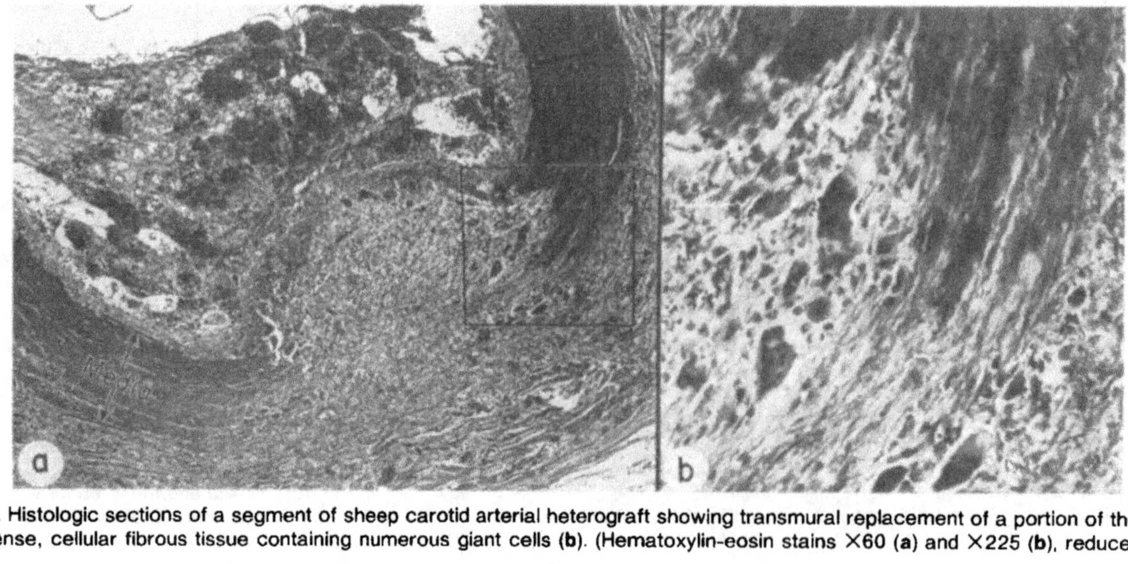

FIGURE 4. Histologic sections of a segment of sheep carotid arterial heterograft showing transmural replacement of a portion of the vessel wall (**a**) by a dense, cellular fibrous tissue containing numerous giant cells (**b**). (Hematoxylin-eosin stains ×60 (**a**) and ×225 (**b**), reduced by 25 percent.)

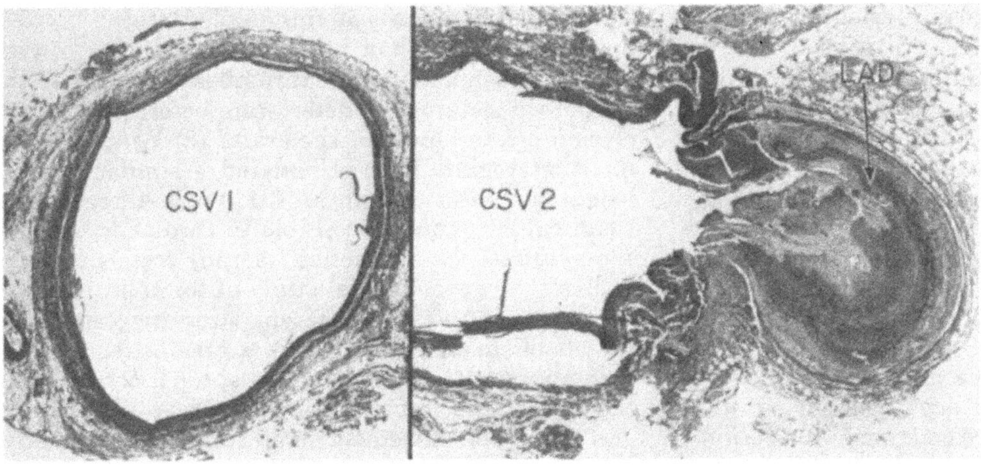

FIGURE 5. Histologic sections through the canine saphenous vein bypass graft (CSV) placed between the aorta and the distal left anterior descending coronary artery (LAD). Proximal to the coronary anastomosis the vein graft was patent (CSV 1), but at the site of anastomosis the left anterior descending coronary artery was occluded by recent thrombus overlying an atherosclerotic plaque (CSV 2). (Movat stain ×13.5, reduced by 23 percent.)

bypass conduits in experimental animals or in man. The experience culled from the use of such material in aortic and femoral reconstruction, however, may be helpful in answering this question and in understanding the observations in our patient.

Previous Experience with Arterial Heterografts and Homografts

For more than 50 years numerous attempts at using arterial heterografts and homografts as vascular transplants met repeated failure.[6-10] Various mammalian arteries were transplanted into the aorta and into segments of the femoral, popliteal or carotid artery of both man and animals. The grafts clotted or became aneurysmally dilated or their walls degenerated. Histologic study of the heterografts suggested that two processes, one degenerative and the other reparative, acted within a short time of the transplantation procedure. The degenerative changes included necrosis of the intima, loss of smooth muscle cells and other components of the media, and inflammation of the adventitia. Simultaneously, host connective tissue covered the degenerating inner surface of the transplanted vessel and endothelial cells and host connective tissue and blood vessels infiltrated adventitia, creating a new host vessel that virtually replaced the original graft.[9-11]

This pattern of degeneration, repair and replacement occurred in both homologous and heterologous arterial transplants.[11-15] The evolution of the heterografts, however, differed from that of the homografts in a few important respects. Host response to the heterografts was generally more vigorous and rapidly destructive, allowing less time for reparative processes to intercede. Also, the degenerating heterologous arteries lost elastic tissue that remained intact in homologous grafts. Heterografts therefore formed less sturdy scaffolds for host connective tissue ingrowth and were more susceptible to dilatation, aneurysmal formation and rupture than homografts. Nevertheless, the far greater availability of the intact viable and nondiseased arteries of animals made the heterologous grafts more feasible in the long term and led to continued attempts to overcome the problems of the heterograft, particularly at a time when synthetic grafts were not widely used.

Newer methods of preparation and fixation of grafts: Advances in the use of heterologous vessels for vascular reconstruction have been due mainly to newer methods of preparation and fixation of the grafts. Through the years, vascular grafts have been used fresh[16,17] and after cold storage,[6,18] freeze drying[19] and formalin fixation.[11] Comparative studies have shown that these various methods of fixation delayed by up to 2 years, but did not eliminate, failure of the grafts from thrombosis or aneurysmal dilatation.

Recently Rosenberg et al.[20,21] have developed a newer method of preparing bovine carotid arterial heterografts and their technique has been applied in a few patients with apparently good results. Preparation of these heterografts includes partial digestion of the vessel with the proteolytic enzyme ficin and subsequent fixation with dialdehyde starch or glutaraldehyde. Enzymatic digestion removes most of the elastic tissue and smooth muscle fibers, the latter

TABLE I

Acceptable Conduits for Arterial Repair or Bypass

Native Vessel	Conduit
Large artery (>12 mm diameter) Aorta Iliac	Synthetic tube (knit Dacron)
Small artery (8–12 mm diameter) Femoral Popliteal Carotid	Autogenous vein Synthetic tube (knit Dacron) Heterograft (bovine carotid artery)
Small artery (<8 mm diameter) Coronary	Autogenous vein Saphenous Cephalic Brachial Autogenous artery Internal mammary ? Heterograft Arterial Venous

presumed to be the most antigenic element of the arterial wall. The residual collagen tube is then strengthened and made less antigenic by cross linking of the collagen molecules by a tanning agent. Initially, formaldehyde was used for this purpose but it produced a less stable end product and was replaced by dialdehyde starch or glutaraldehyde, the tanning agent used in the preparation of leather. These tanning agents also have been demonstrated to shift the electropotential of the intimal surface of the vessel to a net negative charge that is believed to inhibit mural thrombosis.[22-23]

Immunologic studies of these modified bovine arterial heterografts inserted in dogs have shown little[24] or no[25] immunogenicity. Aneurysmal formation and thrombosis have occurred with the modified heterograft, but less frequently than with heterografts used earlier.[26] Thoracoabdominal aortic reconstructions in dogs performed with use of these modified bovine heterografts have been followed up for up to 7 years with apparently good results.[27] A femoral-popliteal bypass bovine heterograft in a patient has been followed up for nearly 7 years. The overall 2 to 4 year patency rate of such heterografts in man has been about 50 percent.[5,28] To our knowledge, there is no reported experience in man or animals with use of modified bovine carotid heterografts as aortocoronary bypass conduits.

Unsuccessful Application in Our Patient

Glutaraldehyde-fixed vascular heterografts (prepared by Hancock Laboratories, Anaheim, Calif.) were used as aortocoronary bypass conduits in our patient, to our knowledge, the first reported instance of such use. The vascular heterografts used in our patient differed from those prepared by the method of Rosenberg et al. in at least two respects: The vessels were not enzymatically predigested; hence the media and elastic fibers remained intact and the arteries were harvested from sheep and the vein from dogs. Although there is evidence that porcine arterial heterografts prepared by the Hancock method are only mildly antigenic,[24] there are no published data on their use in man or animals for any type of arterial reconstruction.

The failure of the glutaraldehyde-fixed vascular heterografts for coronary bypass in our patient raises many questions: (1) Was the vigorous destructive granulomatous reaction seen in the sheep carotid arteries after 30 months an immunologic rejection phenomenon, or was it a host response of the foreign body type against an inert thrombosed tube? Did the wall of the heterograft deteriorate before or after occlusion of the lumen of the graft? (2) Would the canine heterograft have stimulated a similar or even heightened host response? (3) Are heterografts of small caliber more susceptible to thrombosis, in the same way as the synthetic (Dacron) vessels of small caliber? An experimental study of formalin-fixed arterial heterografts of different sizes suggested that vessels of smaller caliber show a greater tendency to thrombosis.[11] (4) Did luminal disproportion between the size of the larger sheep carotid arterial heterografts and the extremely small lumens of the native coronary arteries contribute to the graft thrombosis? The failure of patency of relatively large modified bovine carotid arteries when grafted to smaller canine femoral and renal arteries has been attributed to such luminal disproportion.[23] Sheep or bovine carotid arteries that measure 10 to 12 mm in diameter may never be suitable conduits for grafting into atherosclerotic coronary arteries with lumens 5 to 6 mm in diameter or less. (5) Are species differences important in choice of vascular heterograft? Heterografts that have been utilized in man for vascular reconstruction have included those from pigs, cows, sheep, horses, and dogs. It has been suggested that the pig and cow may be closer to man immunologically and, hence, a better source than other species for human heterografts.[24] Sheep heterografts, in particular, appear to do poorly. Whether this is due to immunologic species differences[24] or to gross structural differences in the vessel wall that promote clotting[19] is uncertain, but current evidence shows that arterial heterografts from sheep have a far greater rate of failure than those of porcine or bovine origin.[23] The canine heterografts also do poorly in man.[23]

Glutaraldehyde-fixed sheep carotid arteries failed as aortocoronary bypass conduits in our patient soon after implantation, and 30 months after operation were virtually destroyed by a vigorous host response. Possibly, the canine saphenous vein graft may have had a similar fate. There are no published data on the use of stabilized glutaraldehyde-fixed vascular heterografts for aortocoronary bypass in man or in animals, but the results in our patient strongly suggest that more information is needed before such heterografts are again utilized for this procedure.

References

1. **Sawyer PN, Srinivasan S:** Metallic and plastic prosthetic devices as vascular wall substitutes: biophysical criteria and methods for evaluation. J Biomed Mater Res 1:83–101, 1967
2. **Dale WA, Niguidula FN:** Study of elasticized Dacron as arterial prosthesis. Arch Surg 72:246–259, 1959
3. **Benjamin RB, Turbak CE, Hannon DW, et al:** Polyvinyl sponge in experimental surgery. Ann Surg 145:509–516, 1957
4. **Harrison JH:** Synthetic materials as vascular prostheses. I. A comparative study in small vessels of nylon, dacron, orlon, ivalon sponge and teflon. Am J Surg 95:3–15, 1958
5. **Rosenberg N:** The modified bovine arterial graft. Arch Surg 105:547–548, 1972
6. **Carrel A:** Heterotransplantation of blood vessels preserved in cold storage. J Exp Med 9:226–228, 1907
7. **Carrel A:** Ultimate results of aortic transplantation. J Exp Med 15:389–392, 1912
8. **Guthrie CC:** Heterotransplantation of blood vessels. Am J Physiol 19:482–487, 1907

9. **Schloss G, Shumacker HB:** Studies in vascular repair. The use of free vascular transplants for bridging arterial defects. A historical review with particular reference to histologic observations. Yale J Biol Med 22:273–290, 1950
10. **Deterling RA Jr:** Transplantation of blood vessels. In, Transplantation of Tissues vol 2, chap 11 (Peer LA, ed). Baltimore, Williams & Wilkins, 1959, p 313–397
11. **Creech O Jr, DeBakey ME, Self M, et al:** The fate of heterologous arterial grafts: an experimental study. Surgery 36:431–444, 1954
12. **Swan H, Robertson HT, Johnson ME:** Arterial homografts. I. The fate of preserved aortic grafts in the dog. Surg Gynecol Obstet 90:568–579, 1950
13. **DeBakey ME, Creech O Jr, Cooley DA, et al:** Structural changes in human aortic homografts. A study of ten cases. Arch Surg 69:472–482, 1954
14. **Szilagyi DE, McDonald RT, Smith RF, et al:** Biologic fate of human arterial homografts. Arch Surg 75:506–529, 1957
15. **Payne WS, Edwards JE, Grindlay JH, et al:** The ultimate fate of implanted aortic homografts preserved in acid-buffered formalin. Arch Surg 80:61–70, 1960
16. **Guthrie CC:** Heterotransplantations of blood vessels. Am J Physiol 19:482–487, 1907
17. **Klotz O, Permar HH, Guthrie CC:** End results of arterial transplants. Ann Surg 78:305–320, 1923
18. **Carrel A:** Ultimate results of aortic transplantation. J Exp Med 15:389–396, 1912
19. **Hufnagel CA, Rabil PJ, Reed L:** A method for the preservation of arterial homo- and heterografts. Surg Forum 4:162–168, 1953
20. **Rosenberg N, Henderson J, Lord G, et al:** An arterial prosthesis of heterologous vascular origin. JAMA 187:741–743, 1964
21. **Rosenberg N, Martinez A, Sawyer PN, et al:** Tanned collagen arterial prostheses of bovine carotid origin in man. Ann Surg 164:247–256, 1966
22. **Bothwell JW, Lord GH, Rosenberg N, et al:** Modified arterial heterografts: relationship of processing techniques to interface characteristics. In, Biophysical Mechanisms in Vascular Homeostasis and Intravascular Thrombosis (Sawyer PN, ed). New York, Appleton-Century Crofts, 1965, p, 306–313
23. **Dale WA, Lewis MR:** Modified bovine heterografts for arterial replacement. Ann Surg 169:927–946, 1969
24. **Mattila SP, Fogarty TJ:** Antigenicity of vascular heterografts. J Surg Res 15:81–86, 1973
25. **DeFalco RJ:** Immunologic studies of untreated and chemically modified bovine carotid arteries. J Surg Res 10:95–100, 1970
26. **Dillon ML, Scott SM, Vasquez MD, et al:** Tissue response to an arterial substitute of bovine origin. Arch Aurg 105:547–548, 1972
27. **Rosenberg N, Lord GH, Henderson J, et al:** Collagen arterial graft of bovine origin: seven-year observations in the dog. Surgery 67:951–956, 1970
28. **Keshishian JM, Adkins PC, Camp F, et al:** Surgical techniques using the bovine arterial graft. Surg Gynecol Obstet 133:268–272, 1971

Tension on coronary bypass conduits

A neglected cause of real or potential obstruction of saphenous vein grafts

Of 41 saphenous vein aorta-coronary bypass grafts from 21 patients, abnormal graft tension was judged to be present at necropsy in 6 grafts (15 per cent) from 5 patients (24 per cent). Five (33 per cent) of 15 grafts placed to the right coronary system and one (3 per cent) of 26 grafts to the left coronary system were under excess tension. The abnormal tension appeared to result from the insertion of grafts too short to accommodate normal or abnormal distention of the right atrium and ventricle (graft to distal right coronary or posterior descending coronary artery) or of the pulmonary trunk (graft to left coronary system) after discontinuation of cardiopulmonary bypass or development of acute congestive cardiac failure.

Thomas L. Spray, M.D., and William C. Roberts, M.D., *Bethesda, Md.*

Many causes of obstruction to flow of blood in coronary bypass conduits have been described (Fig. 1). A possible but neglected cause of graft obstruction is excessive tension on the bypass conduit. Observations in five patients who died early after aorta-coronary bypass procedures in whom excessive graft tension appeared to be present at necropsy are described in this report.

Patients studied, methods, and results

The hearts of 21 necropsy patients who had undergone aorta-coronary bypass procedures and had died within a month of operation were re-examined. Only cases in which the hearts were available for re-examination and the aorta-coronary bypass grafts were more or less intact were included in this analysis. A total of 41 saphenous vein bypass grafts had been inserted: 19 to the left anterior descending, 9 to the right, 6 to the posterior descending (each arising from the right), and 7 to other branches of the left coronary artery. Excessive graft tension, as indicated by grooving of the right atrial wall or right atrioventricular sulcus (Figs. 2 and 3) or by flattening of the graft passing anterior to the pulmonary trunk (Fig. 2), occurred in 5 (24 per cent) of the 21 patients or in 6 (15 per cent) of the 41 grafts. The excess tension involved 5 (33 per cent) of the 15 grafts placed to the distal right or proximal posterior descending coronary artery and one (3 per cent) of the 26 grafts placed to a left coronary artery. Among the 5 patients with excess graft tension as judged at necropsy, death occurred either in the operating room or within 24 hours after operation in 3 patients, on Day 4 postoperatively in one, and on Day 18 in one. All 6 grafts were flattened at necropsy: one contained a thrombus; the lumina of the other 5 were patent. None of the 5 patients with graft tension had myocardial necrosis.

From the Section of Pathology, National Heart and Lung Institute, National Institutes of Health, Bethesda, Md. 20014.

Received for publication March 3, 1976.

Accepted for publication June 3, 1976.

Comments

The present study provides necropsy evidence suggesting that abnormal graft tension may be a significant technical factor affecting graft function. Several explanations for the occurrence of this tension are probable. In some centers, the aortic anastomoses of the vein grafts are performed with the patient not supported by cardiopulmonary bypass, but the distal coronary anastomoses usually are completed with cardiopulmonary bypass. Thus, at the time of graft trimming and final anastomosis, the right atrium is relatively empty and the left ventricle is not beating (Fig. 4, *A*). Furthermore, the apex of the heart may have to be retracted superiorly or to either side to facilitate exposure of the distal right coronary artery or distal

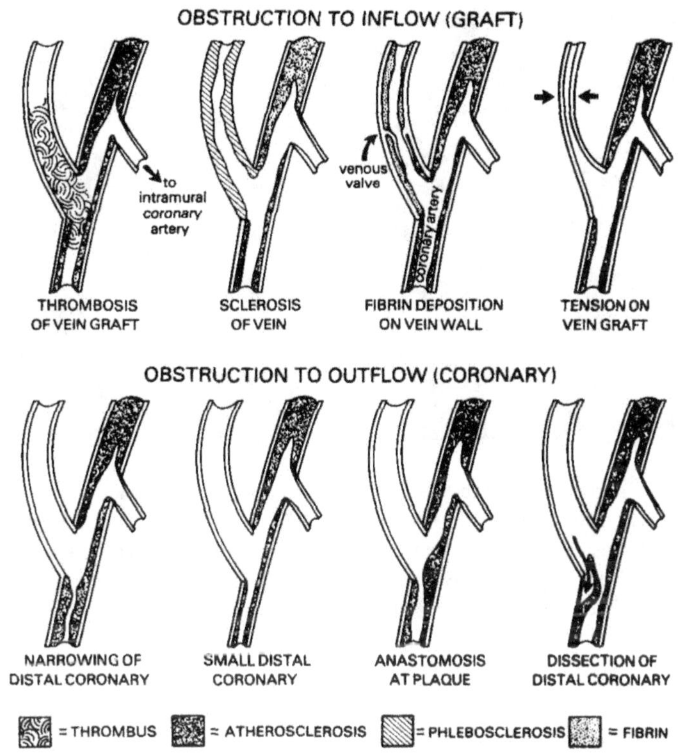

Fig. 1. Anatomic and technical factors that affect flow in the coronary arteries following aorta-coronary bypass.

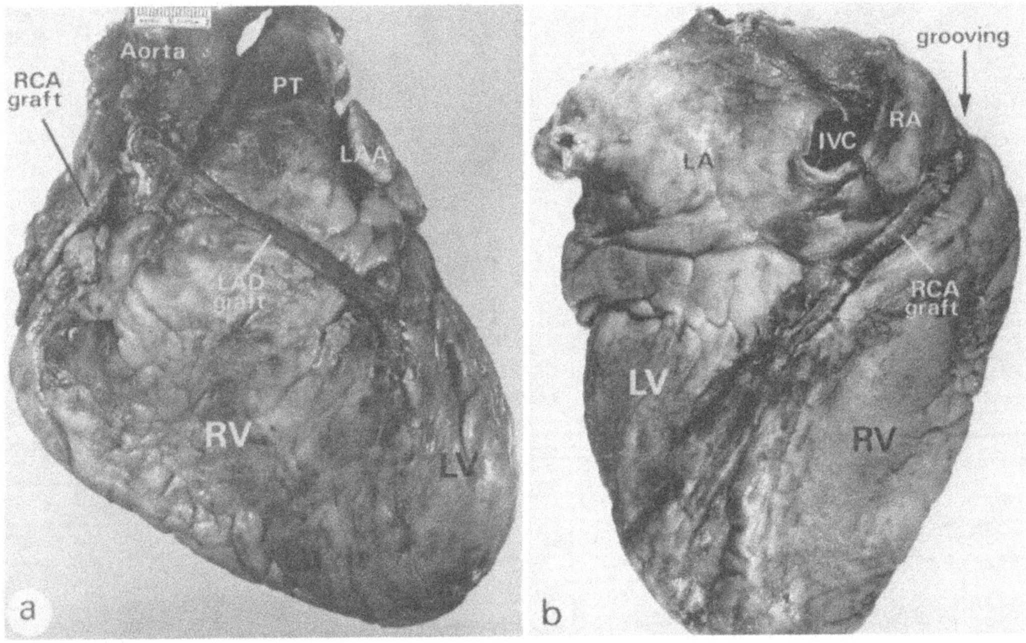

Fig. 2. The heart in one patient with graft tension. *a, Anterior view.* Mild flattening is present in a saphenous vein graft to the left anterior descending *(LAD)* coronary artery. The patient was a 66-year-old woman (A75-109) who died 4 days after double vein bypass grafting and aortic valve replacement for aortic stenosis. Postoperatively, she had congestive heart failure and hypotension. *b, Posterior view.* Grooving of the right atrium *(RA)* by the vein graft placed to the posterior descending branch of the right coronary artery *(RCA)* is present. The grooving is indicative of excess tension on the graft. *LA,* Left atrium. *LV,* Left ventricle. *RV,* Right ventricle. *PT,* Pulmonary trunk. *IVC,* Inferior vena cava orifice in RA. *LAA,* Left atrial appendage.

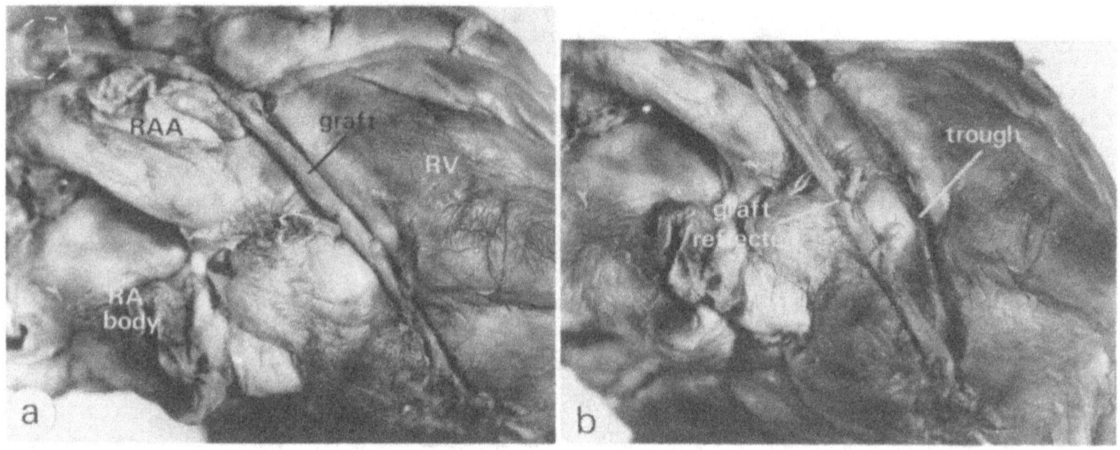

Fig. 3. Saphenous vein aorta-coronary bypass graft from the aorta *(dashed circle)* to the right posterior descending coronary artery in a 49-year-old man (75A-107) who died 2 hours after operation from persistent hypotension. *a,* The graft passes along the right atrioventricular sulcus below the ligated right atrial appendage *(RAA)* and the right atrial *(RA)* body. *b,* A view of the graft after it has been reflected. A deep trough is present in the atrioventricular sulcus, indicating that the graft was under tension. *RV,* Right ventricle.

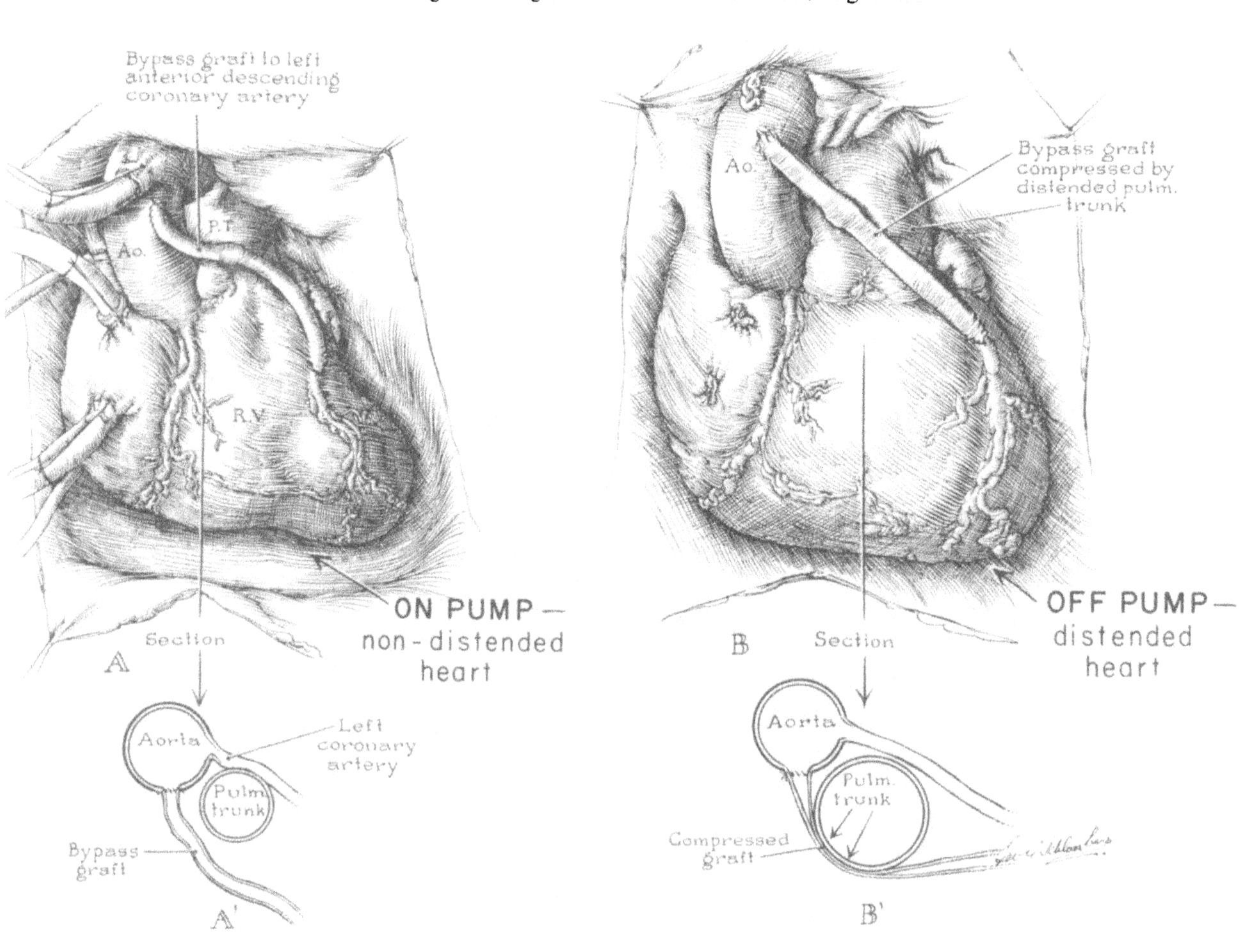

Fig. 4. See comments section of text for explanation.

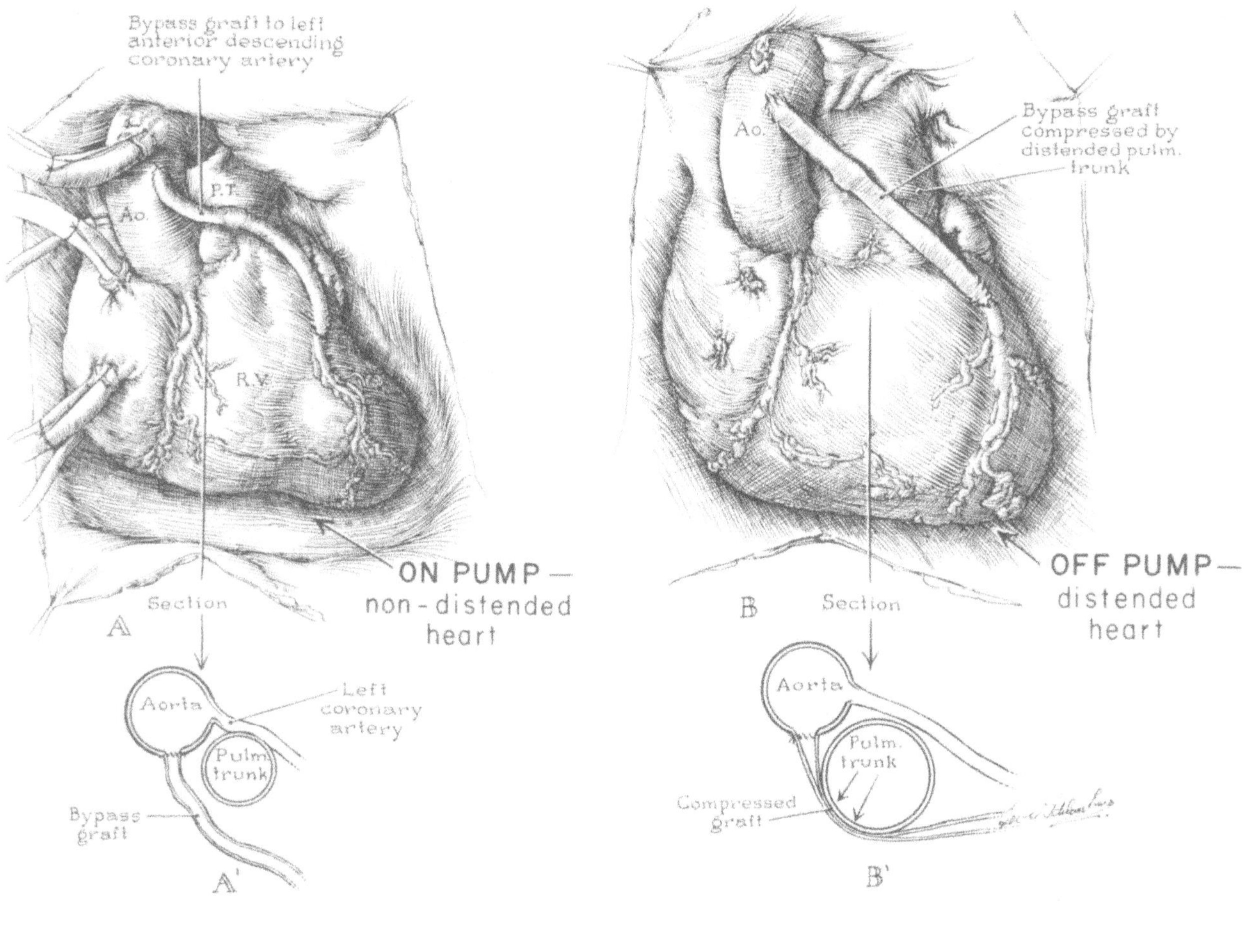

Fig. 5. See comments section of text for explanation.

portions of the left circumflex coronary artery. Although the distal anastomoses are completed with the graft under no tension, when the heart is re-placed in the pericardial sac, significant tension may be placed on the graft. Grafts to the distal right coronary artery and the posterior descending branch are generally placed in the atrioventricular sulcus. As the patient is weaned from bypass, the right atrium dilates and the right ventricle fills, so that outward-directed tension is imposed on the graft and transmitted tension on the anastomoses (Fig. 4, *B*). Although hemodynamic evidence is lacking, the tension on the graft would be expected to decrease flow through the graft. Although the right atrial and right ventricular distending pressures can be expected to be less than the intraluminal pressure in the graft, the leverage produced at or near the midpoint of the graft by the outward pressure when both ends of the graft are fixed could significantly narrow the lumen. Anatomic evidence for this graft tension is seen by a deep trough in the right atrium or right atrioventricular sulcus at necropsy, with flattening of the vein graft itself (Fig. 3).

A mechanism similar to that described herein may occur in grafts placed to the left anterior descending or left circumflex coronary system, since these grafts must cross over the pulmonary trunk or right ventricular outflow tract and since the distal anastomosis is performed at a time when there is little pulmonary blood flow (Fig. 5, *A*). Since retraction of the heart is necessary for exposure of the distal left circumflex or obtuse marginal coronary arteries, grafts to these vessels are more likely to be placed under tension when the cardiac apex is later released. Indeed, the problem of kinking of a graft to the left circumflex coronary artery as it crosses the left atrial appendage has prompted several authors[1, 2] to suggest placement of the left circumflex graft through the transverse pericardial sinus posterior to the aorta and pulmonary trunk.

Even when the distal anastomosis is created first and when the grafts are observed to be under no noticeable

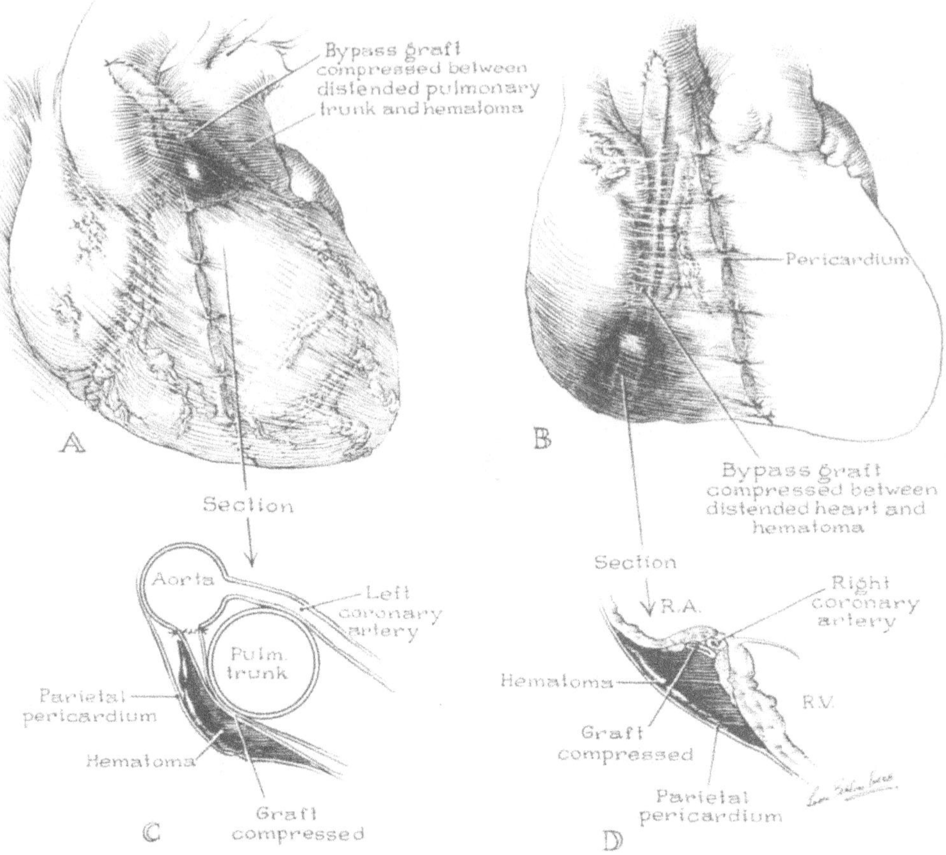

Fig. 6. Localized pericardial hematoma compressing a bypass graft. *A and C*, Hematoma in the sulcus between the aorta and pulmonary trunk affecting graft to a left coronary artery. *B and D*, Compression of a vein graft to the right coronary artery by hematoma formation in the atrioventricular sulcus. Although in this diagram the parietal pericardium is seen as loosely approximated, similar events could occur when the pericardium is not closed if sufficient hematoma is present. *R.A.*, Right atrium. *R.V.*, Right ventricle.

tension at the completion of the bypass procedure, several subsequent events may alter the cardiac anatomy to create tension on the graft. Left ventricular failure from perioperative myocardial infarction or other causes may result in retrograde distention of the pulmonary outflow tract (Fig. 5, *B*). This produces unanticipated tension on a graft to the left coronary system. Right ventricular failure or transmitted failure of the left ventricle may result in right ventricular and right atrial dilatation with resulting tension on a graft to the right coronary system. In addition, graft length has been shown to decrease significantly as the injured vein heals, so that further tension may develop on the graft and the anastomosis.[3] Segmental flattening or stenosis of a vein graft may result from localized hematoma formation and tamponade as diagrammed in Fig. 6.

Significant tension appears to be most pronounced in grafts placed to the distal right or to the proximal posterior descending coronary arteries. In this study, 5 (33 per cent) of 15 grafts to the right coronary system and one (3 per cent) of 26 grafts to the left coronary system were judged to be taut. Problems with kinking and determination of appropriate graft length in grafts to the left circumflex system have prompted Flemma and his associates[1] to create the coronary anastomosis first, with final graft trimming and anastomosis to the aorta being done with the patient not supported by bypass. Other authors[4, 5] have used a similar approach with grafts to the right coronary system. The surprisingly high frequency of evidence for significant tension on saphenous vein aorta-coronary bypass grafts seen at necropsy in this study suggests that determination of graft length while the patient is supported by cardiopulmonary bypass is inaccurate. Creation of the venocoronary anastomosis first, and measurement of graft length before institution of cardiopulmonary bypass or after partial occlusion of venous return lines to distend the right atrium and right ventricle, should prevent underestimation of graft length in most patients.

REFERENCES

1 Flemma, R. J., Singh, H. M., and Tector, A. J.: A Method for Revascularization of Circumflex Marginal Coronary Arteries, Ann. Thorac. Surg. **20:** 706, 1975.

2 Cheanvechai, C., Groves, L. K., Surakiatchanukul, S., Tanaka, N., Effler, D. B., Shirey, E. K., and Sones, M. F., Jr.: Bridge Saphenous Vein Graft, J. THORAC. CARDIOVASC. SURG. **70:** 63, 1975.

3 Cody, M. C., Smith, H. C., Frye, R. L., Danielson, G. K., Pluth, J. R., and Wallace, R. B.: Long-Term Followup of Flow and Dimension Changes in Saphenous Vein Bypass Grafts to the Coronary Arteries (Abstr.), Circulation **50:** 132, 1975 (Suppl III).

4 Cohn, L. H.: The Surgical Treatment of Acute Myocardial Ischemia, Mt. Kisco, N. Y., 1973 Futura, 172 pp.

5 Urschel, H. C., Razzak, M. A., Wood, R. E., and Paulson, D. L.: Factors Influencing Patency of Aortocoronary Artery Saphenous Vein Grafts, Surgery **72:** 1048, 1972.

Histologic changes in saphenous vein aorta-coronary bypass grafts

The effect of the angle of the aortic anastomosis

Thirteen dogs were subjected to bypass grafting from the aorta to the left circumflex coronary artery with the saphenous vein to determine whether the angle of insertion of the saphenous vein into the aorta influences the functional and histologic fate of the grafts. The angle of the aortic anastomosis was obtuse in 6 dogs, acute in 5, and perpendicular in 2. Histologic examination of all 13 grafts 6 to 19 months (mean 9.4) postoperatively showed fibrous intimal proliferative lesions of variable severity along the entire length of the grafts, occasionally with extension into the native coronary arteries. Loss of medial smooth muscle and adventitial fibrosis also occurred in all 13 grafts. The extent and severity of these changes, however, were not *related to the angle of the aortic anastomosis.*

Robert H. Breyer, M.D.,* Thomas L. Spray, M.D., David G. Kastl, M.D., and William C. Roberts, M.D., *Bethesda, Md.*

Intimal fibrous proliferation (IFP), medial smooth muscle degeneration and fibrous tissue replacement, and adventitial fibrosis are common late findings in saphenous veins used for aorta-coronary bypass.[1-9] The relative contributions of ischemia, arterial pressure, and poor distal coronary runoff to the development of these changes have been reported.[10-12] Additional factors, including vein handling during "harvesting," vein length and diameter, and the geometry of the proximal and distal anastomoses may influence the fate of autogenous vein grafts.[13-16] Although a theoretical and hydraulic basis for such an effect has been reported,[17] it has not been determined whether the angle of the aorta-vein anastomosis of an aorta-coronary bypass graft can influence late graft changes. This possibility was examined in the present experimental study.

From the Clinic of Surgery and the Pathology Branch, National Heart, Lung and Blood Institute, National Institutes of Health, Bethesda, Md. 20014.

Received for publication July 13, 1976.

Accepted for publication Aug. 26, 1976.

Address for reprints: William C. Roberts, M.D., NIH Bldg. 10A, Room 3E30, Bethesda, Md. 20014.

*Present address: Department of Surgery, University of Chicago Medical Center, Chicago, Ill.

Material and methods

Thirteen foxhounds (14 to 25 kilograms) underwent a bypass graft from the aorta to the left circumflex coronary vessel with autogenous saphenous vein. Standard techniques were used. The veins were transiently distended with saline and maintained in saline at room temperature until used. The coronary artery proximal to the site of bypass was ligated. The proximal anastomosis was constructed by one of three methods (Fig. 1). In 2 dogs, the vein graft was cut at a 90 degree angle and sutured to a circular ostium in the aortic wall, so that an aorta-graft angle of approximately 90 degrees was created (perpendicular, Group A). In 11 dogs, the vein graft was cut at a 45 degree angle and sutured to a longitudinal slit in the aortic wall. In 5 of these dogs, the vein graft was directed distally toward the circumflex artery, so as to create an angle of 45 to 60 degrees with the ascending aorta (acute, Group B). In the remaining 6 dogs, the vein graft was directed cephalad and then looped gently back toward the circumflex artery, so that an aorta-graft angle of 120 to 135 degrees was created (obtuse, Group C).

All 13 dogs underwent aortic root angiograms to determine graft patency from 2 to 28 days (average 13 days) after operation and again from 5 to 20 months (average 8 months) postoperatively (Fig. 1). The animals were put to death 6 to 19 months following opera-

Table I. *Histologic changes (0-4+) in saphenous vein aorta-coronary bypass grafts*

Dog No.	Graft angle	Graft age (mo.)	Graft length (cm.)	IFP in graft at aortic anastomosis	Graft at midportion		Graft and CA at CA anastomosis	
					IFP	SM loss	IFP vein	IFP CA
Group A								
12	Perpendicular	21	5.5	+	+	+	+	++
13	Perpendicular	21	5.5	++	+++	++	++	0
Group B								
7	Acute	6	5.5	0	0	0	0	+
8	Acute	8	5.5	++	+	++	+	++
9	Acute	8	4.5	+	+	+	+	0
10	Acute	8	6	+	++	+	++	+++
11	Acute	9	5	+	+	0	++	++
Group C								
1	Obtuse	6	6	++	++	+	++	+
2	Obtuse	6	6	0	++	++	++	++
3	Obtuse	8	6	+	++	+	+	+
4	Obtuse	6	6	+	+	+++	0	0
5	Obtuse	10	7.5	+	+	+++	0	+++
6	Obtuse	6	6	++	+	+	++	+

Legend: CA, Coronary artery. IFP, Intimal fibrous proliferation. SM, Smooth muscle in media.

tion (average 9.4 months) and the hearts perfused with 10 per cent buffered formalin. The venous bypass grafts, both anastomoses, and the distal coronary artery were subserially sectioned, processed in alcohol and xylene, embedded in paraffin, and sectioned for light microscopy. The remaining saphenous vein from each animal was removed at the time of sacrifice and processed to serve as a control.

Results

Initial angiographic evaluation demonstrated patent grafts in 12 of the 13 dogs; occlusion in the midportion of the graft was visualized in one of the six Group C (obtuse angle) dogs. The status of all grafts was unchanged at a second angiographic study performed just before the animal was killed. The angle of takeoff of the vein graft from the aorta was confirmed by postmortem angiography.

Gross observations. Vein grafts in all three groups showed marked adventitial fibrosis. In all cases, the grafts were bound down to epicardium throughout their length by fibrous tissue.

Microscopic observations. Control saphenous veins from all dogs were normal (Fig. 2). Each consisted of multiple layers of medial smooth muscle (generally oriented in a circular direction), thin intima, and vascular adventitia. No intimal thickening was observed.

Observations on the vein grafts are summarized in Table I.

Group A (perpendicular). Both grafts in this group measured 5.5 cm. in length. Mild-to-moderate IFP was seen in one graft with no increase in amount at or near the aortic anastomosis. These lesions consisted of thickening of the intimal layer, primarily by fibrous tissue, and an increase in mucopolysaccharide ground substance (Fig. 3). The other graft had moderately severe IFP at the midpoint of the graft but less change at the aortic anastomosis. IFP was variable throughout the length of both grafts. Moderate loss of medial smooth muscle and marked adventitial fibrosis were present. In one graft, the distal (coronary) anastomosis showed mild IFP in the vein but moderate IFP in the coronary artery at the anastomosis. In the other graft, moderate IFP of the vein was seen but none was present in the coronary artery. Fibrin was absent in the intimal lesions (phosphotungstic acid hematoxylin stain).

Group B (acute). Vein graft length in these 5 dogs averaged 5.3 cm. Mild-to-moderate IFP was seen at the aortic anastomosis in four grafts, and in each it extended the length of the graft with variable medial smooth muscle loss. Often subendothelial collections of cells resembling myocytes were present (myointimal cells) (Fig. 4). One vein graft had a minimal amount of intimal proliferation, yet mild IFP was present in the circumflex coronary at the distal anastomosis (Fig. 5). Of the remaining four grafts, the distal coronary artery had IFP in three; in one graft the fibrous proliferation in the coronary was greater than that in the vein graft itself

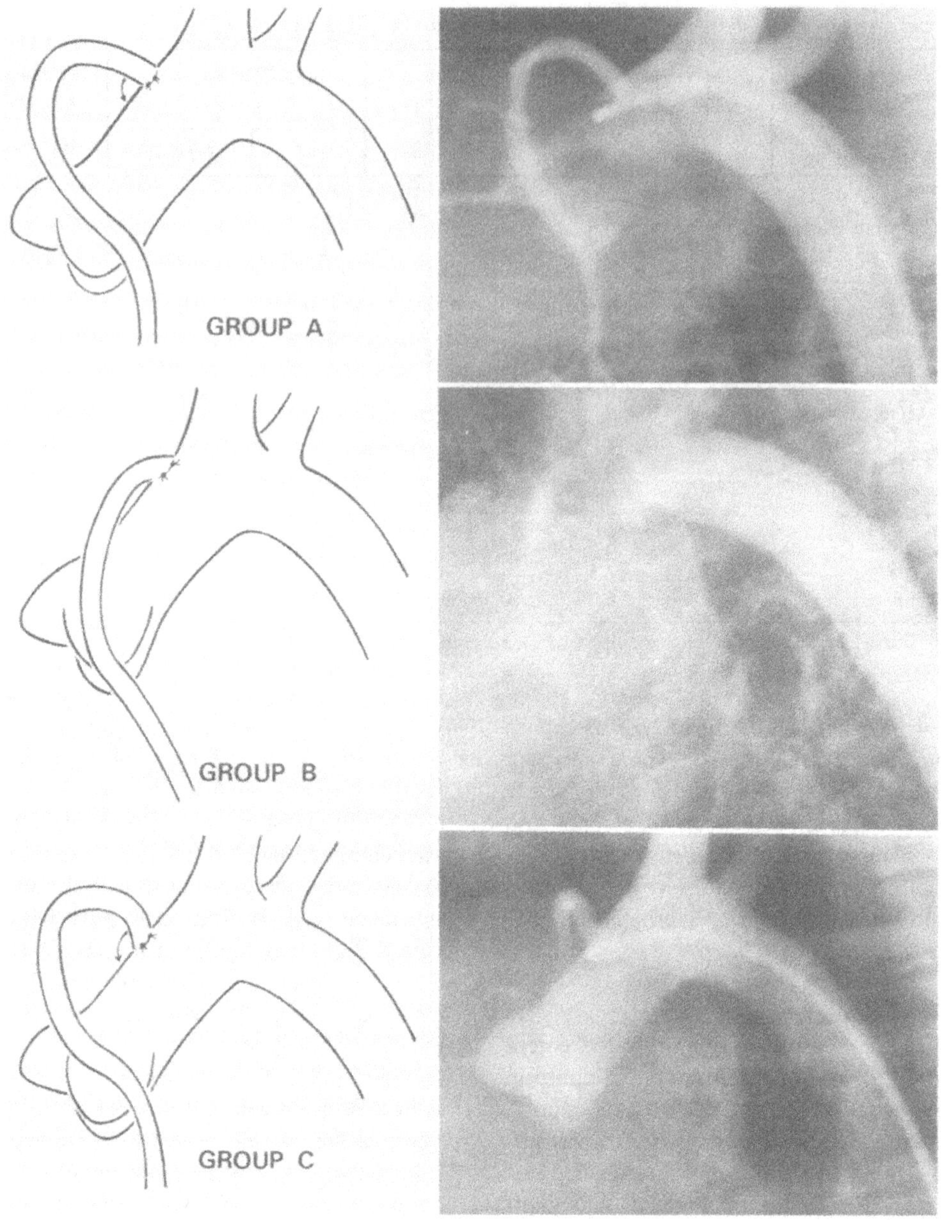

Fig. 1. Diagrams *(left)* and postoperative angiograms *(right)* of the angle of takeoff of the vein grafts. Group A, The vein graft emerges from the aorta at a 90 degree angle (perpendicular). Group B, The vein graft takes off at an acute angle. Group C, The graft takes off at an obtuse angle.

(Fig. 6). The fibrous lesions in the coronary arteries were localized to within 5 mm. of the anastomosis in each case and did not extend down the vessel.

Group C (obtuse). The mean length of these six grafts was 6.2 cm. Mild-to-moderate IFP was present in five of the six grafts at the aortic anastomosis, but moderate intimal thickening was present in the more distal portions of the graft. All six vein grafts had some (usually small) degree of intimal thickening at some point along their length and moderately severe loss of smooth muscle in the media. Four of the six grafts had lesions of IFP in the vein at the distal (coronary) anastomosis. In 5 of 6 dogs, intimal lesions were present in the coronary artery itself at the anastomosis (Fig. 7), and in 2 they extended for up to 1.0 cm. in the distal vessel. In one graft, no IFP of the vein at the distal

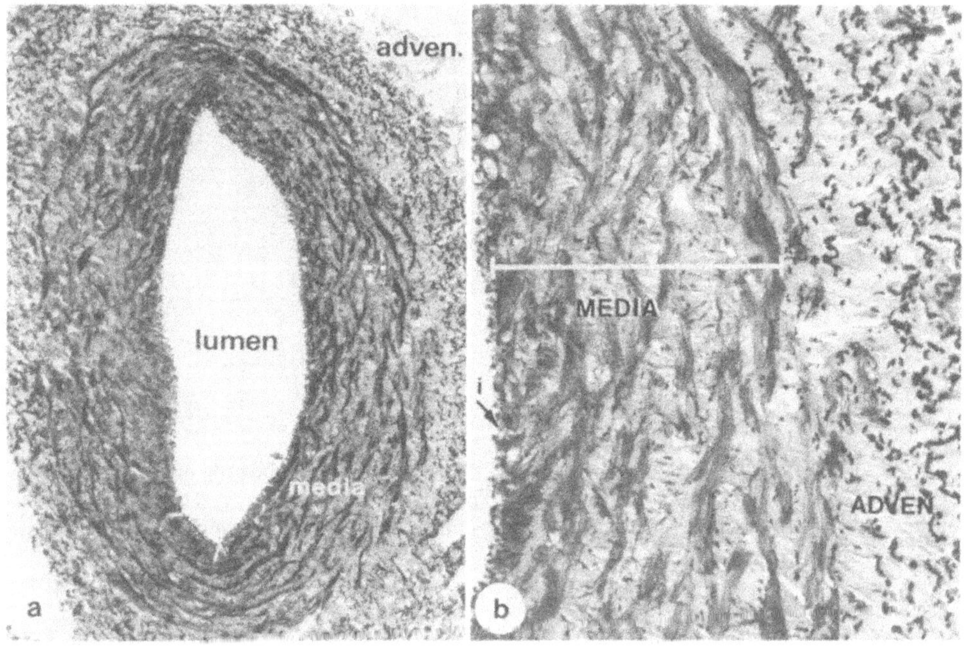

Fig. 2. Normal dog saphenous vein. *a,* Multiple lamina of circularly oriented smooth muscle compose the media. The adventitia *(adven.)* contains many short, broad elastic fibers. *b,* A higher power view shows the intima *(i)* composed of almost a unicellular layer and basement membrane. The relatively thick media is seen in contrast. (Movat stains: orig. mag.; *a* × 72, *b* × 220.)

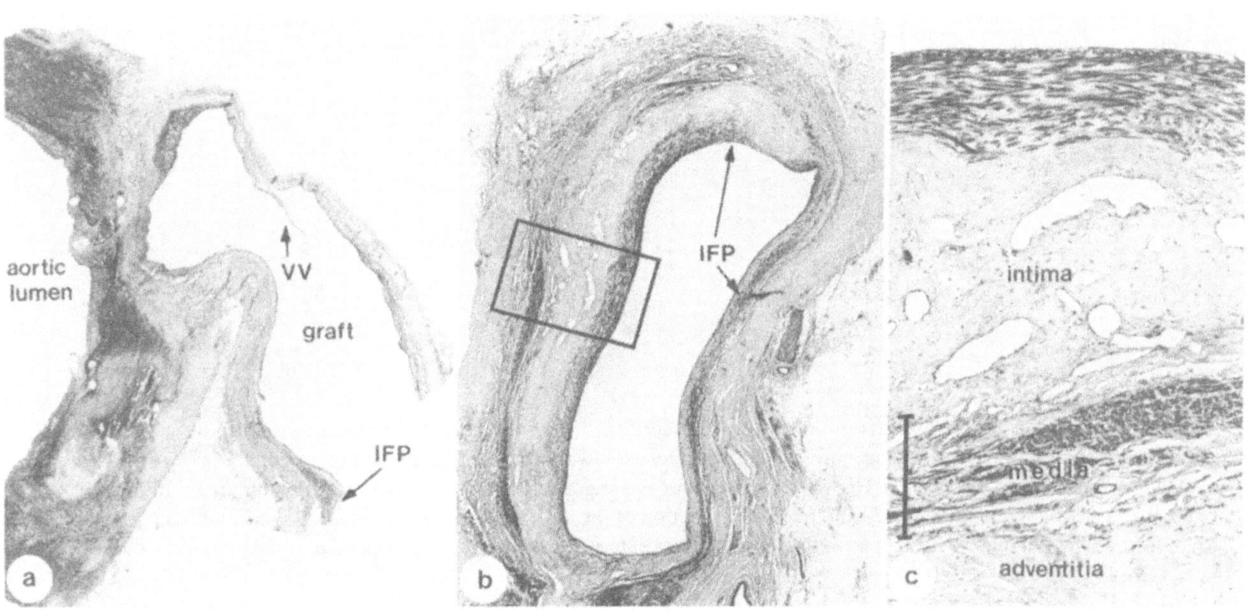

Fig. 3. Group A (perpendicular) grafts. *a,* Oblique section through the aortic anastomosis of one graft showing little intimal fibrous proliferation *(IFP)* near the anastomosis. One leaflet of a thin, delicate venous valve *(vv)* projects into the lumen of the graft close to the takeoff from the aorta. *b,* Distal vein graft from a second dog showing moderately severe IFP. *c,* Higher power view of area enclosed in box in *b,* showing the similarity of IFP to organized thrombus and the thickness of the IFP in relation to the media, which shows moderate loss of smooth muscle cells. (Movat stains: orig. mag.; *a* × 10, *b* × 14, *c* × 80.)

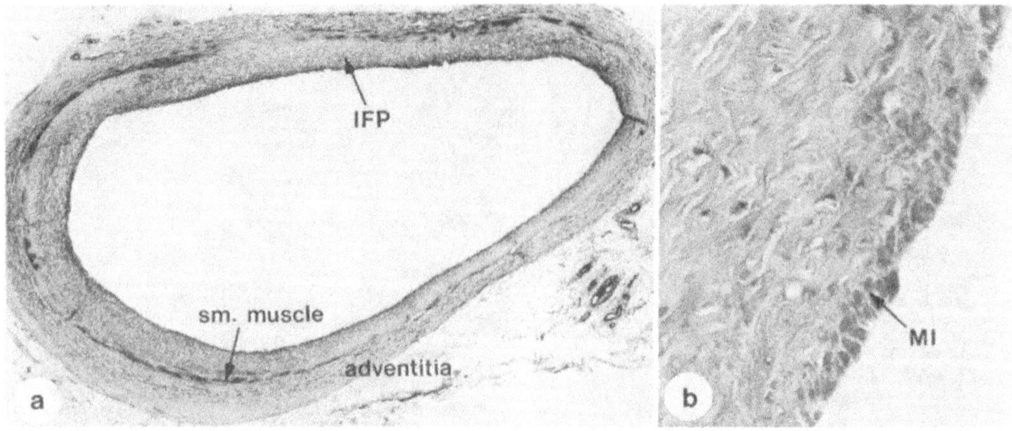

Fig. 4. *a*, Midportion of vein graft from a Group B (acute angle) dog showing moderate intimal fibrous proliferation *(IFP)* and severe loss of smooth muscle. The adventitia is fibrotic. *b*, Higher power view of the luminal surface showing subendothelial collections of myointimal *(MI)* cells. (Movat stains: orig. mag.; *a* × 20, *b* × 330.)

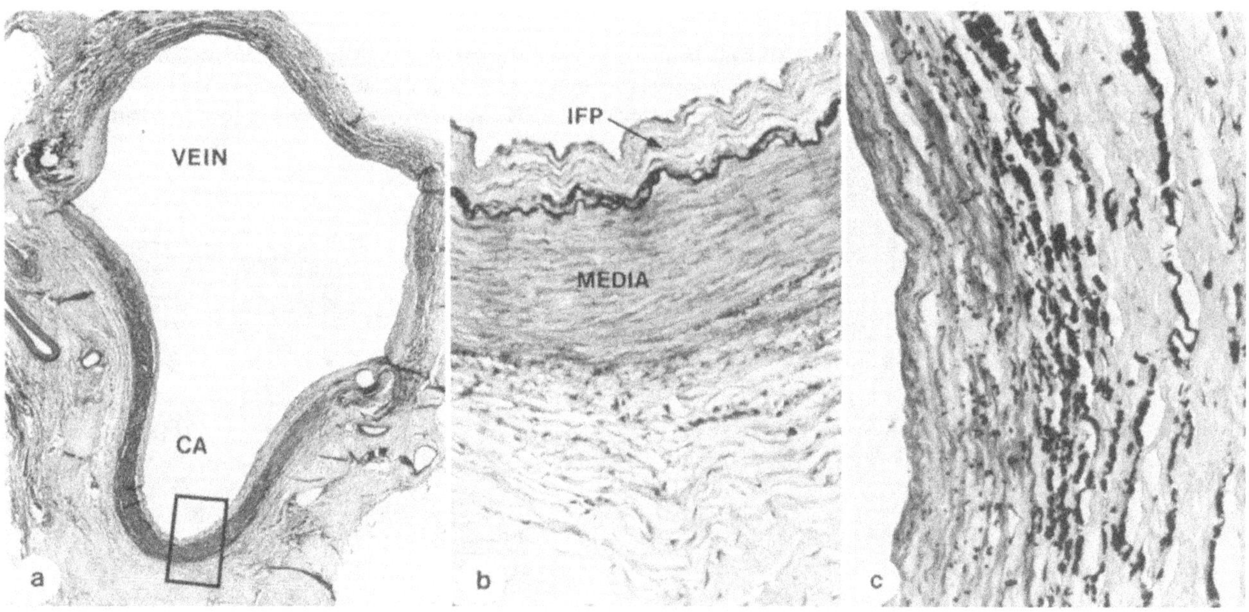

Fig. 5. Intimal fibrous proliferation *(IFP)* in the coronary artery *(CA)* at the distal anastomosis in a Group B (acute angle) dog. *a*, Section of the venocoronary anastomosis. Mild IFP is seen in the coronary artery *(CA)* but little is present in the vein. *b*, Higher power view of the area enclosed in the box in *a*, showing the small layer of IFP covering the internal elastic membrane. *c*, Section of the vein graft at a higher magnification showing marked medial smooth muscle loss, but minimal intimal thickening. (Movat stains: orig. mag.; *a* × 23, *b* and *c*, × 220.)

anastomosis was present, but moderately severe luminal narrowing of the coronary artery by intimal proliferation was seen.

One vein graft in a Group C dog was almost occluded. Sections showed a recanalized lumen (Fig. 8), suggesting earlier thrombotic occlusion of the graft. The luminal surfaces of the recanalized channels had cellular collections typical of intimal proliferative lesions, and sections of graft proximal to the recanalized lesions showed changes consistent with moderately severe IFP. No residual fibrin was seen in the recanalized thrombus or in the IFP lesions.

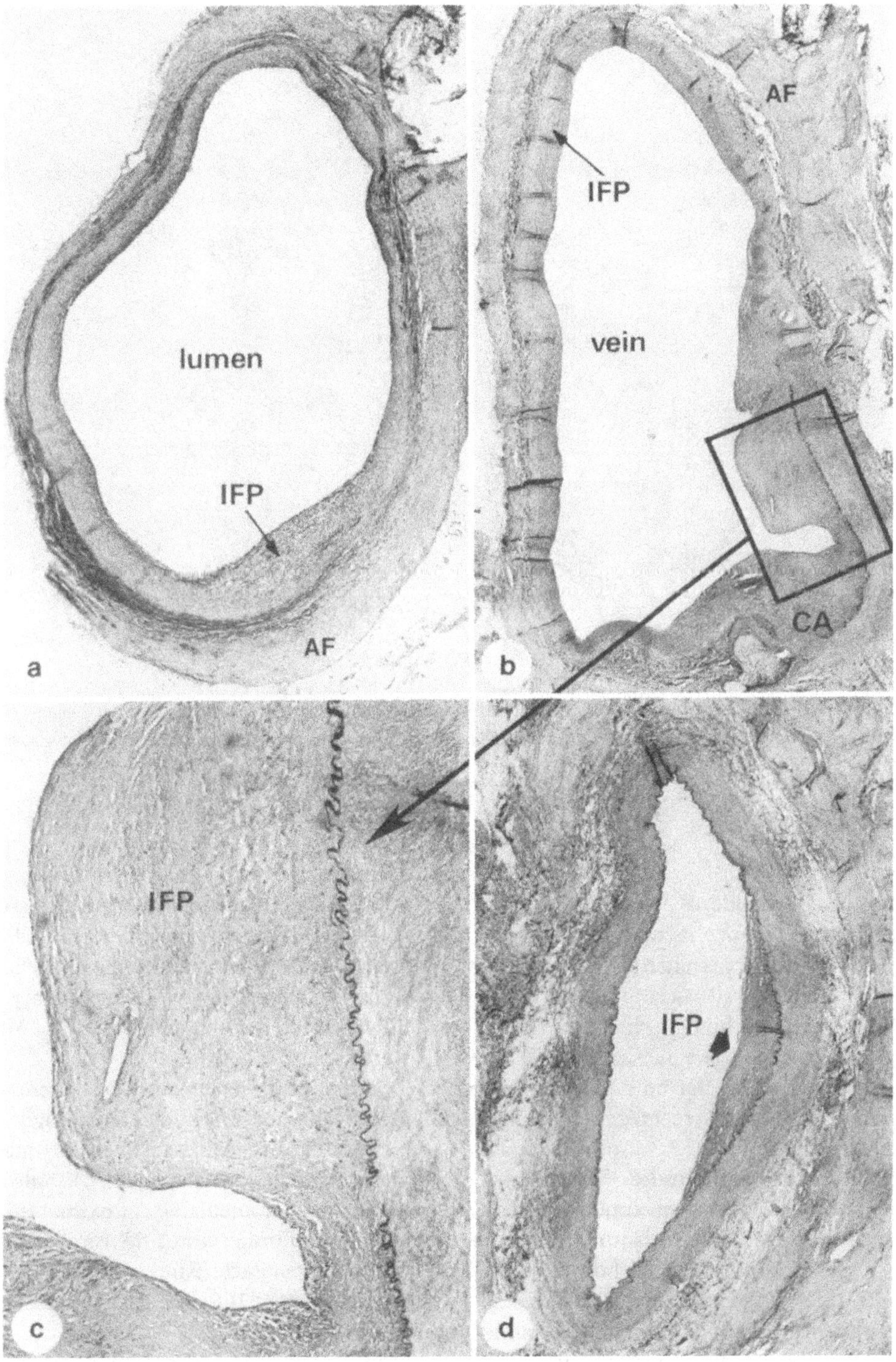

Fig. 6. Severe intimal fibrous proliferation *(IFP)* in the coronary artery *(CA)* at the distal anastomosis in a Group B (acute angle) dog. *a,* Section of vein graft at midportion, showing moderate IFP and adventitial fibrosis *(AF)*. Variable medial smooth muscle loss is present. *b,* Section of the distal anastomosis shows IFP extending from the vein across the suture line into the coronary artery (CA). *c,* Higher power view of area enclosed in the box in *b,* showing the thick layer of IFP and its histologic similarlity to that seen in the vein graft. *d,* Section of coronary artery less than 5 mm. distal to *b,* showing continuance of the IFP lesion for a short length down the native artery. (Movat stains: orig. mag.; *a* and *b* × 20, *c* × 80, *d* × 35.)

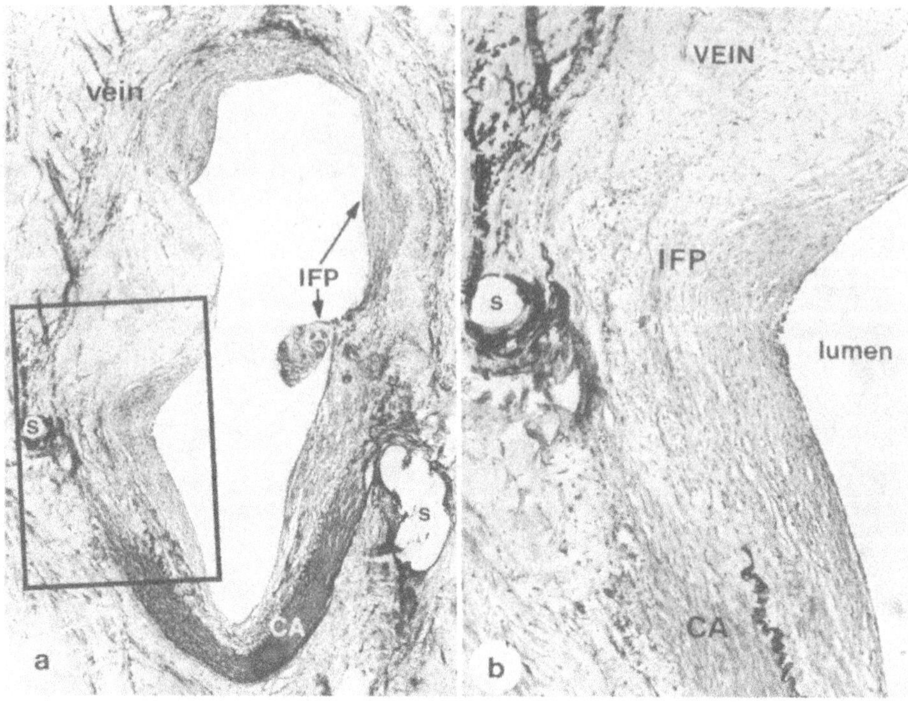

Fig. 7. *a*, Intimal fibrous proliferation *(IFP)* extending across suture line *(s)* into the coronary artery *(CA)* at the distal anastomosis in a Group C (obtuse angle) dog. *b*, Higher power view of area enclosed in box in *a*, showing IFP continuous across the anastomosis. (Movat stains: orig. mag.; *a* × 34, *b* × 80.)

Discussion

Evidence that the magnitude of flow through a venous bypass graft may influence its ultimate histologic fate[12, 18] suggests that variables altering the hemodynamics of coronary bypass grafts may affect the development of IFP and other morphologic changes. Increasing graft length only mildly decreases flow.[19] The important effects of vein diameter on both magnitude and velocity of flow have been recognized clinically[15] and demonstrated experimentally.[19–21] Low velocity of flow predisposes to thrombotic closure. Mathematical and hydraulic models predict that maximum hemodynamic efficiency is achieved with an aorta-graft angle of 90 degrees.[17] In clinical practice, however, this angle is often 45 to 60 degrees. Kennedy[17] has suggested that turbulent flow secondary to an acute aorta-graft angle may contribute to the development of IFP. This was not confirmed by our study. Saphenous vein aorta-coronary bypass grafts constructed with acute, perpendicular, or obtuse aorta-graft angles all had similar histologic changes comparable to those reported by others. The degree of IFP, in addition, was variable along the length of the graft, and occasionally IFP was absent at the aortic anastomosis, the suggestion being that turbulent flow at or near the anastomosis was not its cause. The common finding of IFP in the coronary artery at the site of anastomosis indicates that jet lesions may be produced in the coronary arteries by local flow characteristics as suggested by Vlodaver and Edwards.[5]

Early graft occlusion was demonstrated angiographically in one dog. Histologic examination 6 months later revealed recanalized thrombus. Interestingly, lesions consistent with IFP also were observed in sections immediately proximal to this organized thrombus. Furthermore, the recanalized thrombus had histologic characteristics similar to those of the IFP lesions, so that IFP also may represent organization of mural thrombi.

In conclusion, characteristic histologic changes occur in the intima, media, and adventitia of saphenous veins used as aorta–coronary arterial conduits in dogs, but the angle of the aorta–vein graft anastomosis does not appear to influence the magnitude, location, or frequency of these changes, provided that reasonable flow through the graft is achieved.

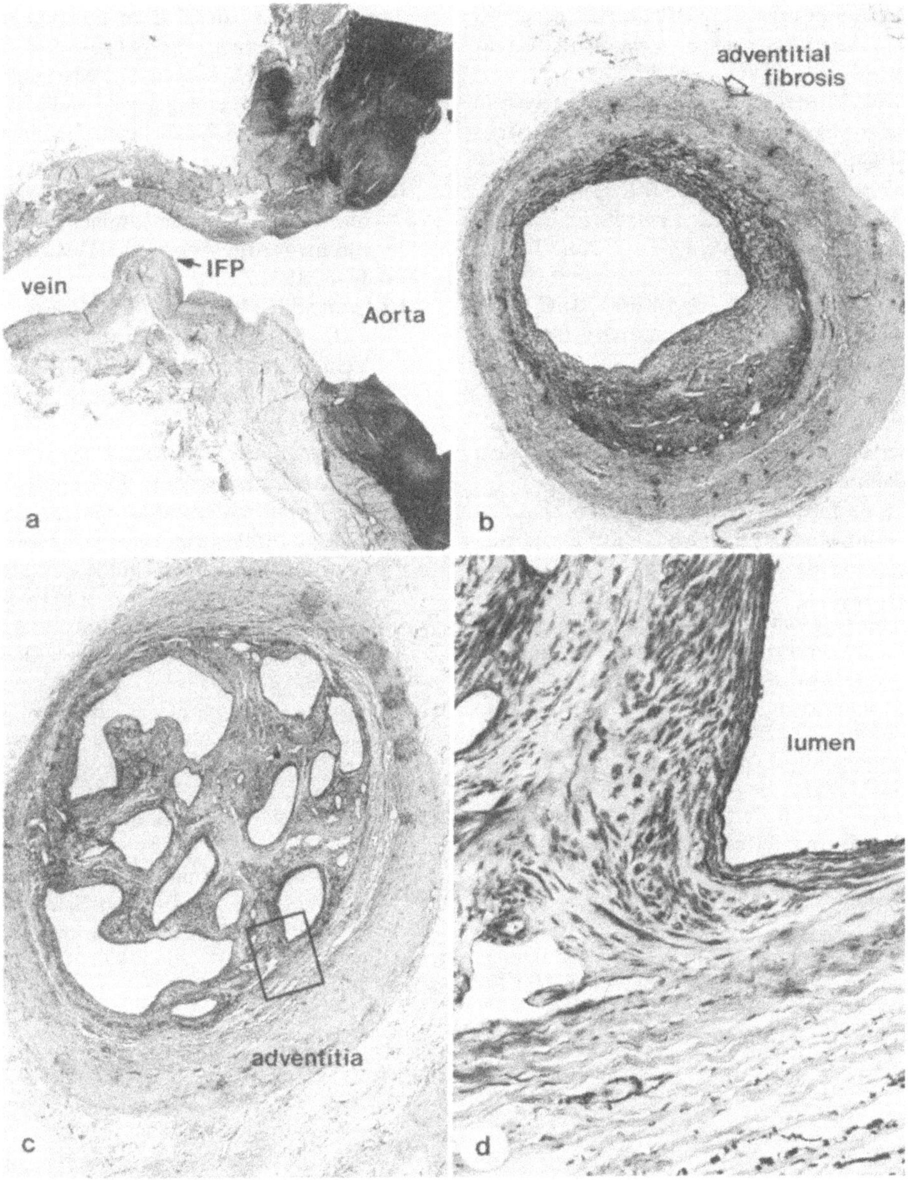

Fig. 8. Recanalized thrombus in a Group C (obtuse angle) dog. Graft occlusion was confirmed by angiography less than 2 weeks after operation. *a,* Section of aortic anastomosis showing obtuse angle of takeoff and moderate intimal fibrous proliferation *(IFP). b,* Proximal vein graft showing recanalized thrombus which has histologic characteristics of IFP. *c,* Section of graft more distal than *b,* showing obvious recanalized channels. *d,* Higher power view of area enclosed by box in *c,* showing similarity of the recanalized thrombus to IFP. (Movat stains: orig. mag.: *a* × 10, *b* × 31, *c* × 32, *d* × 130.)

REFERENCES

1 Johnson, W. D., Auer, J. E., and Tector, A. J.: Late Changes in Coronary Vein Grafts (Abstr.), Am. J. Cardiol **26:** 640, 1970.

2 Grondin, C. M., Meere, C. M., Castonguay, Y., Lepage, G., and Grondin, P.: Progressive and Late Obstruction of an Aorto-coronary Venous Bypass Graft, Circulation **43:** 698, 1971.

3 Hamaker, W. R., Doyle, W. F., O'Connell, T. J., and Gomez, A. C.: Subintimal Obliterative Proliferation in Saphenous Vein Grafts, Ann. Thorac. Surg. **13:** 488, 1971.

4 Vlodaver, Z., and Edwards, J. E.: Pathologic Changes in Aorta–Coronary Arterial Saphenous Vein Grafts, Circulation **44:** 719, 1971.

5 Vlodaver, Z., and Edwards, J. E.: Pathologic Analysis in Fatal Cases Following Saphenous Vein Coronary Arterial Bypass, Chest **64:** 555, 1973.

6 Unni, K. K., Kottke, B. A., Titius, J. L., Frye, R. L., Wallace, R. B., and Brown, A. L.: Pathologic Changes in Aortocoronary Saphenous Vein Grafts, Am. J. Cardiol. **34:** 526, 1974.

7 Brody, W. R., Angell, W. W., and Kosek, J. C.: Histologic Fate of the Venous Coronary Artery Bypass in Dogs, Am. J. Pathol. **66:** 111, 1972.

8 Jones, M., Conkle, D. M., Ferrans, V. J., Roberts, W. C., Levine, F. H., Melvin, D. B., and Stinson, E. B.: Lesions Observed in Arterial and Autogenous Vein Grafts, Circulation **47:** 198, 1973, (Suppl. III).

9 Silver, M. D., MacGregor, D. C., Agarwal, V. K., and Lifield, W.: Aortocoronary Bypass Graft: Early Histologic Changes in Dogs, Can. J. Surg. **16:** 246, 1973.

10. Brody, W. R., Kosek, J. R., and Angell, W. W.: Changes in Vein Grafts Following Aorto-coronary Bypass Induced by Pressure and Ischemia, J. THORAC. CARDIOVASC. SURG. **44:** 847, 1972.

11 McCabe, M., Cunningham, G. J., Wyatt, J. P., Rothnie, N. G., and Taylor, G. W.: A Histological and Histochemical Examination of Autogenous Vein Grafts, Br. J. Surg. **54:** 147, 1967.

12 Faulkner, S. L., Fisher, R. D., Conkle, D. M., Page, D. L., and Bender, H. W.: Effect of Blood Flow Rate on Subendothelial Proliferation in Venous Autografts Used as Arterial Substitutes, Circulation **51:** 163, 1975 (Suppl. I).

13 Storm, F. K., Gierson, E. D., Sparks, F. C., and Barker, W. F.: Autogenous Vein Bypass Grafts: Biological Effects of Mechanical Dilatation and Adventitial Stripping in Dogs, Surgery **77:** 261, 1975.

14 Ramos, J. R., Berger, K., Mansfield, P. B., and Sauvage, L. R.: Histologic Fate and Endothelial Changes of Distended and Nondistended Vein Grafts, Ann. Surg. **183:** 205, 1976.

15 Urschel, H. C., Razzuk, M. A., Wood, R. E., and Paulson, D. L.: Factors Influencing Patency of Aorto–coronary Artery Saphenous Vein Grafts, Surgery **72:** 1048, 1972.

16 Grondin, C. M., Lepage, G., Castonguay, Y. R., Meere, C. P., Martineau, J. P., and Grondin, P.: Aorto-coronary Vein Graft: Technical Modifications That May Improve Short- and Long-Term Results, Can. J. Surg. **16:** 261, 1973.

17 Kennedy, J. H., Wieting, D. W., Hwang, N. H., Anderson, M. S., Bayardo, R. J., Howell, J. F., and De Bakey, M. E.: Hydraulic and Morphologic Study of Fibrous Intimal Hyperplasia in Autogenous Saphenous Vein Bypass Grafts, J. THORAC. CARDIOVASC. SURG. **67:** 805, 1974.

18 Walker, J. A., Friedberg, H. D., Flemma, R. J., and Johnson, W. D.: Determinants of Angiographic Patency of Aorto-coronary Vein Bypass Grafts, Circulation **15:** 86, 1974 (Suppl. I).

19 Furuse, A., Klopp, E. H., Brawley, R. K., and Gott, V. L.: Hemodynamics of Aorta-to-Coronary Artery Bypass, Ann. Thorac. Surg. **14:** 282, 1972.

20 Szilagyi, D. E., Whitcomb, J. G., Schenker, W., and Waibel, P.: The Laws of Fluid Flow and Arterial Grafting, Surgery **47:** 55, 1960.

21 Overton, J. B., Smith, J. C., Robel, S. B., Spencer, M. P., Mansfield, P. B., and Sauvage, L. R.: Origin of Downstream Flow in Nonobstructed Coronary Arteries, Arch. Surg. **107:** 764, 1973.

Status of the Grafts and the Native Coronary Arteries Proximal and Distal to Coronary Anastomotic Sites of Aortocoronary Bypass Grafts

THOMAS L. SPRAY, M.D., AND WILLIAM C. ROBERTS, M.D.

SUMMARY **The status of the native coronary arteries at necropsy in the vicinity of the coronary anastomoses of saphenous vein aortocoronary bypass grafts in 20 patients with severe coronary heart disease is presented. Of the 37 graft systems (graft plus coronary artery into which graft inserted) analyzed, the lumina of 44% of the native coronary arteries within the first 2 cm distal to the anastomoses were greater than 75% narrowed in cross-sectional area by atherosclerotic plaques, and the native coronary artery at the site of the anastomosis was greater than 50% narrowed in cross-sectional area already by atherosclerotic plaque in 25% of the graft systems. The mean coronary arterial size distal to the site of the coronary graft anastomosis, even after correction for heart weight, was greater in the 13 men than in the seven women. The residual luminal areas squared per gram of heart weight, however, were similar in both men and women. These results suggest that 1) relative coronary vessel size is greater in men than women; 2) the luminal area squared per gram myocardial mass (a relative estimation of flow) is the same in the two groups of patients; and 3) less atherosclerotic plaque is necessary in women then in men to produce similar limitation to coronary flow. Thus, vessel size alone cannot account for the higher reported frequency of unsuccessful aortocoronary bypass procedures in women.**

ALTHOUGH SEVERAL REPORTS have described morphologic observations in bypass grafts and in native coronary arteries of patients who had died shortly after aortocoronary bypass procedures,[1-10] only one[2] focused on the status of the native coronary arteries at, proximal, and distal to the anastomoses of the conduits.

The present report describes the status of the native coronary arteries in the vicinity of the coronary anastomoses in 20 patients (37 grafts) who died shortly after insertion of one or more saphenous vein conduits between ascending aorta and coronary artery.

Materials and Methods

Only patients in whom the major extramural coronary arteries were well preserved were included. Of the 20 patients, 13 were men aged 34 to 59 years (mean, 49) and seven were women, aged 32 to 73 years (mean, 52). All 20 patients preoperatively had severe angina pectoris (stable in five, unstable in 15) and five had histories of acute myocardial infarcts which had healed. By coronary angiography, all 20 patients had severe (judged to be greater than 75% reduction in luminal diameter) narrowing of two or more of the major extramural coronary arteries. Three of the 20 patients also had associated valvular heart disease: one underwent replacement of the mitral valve; one of the aortic valve; and one of both mitral and aortic valves. Clinical evidence of preoperative congestive cardiac failure was present in only three patients, two of the three with associated valvular heart disease (aortic valve, and aortic and mitral valve) and one patient with associated left ventricular aneurysm. By left ventricular angiography, 18 of the 20 patients had well-contracting left ventricles. One patient had localized dyskinesia and one had diffuse hypokinesia and ventricular aneurysm. Of the 20 patients, 15 died within 24 hours and the other five, from four to 56 days after operation. The heart weights ranged from 300 to 700 g, an average of 412 in the women and 447 in the men.

Each specimen was divided for analysis into "graft systems" defined as the vein graft and the entire extramural coronary artery both proximal and distal to the coronary anastomosis. A total of 37 graft systems were available for study: 25 (68%) in men, and 12 (32%) in women. After fixation, each graft system (graft plus coronary artery) was sectioned at 5 mm intervals at right angles to its longitudinal axis. Each 5 mm segment was processed in alcohols and xylene, embedded in paraffin, cut and stained. At least two sections from each 5 mm segment were examined microscopically.

Each graft system was divided into six *segments* (fig. 1): 1) 2 cm portion of coronary artery immediately *distal* to the anastomosis (segment 1); 2) the remaining portion of coronary artery distal to segment 1 (segment 2); 3) 2 cm portion of coronary artery immediately *proximal* to the graft anastomosis (segment 3); 4) the remaining coronary artery proximal to segment 3 (segment 4); 5) the anastomotic site of the graft to the coronary artery (segment 5); and 6) the entire vein graft (segment 6).

Determining the Size of the Coronary Arteries

The size of the coronary artery in segment 1 of each graft system was determined by planimetry. The *smallest* of the four sections in this 2 cm segment was measured. Each section was stained by Movat's pentachrome method which clearly delineates the artery's internal elastic membrane. The circumferences of both the internal elastic membrane and the lumen were traced after projection at known magnification (fig. 2). Where the internal elastic membrane was artifactually indented or in areas of atherosclerotic plaque where the membrane was fragmented, extrapolation to a circular lumen was performed (fig. 2). Planimetry (KE compensating polar planimeter) was carried out on each tracing, yielding the area contained by the internal elastic membrane and the

From the Pathology Branch, National Heart, Lung, and Blood Institute, National Institutes of Health, Bethesda, Maryland.

Address for reprints: Dr. William C. Roberts, Building 10A, Room 3E-30, NHLBI, NIH, Bethesda, Maryland 20014.

Received August 16, 1976; revision accepted December 21, 1976.

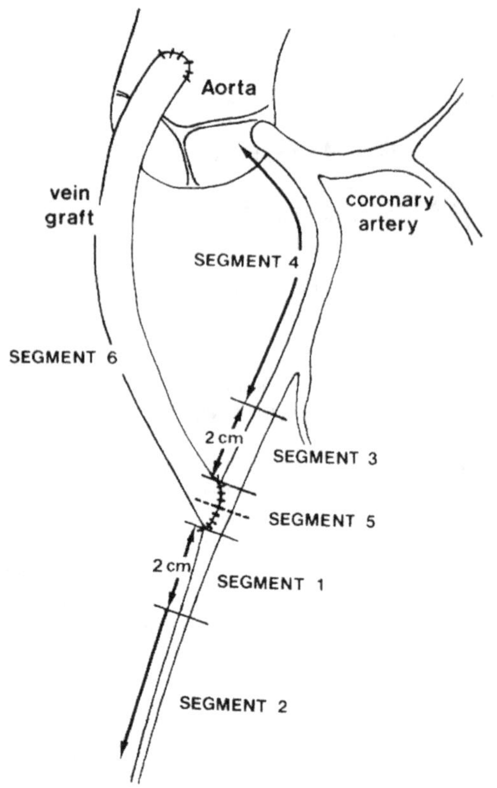

FIGURE 1. *Diagram demonstrating the locations of the six segments of the graft systems studied.*

area contained by the lumen. The area contained by the internal elastic membrane was considered the artery's normal size, and this measurement was used to compare the original size of one vessel to that of another. Percent luminal narrowing by plaque was determined from these calculations in segment 1. The percent luminal narrowing in segments 2–6 was estimated from study by light microscopy of the section of each segment showing the most cross-sectional luminal narrowing and graded as < 25%, 25–50%, 51–75%, and > 75%. In segment 5, where the graft anastomosis distorted the lumen of the native coronary vessel, percent luminal narrowing was estimated after extrapolation to a closed, circular lumen.

Results

The findings of coronary artery narrowings are summarized in table 1.

Segment 1

This segment was greater than 75% narrowed in cross-sectional area in 16 (44%) of 36 graft systems analyzed (fig. 3): in 46% of those in men and in 42% of those in women. This segment in another 11 graft systems (10 in men) was narrowed 51–75%. Thus, in 88% of the graft systems in men and in 50% in women, this segment was greater than 50% narrowed (fig. 4). Only two (6%) of the 36 graft systems showed less than 25% narrowing in this segment. In seven of the 16 (44%) graft systems with greater than 75% narrowing

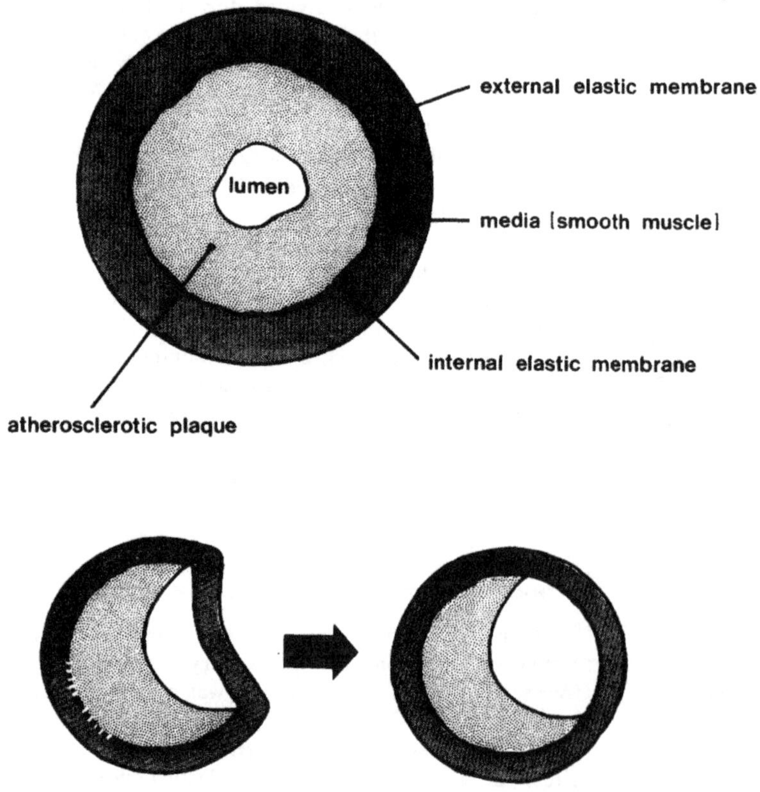

$$\text{\% luminal narrowing [by atherosclerotic plaque]} = 100 \times 1 - \frac{\text{area of lumen}}{\text{area enclosed by internal elastic membrane}}$$

FIGURE 2. *Diagrams of atherosclerotic coronary arteries illustrating the terminology used (above), the means of correcting the artifact (middle left) produced by processing an artery with an eccentric lumen and fragmentation of the internal elastic lamina, and the equation for calculating the percent luminal narrowing (below). Planimetry is performed as if the artery were distended, as shown in the middle right.*

in this segment, less than 75% narrowing was present in the remaining distal coronary artery (segment 2).

Segment 2

This segment was greater than 75% narrowed in eight (24%) of 33 graft systems analyzed: in five (22%) of 23 graft systems in men and in three of ten graft systems in women. In only two patients was this segment 51 to 75% narrowed. Thus, in only 30% (10 of 33) of the graft systems was this segment greater than 50% narrowed.

TABLE 1. *Percent and Location of Narrowings of Native Coronaries Containing a Bypass Graft*

	<25% No. (%)	25-50% No. (%)	51-75% No. (%)	>75% No. (%)	Totals
Segment 1. (*first 2 cm distal to anastomosis*)					
Men	1 (4)	2 (8)	10 (42)	11 (46)	24
Women	1 (8)	5 (42)	1 (8)	5 (42)	12
Totals	2 (6)	7 (19)	11 (31)	16 (44)	36
Segment 2. (*distal to segment 1*)					
Men	10 (43)	6 (26)	2 (9)	5 (22)	23
Women	5 (50)	2 (20)	0 (0)	3 (30)	10
Totals	15 (46)	8 (24)	2 (6)	8 (24)	33
Segment 3. (*immediately proximal to anastomosis*)					
Men	3 (12.5)	3 (12.5)	4 (17)	14 (58)	24
Women	2 (17)	1 (8)	2 (17)	7 (58)	12
Totals	5 (14)	4 (11)	6 (17)	21 (58)	36
Segment 4. (*most proximal portion*)					
Men	0	0	7 (28)	18 (72)	25
Women	0	0	3 (25)	9 (75)	12
Totals	0 (0)	0 (0)	10 (27)	27 (73)	37
Segment 5. (*at anastomosis*)					
Men	7 (32)	10 (45)	4 (18)	1 (5)	22
Women	6 (55)	2 (18)	3 (27)	0 (0)	21
Totals	13 (39)	12 (36)	7 (21)	1 (4)	33

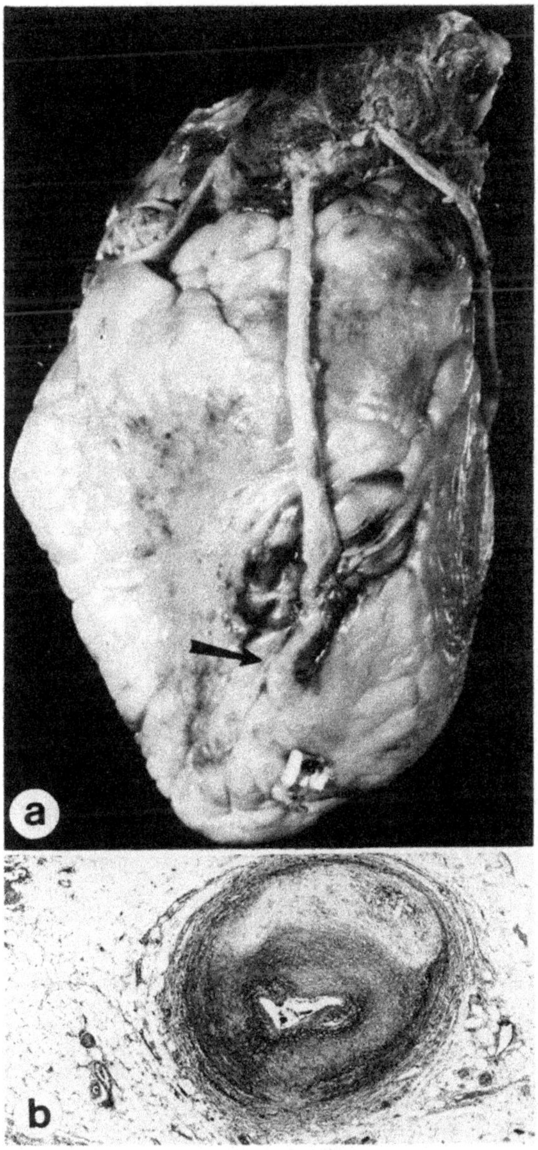

FIGURE 3. *Severe obstruction of coronary artery distal to the site of insertion of a vein bypass graft in a 40-year-old woman (A74-212) who could not be weaned from cardiopulmonary bypass after 3-vessel vein grafting.* a) *Anterior view of heart showing anastomosis of vein graft to the left anterior descending coronary artery (LAD).* b) *LAD at approximate area shown by arrow in* a. *Severe narrowing of the vessel (segment 1) is seen.* b) *Movat stain × 22.*

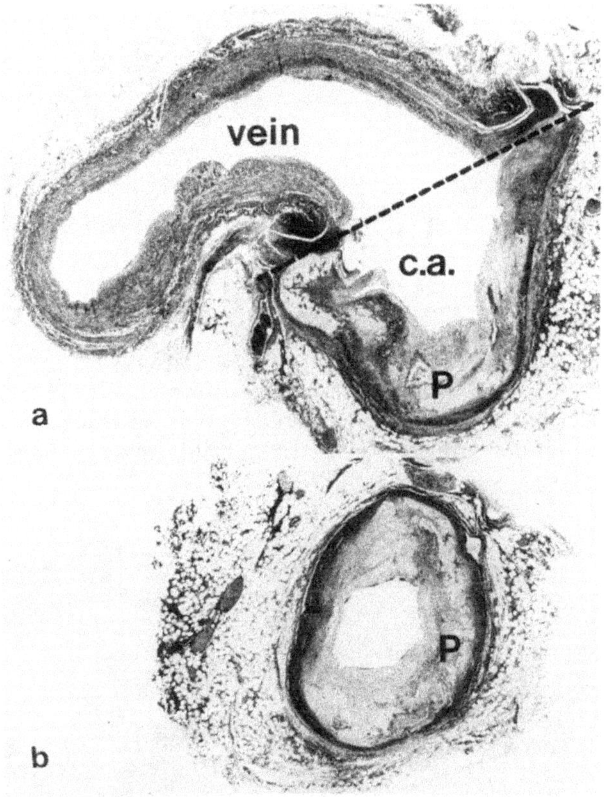

FIGURE 4. *Narrowing of coronary artery distal to insertion of vein graft in a 50-year-old man (MHCMH — 4961) who died less than 24 hours after triple vessel bypass grafting.* a) *Section of the anastomosis of the vein graft to the left anterior descending coronary artery (c.a.) at the site of considerable narrowing by atherosclerotic plaque (p).* b) *Coronary artery section* distal *to the anastomosis showing significant narrowing by plaque. Movat stains, × 11 (a and b).*

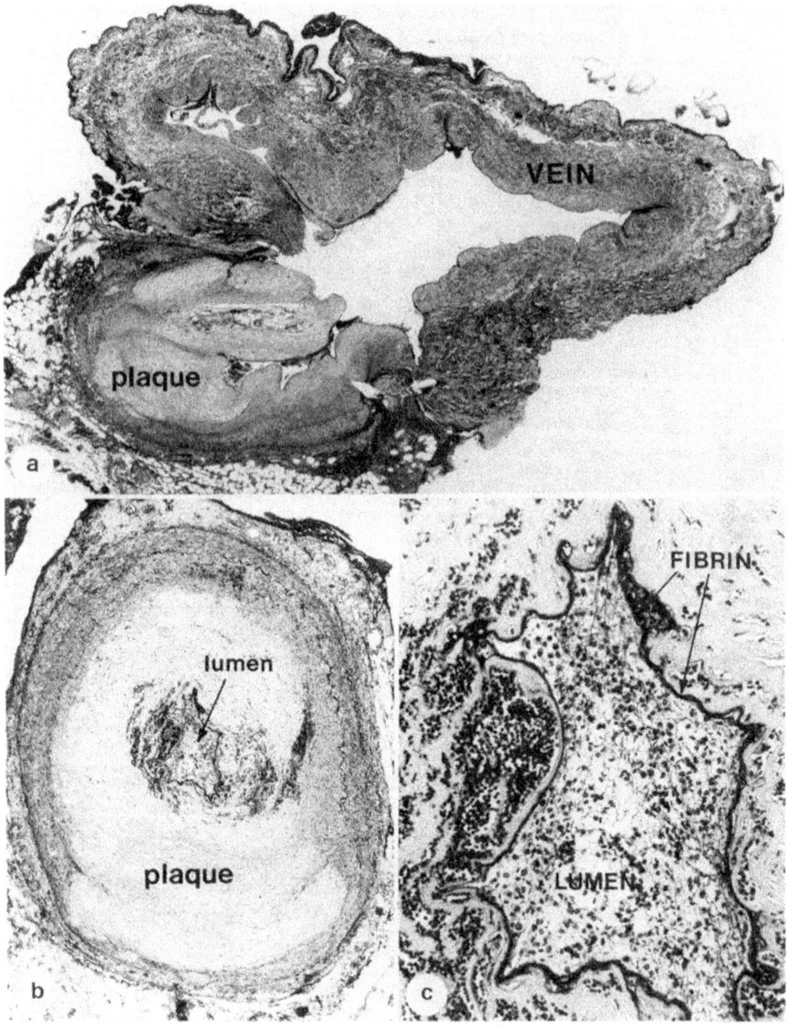

FIGURE 5. *Insertion of vein graft at site of plaque in a 46-year-old man (NA75-107) who died 24 hours after insertion of three grafts.* a) *The vein graft to the right coronary artery is large in relation to the coronary artery into which it inserts. A large atherosclerotic plaque is present at the anastomosis. Postmortem clot present in lumen was eliminated by retouching.* b) *Right coronary artery just* proximal *to the anastomosis in* a *showing hemorrhage into the plaque and fibrin deposition on its luminal surface.* c) *High power view of lumen of* b, *showing fibrin deposition on the luminal surface. Movat stains* × *22.6* (a), × *40* (b), × *184* (c).

Segment 3

This segment was greater than 75% narrowed in 21 (58%) of 36 systems analyzed, 51 to 75% narrowed in six (17%), and less than 50% narrowed in nine (25%). The degree of narrowing of this segment was similar in both men and women.

Segment 4

This segment was greater than 75% narrowed in 27 (73%) and 51–75% narrowed in 10 (27%) of 37 graft systems analyzed. The degree of narrowing was similar in both men and women.

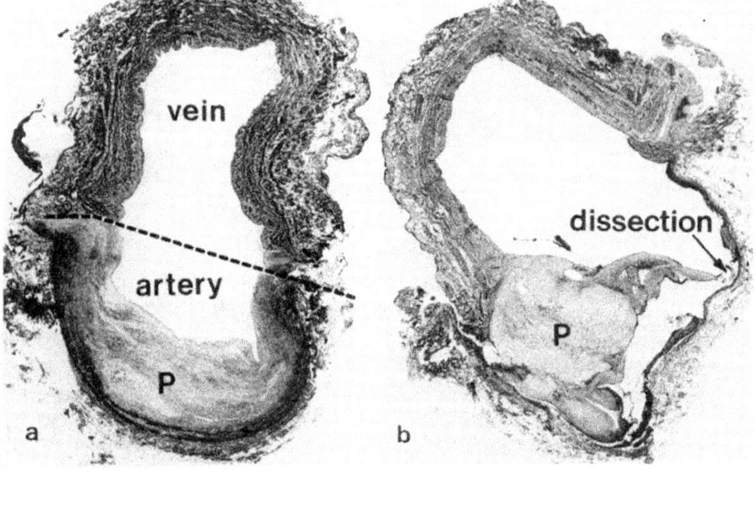

FIGURE 6. *Anastomosis of vein graft at plaque (segment 5).* a) *Anastomosis of vein graft to the proximal right coronary artery in a man (A75-279) who died shortly after operation. Significant narrowing of the coronary artery by plaque (p) at the site of insertion of the graft is seen.* b) *Dissection of atherosclerotic plaque from coronary wall at the anastomosis of the vein graft to the posterior descending coronary artery in the same patient. The dissection extended for 2 cm proximal to the anastomosis. Movat stains;* × *11* (a), × *16* (b).

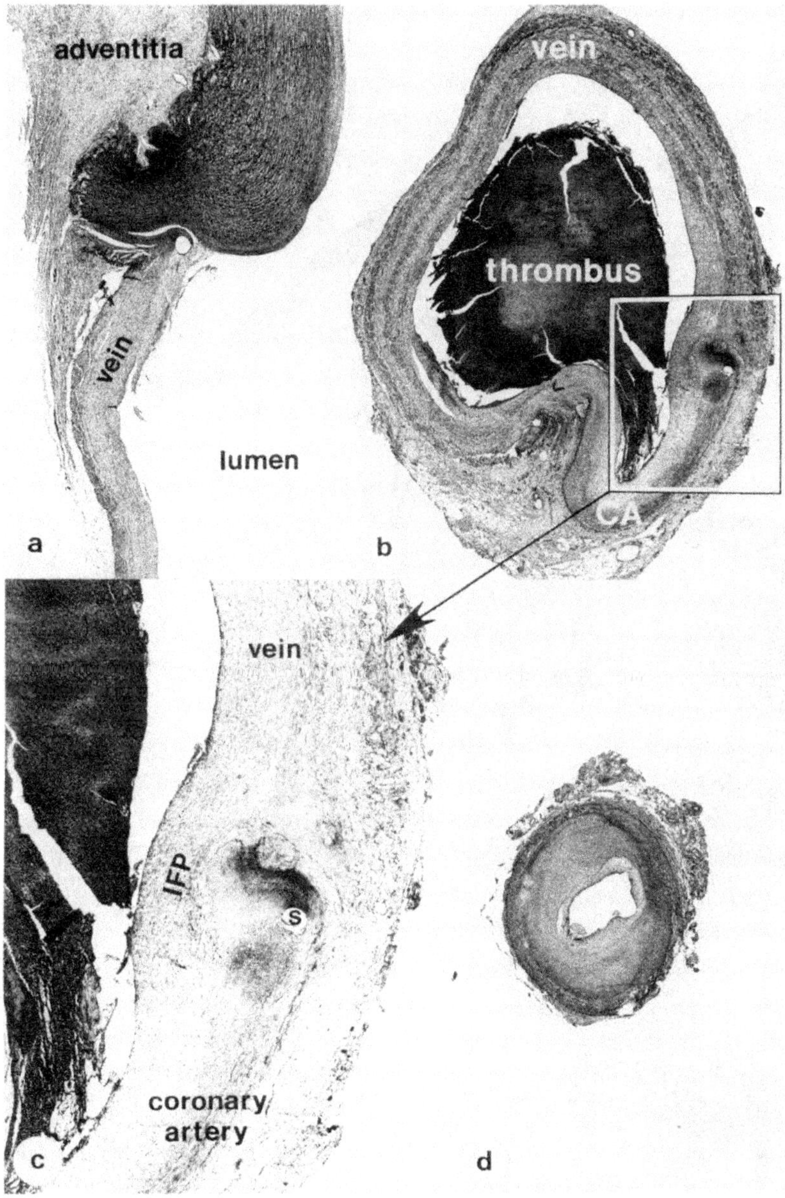

FIGURE 7. *Graft thrombosis and intimal fibrous proliferation (IFP) extending into the coronary artery at the site of vein graft anastomosis in a man (PHWT A73-28) who died suddenly 34 days after bypass grafting to the right coronary artery.* a) *Anastomosis of vein graft to aortic wall, showing intimal proliferation of the vein and adventitial fibrosis extending from the aorta over the exterior of the graft.* b) *Section taken at the venocoronary anastomosis (Segment 5) showing antemortem thrombosis of the vein graft extending into the coronary artery (CA).* c) *Higher power view of area enclosed by box in* b *showing moderate IFP of the vein with extension across the suture line (s) into the coronary artery.* d) *Section of the coronary artery distal to the anastomosis of the graft showing marked narrowing by plaque and fibrous tissue. Movat stains;* × *13* (a), × *11* (b), × *31* (c) × *12* (d).

Segment 5

This segment was greater than 75% narrowed in one (3%), 51–75% narrowed in seven (21%), and less than 50% narrowed in 25 (76%) of 33 graft systems analyzed (figs. 5 and 6).

Segment 6

Of the 37 grafts, 2 (5%) were totally occluded by thrombus (fig. 7); 10 others had mural fibrin deposits (figs. 8 and 9). In 9 of these 12 graft systems, fibrin thrombus also was present in the coronary artery at the anastomosis (table 2), and in 4, the coronary arteries proximal to the graft anastomoses contained fibrin thrombi (fig. 10).

Dissection of Native Coronary Artery at or Near Graft Anastomosis

Dissection occurred in five (14%) of the 37 graft systems. The dissection was confined to the artery within 2 cm of the anastomosis in four graft systems (fig. 6), and in the fifth, it was 8 cm long (fig. 11). In two additional graft systems, the atherosclerotic plaque opposite the site of vein anastomosis was separated from the medial wall (fig. 12). If these two graft systems are included, then disruption of the coronary artery at the anastomosis due to technical factors occurred in seven (19%) of 37 graft systems.

TABLE 2. *Fibrin Present on Walls*

	Graft No. (%)	Coronaries No. (%)	Total Grafts
Males	6 (24)	8 (32)	25
Females	4 (33)	1 (8)	12
Total	10 (27)	9 (24)	37

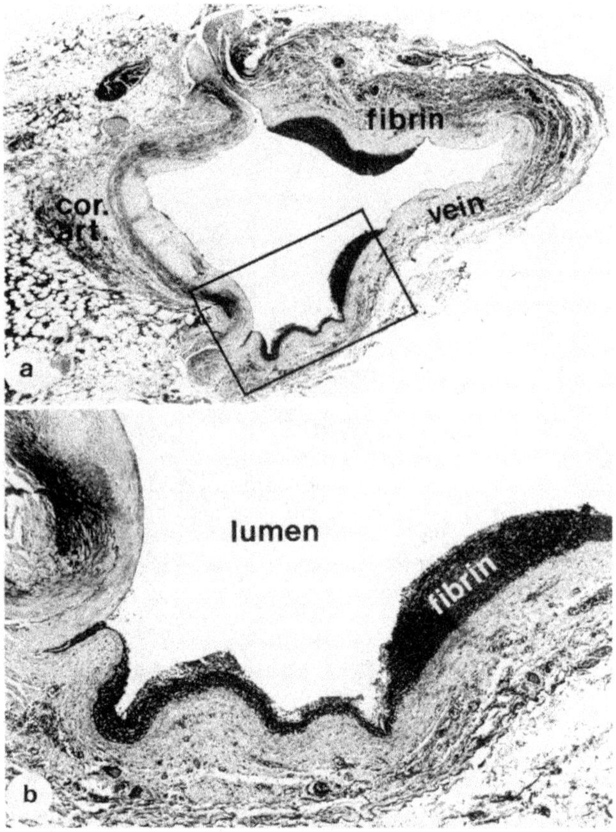

FIGURE 8. *Mural fibrin deposition in a 4-day-old vein graft to the left anterior descending coronary artery (cor. art.) in a woman (A75-109).* a) *Thick fibrin layers are present on the vein wall at the coronary anastomosis.* b) *Higher power view of area enclosed by box in* a. *Deposits of fibrin line the lumen of the vein graft. Movat stain:* × *16* (a) × *54* (b). *Retouched to eliminate artifactual post-mortem clot in lumen.*

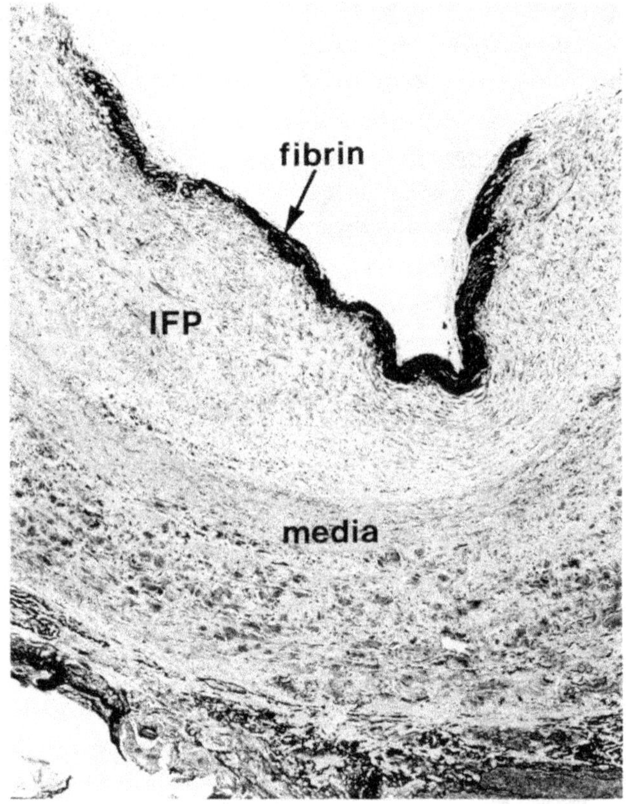

FIGURE 9. *Subendothelial fibrin in a 56-day-old vein bypass graft (male patient). Marked intimal fibrous proliferation (IFP) is present and the smooth muscle in the media is diminished. Phosphotungstic acid-hematoxylin stain;* × *54.*

Size of Coronary Artery Distal to the Anastomosis

Comparison of the areas contained by the internal elastic membrane in the smallest section of the coronary artery within 2 cm distal to the vein graft anastomosis in the 22 graft systems in men and in the 12 graft systems in women is plotted in figure 13. Three graft systems (all in men) were excluded from these comparisons because the grafts were anastomosed to the proximal portions of the coronary arteries and could not be compared with the other 34 grafts which were inserted at, or distal to, the middle portion of the

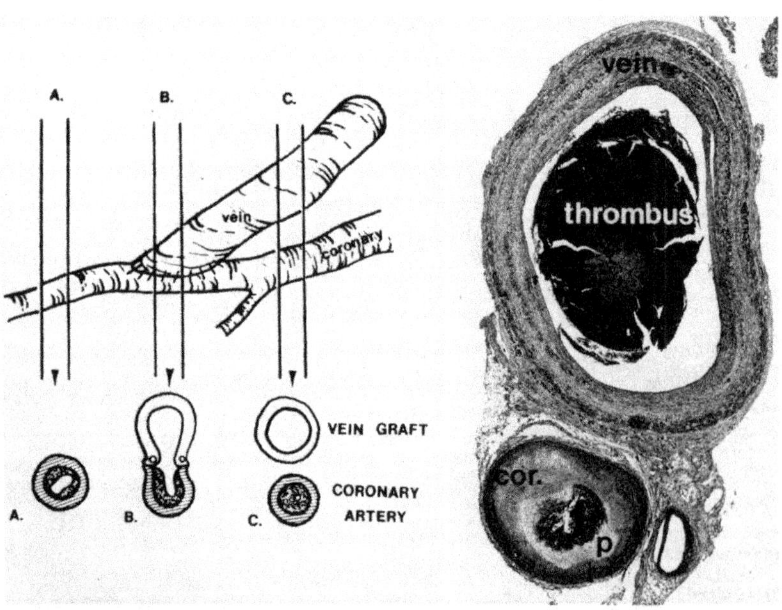

FIGURE 10. *Thrombosis of the coronary artery* proximal *(segment 3) to the site of insertion of a vein bypass graft in a man.* Left) *Diagram showing appearance of histologic sections taken below (A.), above (C.) and at (B.) the level of the venocoronary anastomosis.* Right) *Section of coronary artery (cor.) and thrombosed vein graft taken at level shown in C on left. Large amounts of atherosclerotic plaque (p) are present in the proximal artery, and the residual lumen is filled with thrombus. Movat stain,* × *11.*

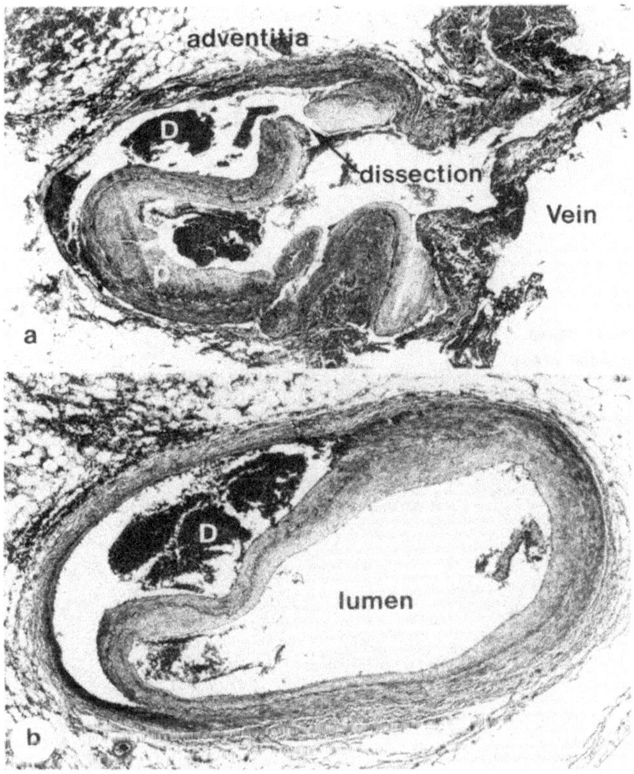

FIGURE 11. *Coronary artery dissection in the left circumflex coronary artery after bypass grafting in a woman who died shortly after operation (A72-209).* a) *Anastomosis of the vein graft to the coronary artery showing entrance site of the dissection. The media of the coronary artery and the associated atherosclerotic plaque (p) are separated from the adventitia by the false lumen (D).* b) *Circumflex coronary artery distal to insertion of the vein graft. The dissection has progressed distally, causing some narrowing of the lumen. Movat stains;* × *38* (a), × *44* (b).

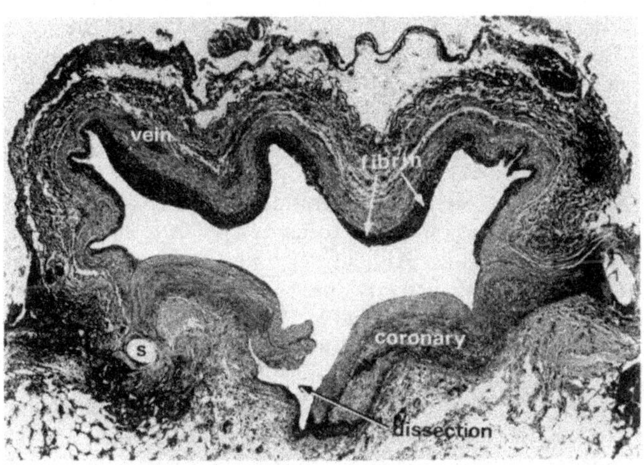

FIGURE 12. *Minimal dissection of the coronary artery immediately beneath the anastomosis in a 4-day-old bypass graft in a woman (A75-109). Incision of the posterior wall of the artery at the time of arteriotomy is the most likely cause of this localized dissection. Fibrin deposition on the vein wall is present. S = suture. Phosphotungstic acid = hematoxylin stain,* × *39. Retouched to eliminate luminal postmortem artifact.*

coronary arteries. Mean cross-sectional area of the arteries in men was 202 × 10^{-4} cm^2, and in women, 124 × 10^{-4} cm^2; mean area of the residual lumens was 63 × 10^{-4} cm^2 in men and 55 × 10^{-4} cm^2 in women (fig. 13). This difference in mean arterial size between men and women cannot be explained by differences in mean heart weights. When the original arterial areas are divided by the cardiac weights for each graft system, the mean values (all × 10^{-4} cm^2/g) were 0.417 in men and 0.316 in women. Luminal size, however, was almost identical in men and women, 0.133 vs 0.131 (× 10^{-4} cm^2/g).

In order to compare the data in men and women on the basis of coronary flow rather than cross-sectional area, the areas of the internal elastic membranes and lumens were squared. This calculation expresses the data in terms of radius to the fourth power (Poiseuille's equation for flow of a

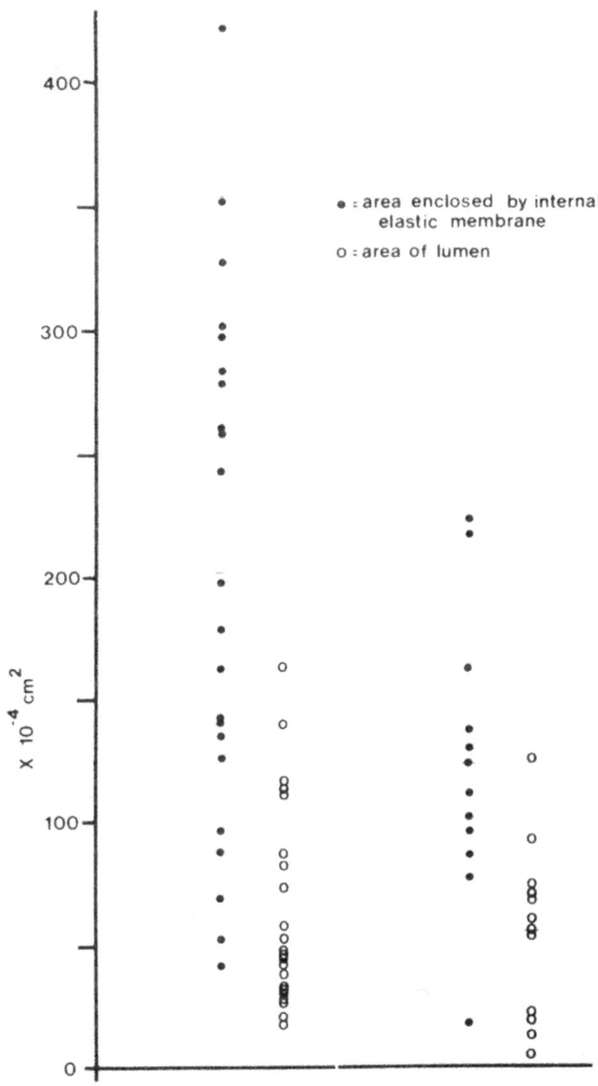

FIGURE 13. *Plot of the area contained by the internal elastic membrane and lumen in the most narrowed section of coronary artery within 2 cm distal to the aortocoronary anastomosis in men and women. The mean area of the internal elastic membrane in the men is larger than that in the women.*

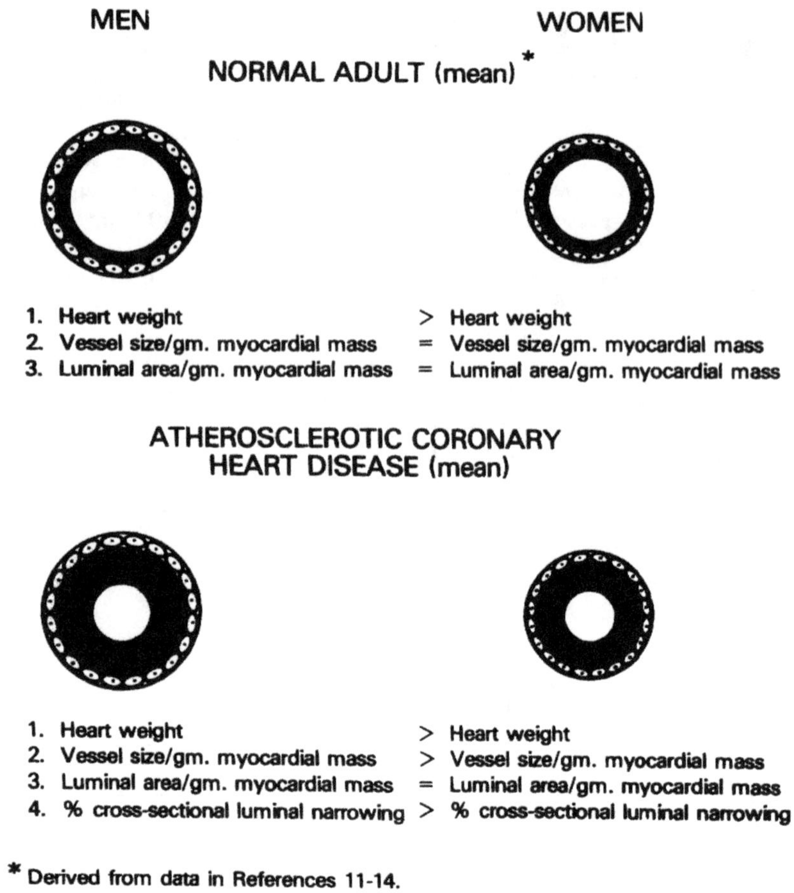

FIGURE 14. *Diagrammatic comparison of heart weight and coronary arterial parameters in normal adult men and women (above) and in men and women with atherosclerotic coronary heart disease (below) who died soon after aortocoronary bypass surgery.*

Newtonian fluid through a nondistensible cylinder) rather than radius squared (area); results were then divided by heart weights and are listed in table 3. The *relative* arterial sizes (expressed as $area^2$) between men and women remained significantly different after correction for differences in heart weight, but the luminal sizes ($area^2$) were similar, suggesting similar limitation to coronary flow in the two groups.

Comments

A high (44%) frequency of significant (> 75%) coronary arterial luminal narrowing by atherosclerotic plaque was found distal to the site of graft insertion in the 37 graft systems studied histologically in our 20 patients. The distal obstructions were due solely to atherosclerotic plaques. Thus, in nearly one-half of the graft systems studied, the bypass grafts failed to bypass significant obstructions. This result suggests that either the grafts were not placed far enough distally or that angiography failed to demonstrate the more distal narrowings or both. Since 44% of the native coronaries which were greater than 75% narrowed within 2 cm distal to the graft anastomosis were less than 75% narrowed in the remaining coronary artery, placement of the graft more distally would have bypassed significant obstructions in these patients, assuming that such anastomoses had been technically feasible. Comparison of men to women in this study disclosed similar degrees of *maximal cross-sectional luminal narrowing* by atherosclerotic plaques in all segments studied in each group. The *mean coronary arterial size,* however, was smaller in the women than in the men. This difference was not explained entirely on the basis of differences in heart weights between the sexes. Residual coronary arterial luminal area squared (which can be taken as a measure of outflow of the graft system), however, was almost identical in men and women after correction for heart weight. Thus, less atherosclerotic narrowing is required to produce a given limitation to blood flow in women than in men[11-14] (fig. 14). Although greater than 50% luminal narrowing of the coronary artery in the segment distal to the graft anastomosis was found in 50% of the women compared to 88% of the men, the mean residual luminal area in each sex was similar because the original vessel size in the women was smaller. Smaller coronary size alone, therefore, cannot account for the slightly higher reported early mortality in women than in men after aortocoronary bypass surgery.[15, 16]

TABLE 3. *Coronary Size Expressed As $Area^2$/Heart Weight**

	Men	Women	
Internal elastic membrane	106.7 ± 22.2	47.1 ± 12.1	$P < 0.025$**
Lumen	11.6 ± 3.1	9.2 ± 2.7	NS**

*Mean ± SEM × 10^{-8} cm^4/g.
**Student's *t*-test.

A relatively high (17%) frequency of coronary arterial dissection at the level of the vein graft anastomosis was found. The length of the dissection, however, was short in all but one patient. The occurrence of this complication appeared to be the result of detachment of atherosclerotic plaque from the coronary wall and was seen most commonly when the anastomosis was created at a site of moderately severe atherosclerotic narrowing. The presence of such plaque at the site of anastomosis was common: greater than 50% narrowing at this location occurred in about 25% of the graft systems studied.

The presence of fibrin deposits on the walls of both grafts and adjacent coronary arteries in many patients may be related to injury to the vessel walls by high flow or "jet" lesions or to relative stasis of blood in these graft systems.[2, 17, 18] If similar deposits occur in successful grafts, organization of the fibrin deposits may result in luminal narrowing of the graft, or increases in the degree of narrowing of the coronary artery at or distal to the anastomoses.[1, 7]

Thrombosis in our patients was occasionally present in the portion of the coronary artery proximal to the graft. In this location, it presumably is the result of relative stasis caused by competitive blood flow due to stenosis in the upstream coronary artery.[19-24]

References

1. Hamaker WR, Doyle WF, O'Connell TJ, Gomez AC: Subintimal obliterative proliferation in saphenous vein grafts. Ann Thorac Surg **13:** 488, 1972
2. Vlodaver Z, Edwards JE: Pathologic analysis in fatal cases following saphenous vein coronary arterial bypass. Chest **64:** 555, 1973
3. Vlodaver Z, Edwards JE: Pathologic changes in aortic-coronary arterial saphenous vein grafts. Circulation **44:** 719, 1971
4. Grondin CM, Dyrda I, Pasternac A, Campeau L, Bourassa MG, Lesperance J: Discrepancies between cineangiographic and postmortem findings in patients with coronary artery disease and recent myocardial revascularization. Circulation **49:** 703, 1974
5. Marti MC, Bouchardy B, Cox JN: Aorto-coronary bypass with autogenous saphenous vein grafts: Histopathologic aspects. Virchow Arch Path Anat **352:** 255, 1971
6. Kennedy JH, Wieting DW, Hwang NH, Anderson MS, Bayardo RJ, Howell JF, DeBakey ME: Hydraulic and morphologic study of fibrous intimal hyperplasia in autogenous saphenous vein bypass grafts. J Thorac Cardiovasc Surg **67:** 805, 1974
7. Jones M, Conkle DM, Ferrans VJ, Roberts WC, Levine FH, Melvin DB, Stinson EB: Lesions observed in arterial autogenous vein grafts. Light and electron microscopic evaluation. Circulation **47, 48** (suppl III): III-198, 1973
8. Unni KK, Kottke BA, Titus JL, Frye RL, Wallace RB, Brown AL: Pathologic changes in aorto-coronary saphenous vein grafts. Am J Cardiol **34:** 526, 1974
9. Kern WH, Dermer GB, Lindesmith GG: The intimal proliferation in aorto-coronary saphenous vein grafts: Light and electron microscopic studies. Am Heart J **84:** 771, 1972
10. Brody WR, Kosek JC, Angell WW: Changes in vein grafts following aorto-coronary bypass induced by pressure and ischemia. J Thorac Cardiovasc Surg **64:** 847, 1972
11. Harrison CV, Wood P: Hypertensive and ischaemic heart disease: A comparative clinical and pathological study. Br Heart J **11:** 205, 1949
12. Lewis BS, Gotsman MS: Relation between coronary artery size and left ventricular wall mass. Br Heart J **35:** 1150, 1973
13. Wilens SL, Plair CM, Henderson D: Size of the major epicardial coronary arteries at necropsy. JAMA **198:** 1325, 1966
14. Milles G, Dalessandro W: The relationship of the weight of the heart and the circumference of the coronary arteries to myocardial infarction and myocardial failure. Am J Pathol **30:** 31, 1954
15. Bolooki H, Vargas A, Green R, Kaiser GA, Ghahramani A: Results of direct coronary artery surgery in women. J Thorac Cardiovasc Surg **69:** 271, 1975
16. Hall RJ, Garcia E, Wukasch DC, Hallman GL, Cooley DA: Aortocoronary bypass (CAB): Long-term follow-up. Circulation **51, 52** (suppl II): II-90, 1975
17. Faulkner SL, Fisher RD, Conkle DM, Page DL, Bender HW Jr: The effect of blood flow rate on subendothelial proliferation in venous autografts used as arterial substitutes. Circulation **51, 52** (suppl I): I-163, 1975
18. Bourassa MG, Lesperance J, Campeau L, Simard P: Factors influencing patency of aorto-coronary vein grafts. Circulation **46** (suppl I): I-79, 1971
19. Stinson EB, Olinger GN, Glancy DL: Anatomical and physiological determinants of blood flow through aorto-coronary vein bypass grafts. Surgery **74:** 390, 1973
20. Kakos GS, Oldham HN Jr., Dixon SH Jr., Davis RW, Hagen P, Sabiston DC: Coronary artery hemodynamics after aorto-coronary vein bypass: An experimental evaluation. J Thorac Cardiovasc Surg **63:** 849, 1972
21. Pasternak R, Cohn K, Selzer A, Langston MF Jr: Enhanced rate of progression of coronary artery disease following aorto-coronary saphenous vein bypass surgery. Am J Med **58:** 166, 1975
22. Rees S: The watershed: A factor in coronary vein graft occlusion. Br Heart J **38:** 197, 1976
23. Maurer BJ, Oberman A, Holt JH Jr, Kouchoukos NT, Jones WB, Russell RO Jr, Reeves TJ: Changes in grafted and nongrafted coronary arteries following saphenous vein bypass grafting. Circulation **50:** 293, 1974
24. Glassman E, Spencer FC, Krauss KR, Weisinger B, Isom OW: Changes in the underlying coronary circulation secondary to bypass grafting. Circulation **49, 50** (suppl II): II-80, 1974

Morphologic Observations in Biologic Conduits Between Aorta and Coronary Artery

Thomas L. Spray, M. D., and William C. Roberts, M. D.

Although numerous reports have described the use of conduits between aorta and coronary artery as a means of increasing myocardial oxygenation, relatively few have focused on structural alterations in the conduits utilized in this position.[1-21] This report describes histologic observations in autogenous saphenous vein, autogenous internal mammary artery, autogenous radial artery, and heterograft veins and arteries used for varying periods as aortocoronary bypass grafts in patients with severe coronary heart disease.

AUTOGENOUS SAPHENOUS VEIN

Before discussing the expected or normal changes and the unexpected or abnormal changes observed in autogenous veins utilized for varying periods of time as aortocoronary arterial conduits, a histologic description of the normal adult human saphenous vein appears appropriate.

Normal Saphenous Vein

The normal human saphenous vein wall is composed of three layers: thin *intima* of relatively acellular fibrous tissue and ground substance covered by a monolayer of endothelial cells; (2) *media,* composed of multiple layers of smooth muscle cells separated by collagen, ground substance and elastic fibers; and (3) *adventitia* composed of bundles of collagen and occasional smooth muscle fascicles and broad loose bands of elastic tissue (Fig. 1). The media is separated from the intima by a rudimentary internal elastic membrane which may or may not be continuous. The medial smooth muscle layers generally have a circular orientation; however, the innermost layers often are longitudinally oriented and in areas near the venous valves, the circular layers have a more oblique or longitudinal alignment. The vasa vasorum are located in the adventitial layer and may extend to varying depths into the outermost portion of the medial smooth muscle. In almost 25 percent[22] of veins used for bypass conduits, the intimal layer is thickened by spindle-shaped fibroblasts and the media is thinned because of loss of muscle cells (phlebosclerosis) (Fig. 2).

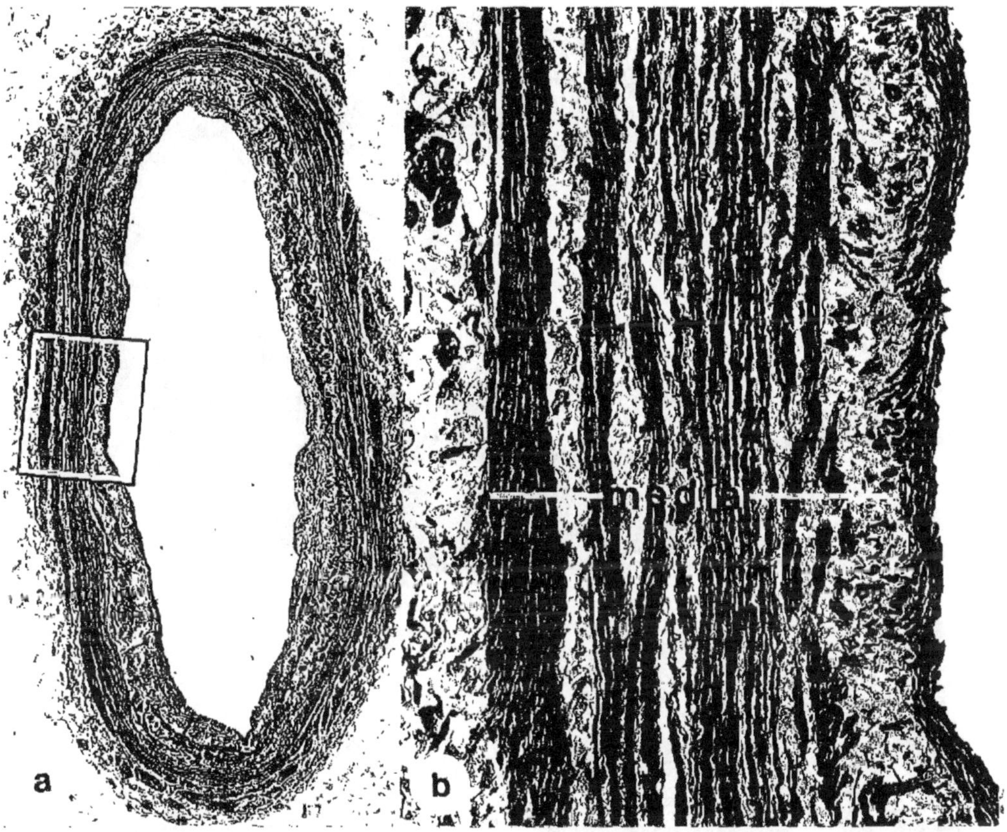

Figure 1. Normal saphenous vein. (a) Low power view showing medial circular and longitudinal smooth muscle layers. (b) High power view of area enclosed in box in (a). Multiple layers of circular smooth muscle separated by layers of fibrous tissue make up the media. Occasional longitudinal smooth muscle fascicles are present near the lumen. Movat stain; × 20 (a), × 130 (b).

Normal or Expected Changes in Saphenous Veins Used as Aortocoronary Conduits

At least seven changes have been observed in veins used as arterial conduits anywhere in the body: (1) *endothelial damage;* (2) *medial necrosis;* (3) *mural fibrosis* (media and adventitia); (4) *intimal fibrous proliferation;* (5) *intimal lipid deposition;* (6) *medial hypertrophy,* and (7) *aneurysm formation.* Of these seven changes, only the first five are of significance in veins used in the aortocoronary position. The first two changes (endothelial damage and medial necrosis) may be considered the stimulus for a reparative process which results in the remaining changes seen, i.e., mural fibrosis and intimal fibrous proliferation. Deposition of lipid in the intima, an infrequent occurrence, up to five years after implantation, may be viewed as a degenerative change after the expected injury and repair processes are complete.[2, 11, 15, 18]

A selected composite of vein grafts from personally studied patients illustrating a normal, unimplanted vein to a vein which was in place for 26 months after operation is shown in Figure 3.[14] In the first few days after implantation, endothelial cells slough and fibrin, with a few inflammatory cells, is deposited on the denuded intima (Fig. 4). The medial smooth muscle layers become edematous and later necrotic. When the necrosis occurs, inflammatory cells also appear within the media (Fig. 5).

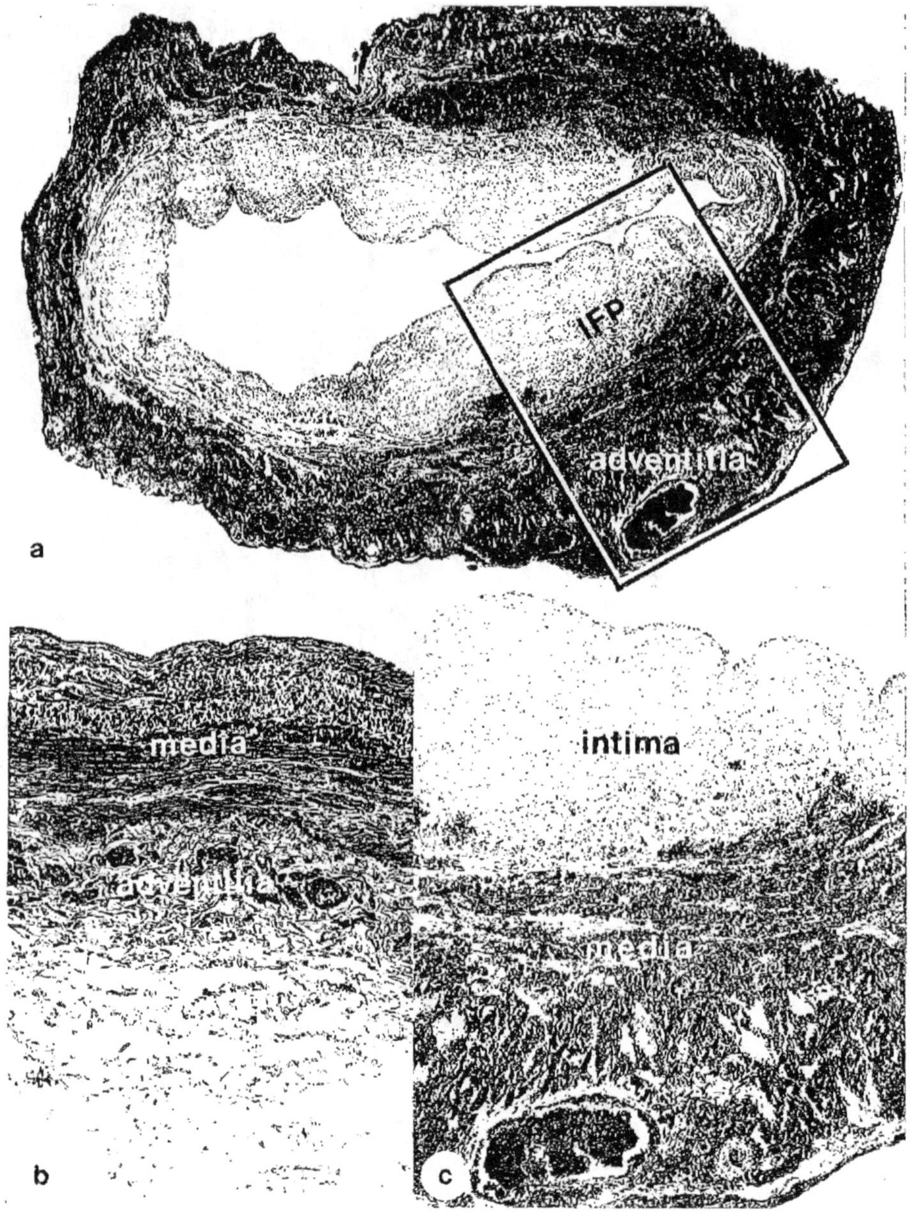

Figure 2. Phlebosclerosis in a saphenous vein used for aortocoronary bypass grafting (N-A75-171). (a) Section of saphenous vein segment left over after use of the major segment for bypass grafting. Phlebosclerosis is present, creating intimal thickening histologically identical to intimal fibrous proliferation (IFP). (b) Normal saphenous vein for comparison. (c) Higher power view of area enclosed in box in a, showing intimal thickening, loss of some medial smooth muscle, and adventitial hemorrhage. Movat stains; reduced 20% from × 28 (a), × 54 (b), × 54 (c).

By three weeks after implantation, the media is thinner and the intima is thicker due to transformation of medial myocytes into myointimal cells and subsequent migration into the intimal layer. Often the myointimal cells are present immediately under the regenerated endothelial layer and are oriented parallel to the direction of blood flow (Fig. 6).

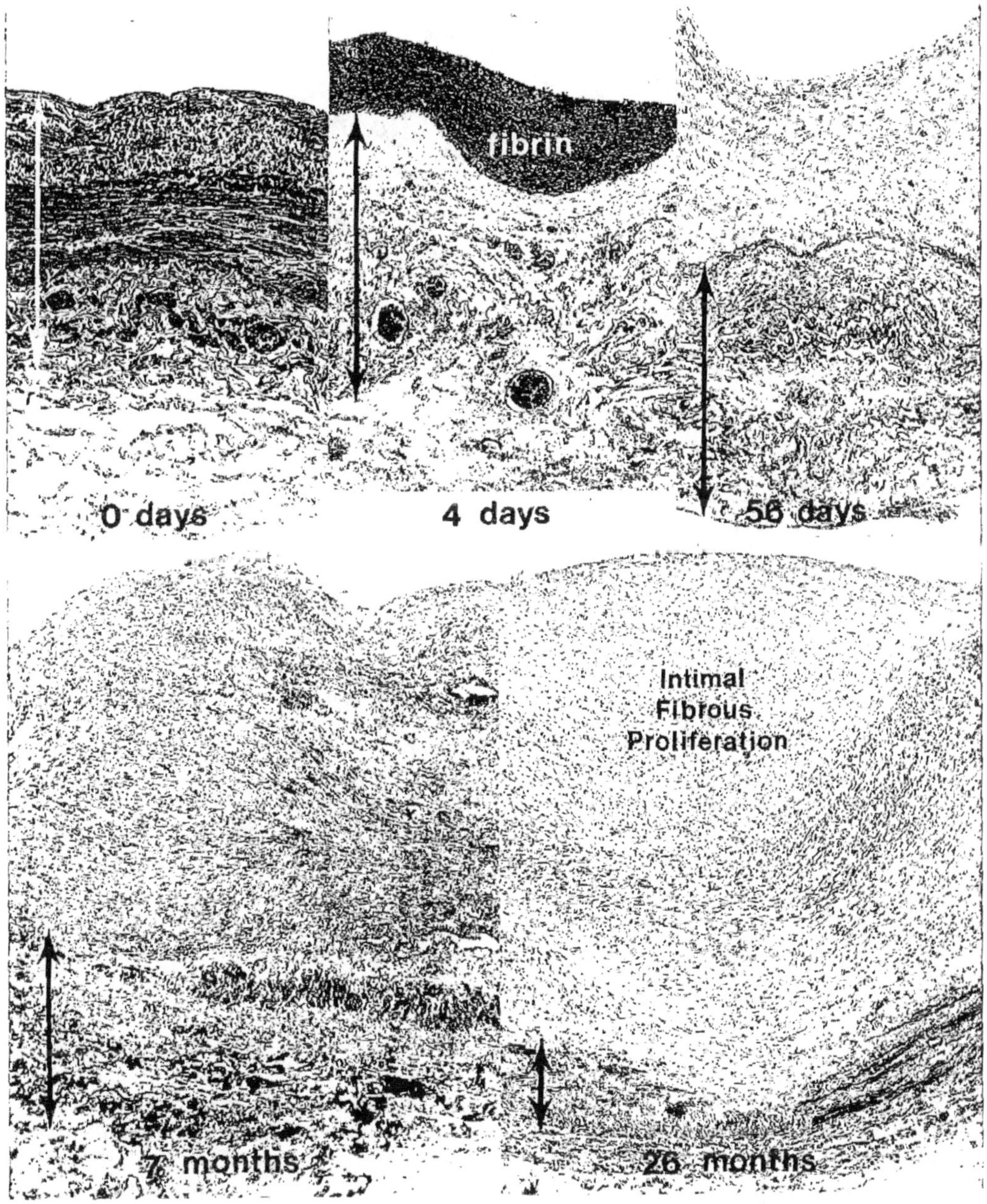

Figure 3. Composite of changes seen in saphenous vein aortocoronary grafts from 0 days (normal vein) to 26 months after implantation *at the same magnification.* Arrows indicate normal wall thickness (media + adventitia). *0 days:* Intima thin, marked medial smooth muscle layers in both circular and longitudinal directions, loose adventitial tissue. *4 days:* Large deposit of fibrin over slightly thickened intima. Marked loss of medial smooth muscle with cellular infiltration. *56 days:* Thickened vein wall with marked intimal fibrous proliferation. The media and adventitia show loss of muscle cells and fibrosis. *7 months:* Severe intimal fibrous proliferation is present, containing some neovascular channels. Marked loss of medial smooth muscle and replacement fibrosis is present. *26 months:* The vein wall has become almost completely replaced by fibrous tissue and intimal proliferation, creating a fibrous tube. Only small areas of medial smooth muscle cells remain. All Movat stains; reduced 20% from × 54.

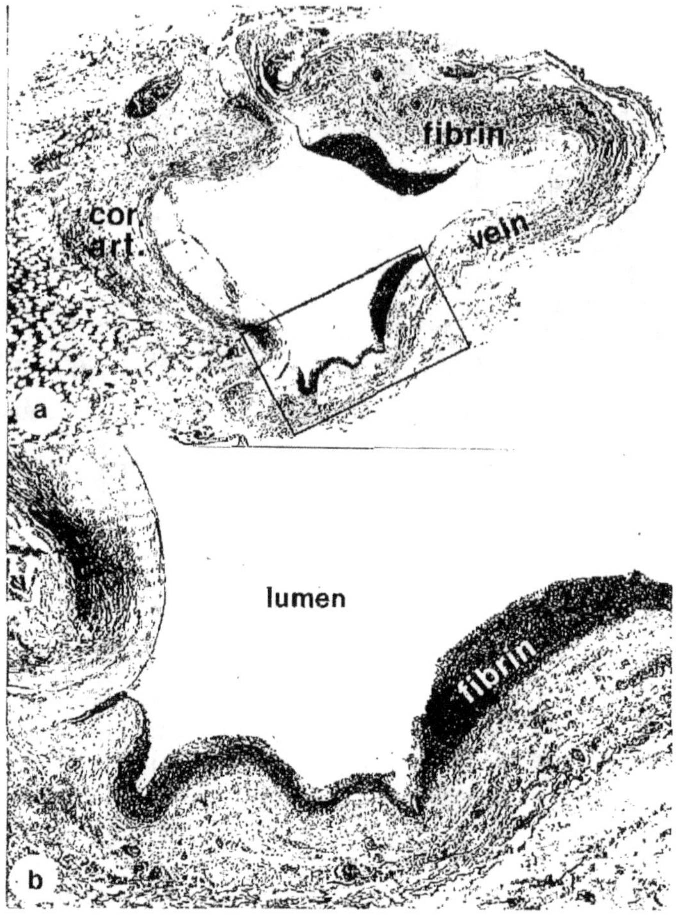

Figure 4. Mural fibrin deposition in a four-day-old vein graft to the left anterior descending coronary artery (cor. art.) in a woman (A75–109). (a) Thick fibrin layers are present on the vein wall at the coronary anastomosis. (b) Higher power view of area enclosed by box in (a). Deposits of fibrin line the lumen of the vein graft. Movat stain; reduced 20% from × 16 (a) × 54 (b).

By 60 days after implantation, some veins show diffuse luminal narrowing by subendothelial fibrous intimal proliferation consisting of relatively acellular fibrous tissue, ground substance, and occasional elastic fibers and vascular channels. Such intimal lesions are common in grafts in place from 2 to 72 months; however, the extent and severity of the proliferative lesions are variable among grafts in the same patient and they also vary in different areas of the same graft (Figs. 7 and 8). Occasionally fibrin deposits are present in the subendothelial areas of late grafts (Fig. 9). In the adventitial layers of the grafts, organization of fibrin deposits and new vascular ingrowth create a fibrous sheath around the graft (Fig. 8). In contrast to the intimal and adventitial fibrous thickening, the media tends to become thinner and the medial smooth muscle cells are replaced with fibroblasts and collagen.

The net result of the fibrous changes in all three vein layers is a tough, relatively inflexible conduit composed of poorly vascularized fibrous tissue lined by endothelium.

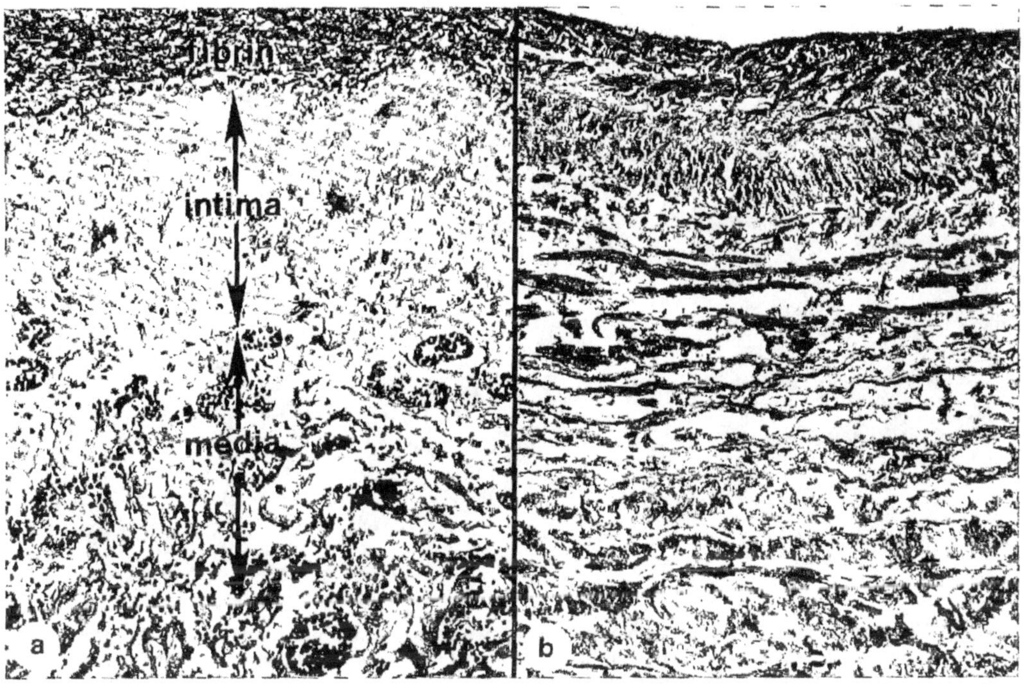

Figure 5. (a) Wall of a vein graft taken four days after implantation. Fibrin deposition on the intimal surface and infiltration of the intima and media with acute inflammatory cells is seen. Necrosis of medial smooth muscle also is present. (b) Vein graft implanted for 18 days showing edema and necrosis of medial smooth muscle cells. Hematoxylin and eosin stains; reduced 20% from × 220 (a and b).

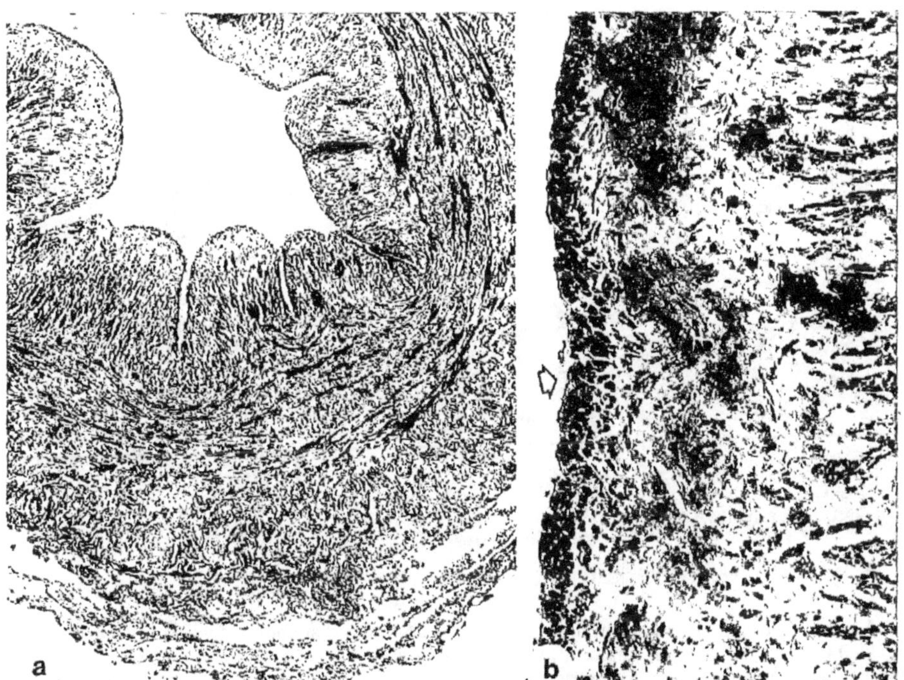

Figure 6. Subendothelial myointimal cell accumulation in a 19-month-old graft to the circumflex coronary artery from a 52-year-old man (GT 75A – 69) who died at reoperation for replacement of an occluded graft to the left anterior descending coronary artery. (a) Marked medial and subendothelial cellularity is noted. (b) Higher power view showing subendothelial collections of myointimal cells (arrow) immediately under the endothelial layer. Beneath these cells is proliferative intimal tissue. Movat stain; reduced 20% from × 54 (a), × 220 (b).

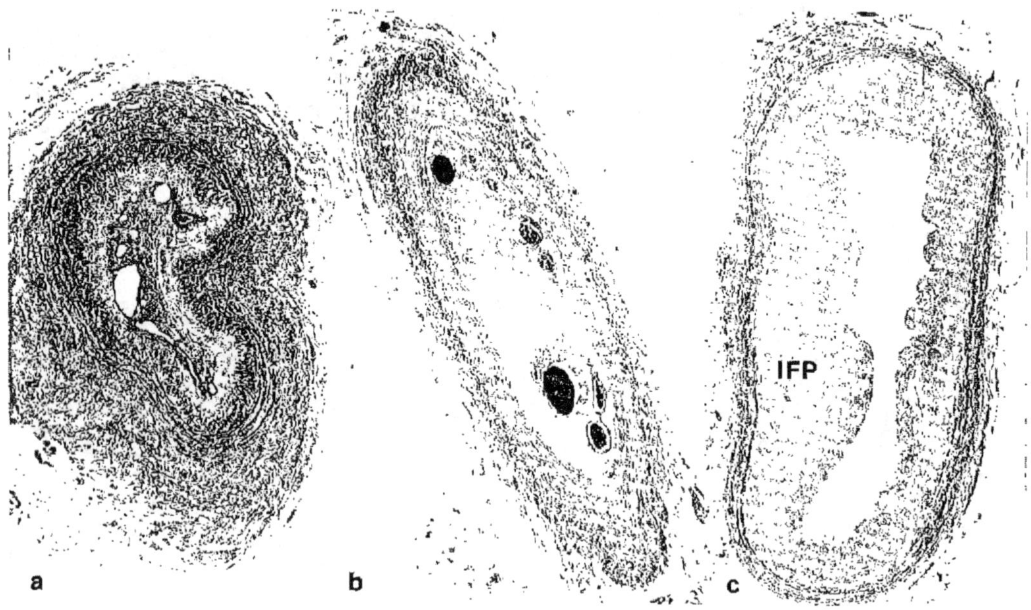

Figure 7. Vein grafts from a 44-year-old woman (7983), who died suddenly at home 26 months after bypass grafting, showing differing histologic fates in three grafts. (a) Graft to the right coronary artery shows mild intimal fibrous proliferation and loss of medial smooth muscle with a recanalized lumen suggesting organizing thrombus. (b) Graft to the left obtuse marginal coronary artery showing occlusion of the lumen by fibrous tissue and recanalization. The presumed cause for the development of the latter lesion is organizing thrombus. (c) Graft to the left anterior descending coronary artery showing severe intimal fibrous proliferation (IFP). The histologic pictures of IFP (c) and thrombus (b) may be similar. Movat stains; reduced 27% from × 27 (a), × 22 (b) × 27 (c).

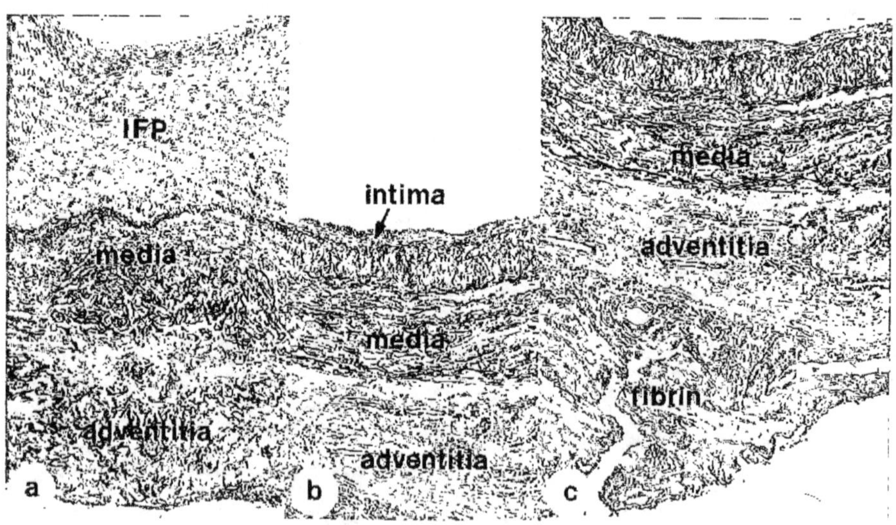

Figure 8. Variable intimal fibrous proliferation (IFP) in a 56-day-old spahenous vein graft from a 46-year-old man (A71–94) who died of renal failure after aortic and mitral valve replacements and vein grafting to the right and left anterior descending coronary arteries. (a) Proximal portion of vein graft. There is marked IFP and smooth muscle loss in the media. (b) Distal part of graft. Minimal IFP is present. (c) Adventitial fibrosis and organizing fibrin in same area of graft as (b). Movat stains; reduced 20% from each × 54.

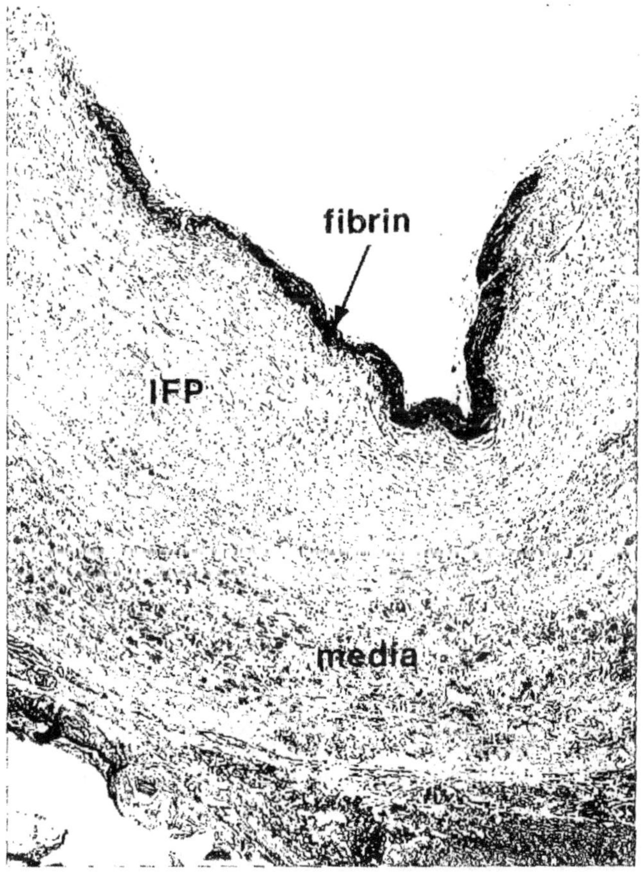

Figure 9. Subendothelial fibrin in a 56-day-old vein bypass graft. Marked intimal fibrous proliferation (IFP) is present and the amount of smooth muscle in the media is diminished. Phosphotungstic acid-hematoxylin stain; × 54.

Abnormal or Unexpected Changes in Saphenous Veins Used as Aortocoronary Conduits

As noted, certain changes occur normally in all saphenous veins used as aortocoronary conduits. Additional changes, however, may occur in some of these venous bypass grafts, and these changes are considered abnormal. There are three major ones: (1) *luminal obliteration,* either partial or complete, secondary to *thrombus formation* or *intimal fibrous proliferation* (this may also be the result of organization of thrombus) (Figs. 10 and 11) or *atherosclerosis* or a combination of these; (2) *luminal dilatation* or aneurysm formation of uncertain cause;[16, 23] and (3) *atherosclerosis* not resulting in significant luminal narrowing.[3, 11, 15, 18]

Causes of Normal and Abnormal Changes in Saphenous Veins Used as Aortocoronary Conduits

Although the causes of the above described changes in saphenous vein grafts are unclear, several possible mechanisms have been proposed (Table 1).[4-7, 10, 19, 24-30] Similar

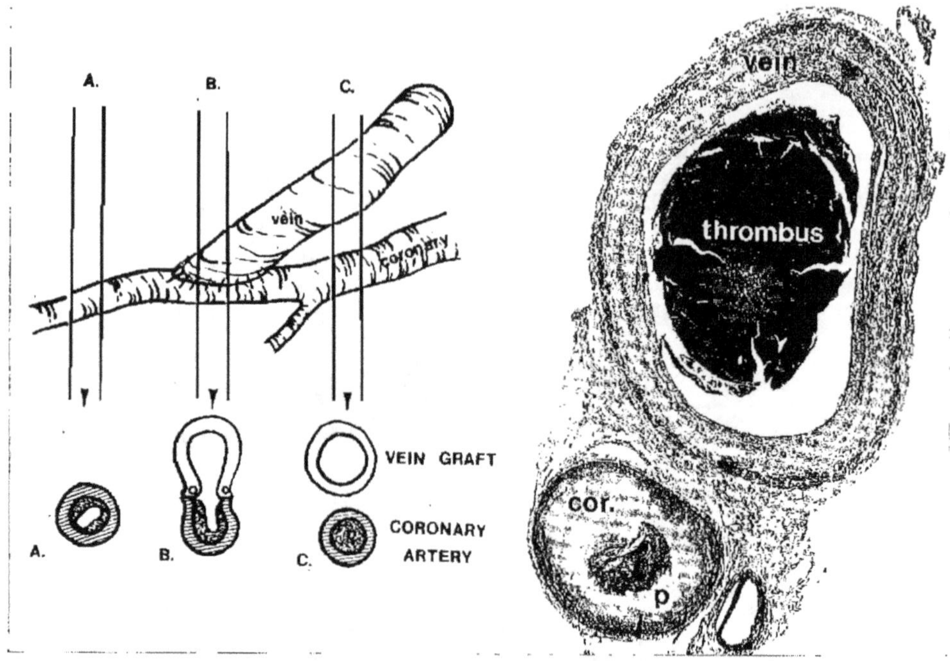

Figure 10. Thrombosis of the coronary artery *proximal* to the site of insertion of a vein bypass graft in a man. *Left:* Diagram showing appearance of histologic sections taken below. (A), above (C) and at (B) the level of the venocoronary anastomosis. *Right:* Section of coronary artery (cor.) and thrombosed vein graft taken at level shown in C on left. Large amounts of atherosclerotic plaque (p) are present in the proximal artery, and the residual lumen is filled with thrombus. Movat stain; reduced 20% from × 11.

subendothelial proliferation of smooth muscle cells resulting in intimal fibrosis has been observed in several situations in the vascular system. The phlebosclerosis observed in venous varicosities is presumably the response of the vein to increases in hydrostatic pressure.[31] Arteriovenous shunts (congenital, traumatic, or iatrogenic) often show intimal thickening. This response is presumably due to increased flow and elevated pressure.[8, 32] Subendothelial proliferative lesions also occur in the small pulmonary arteries of patients with pulmonary hypertension,[33, 34] in vena cava and portal veins in patients with chronic right sided congestive cardiac failure or portal hypertension,[35, 36] and in peripheral arteries of some patients with systemic hypertension.[37] In some patients, the intimal lesions are histologically similar to the fibrous and musculoelastic plaques of atherosclerosis[38-43] (Fig. 12).

Elevation of intravascular pressure or magnitude of flow or both, or a decreased velocity of flow, with resulting increased shear stress on the vascular walls,[2, 24, 44-45] appears to be a common element in each of the above examples. In experimental studies, Brody and colleagues[26] have attempted to differentiate the effects of pressure and ischemia on vein grafts in dogs. Femoral vein segments were either left intact or were dissected free from their adventitia, thereby interrupting the vasa vasorum and producing medial ischemia. Next, the vein segments were either left in the low pressure venous system or were subjected to higher pressure and flow by creation of an arteriovenous fistula. The presence of medial ischemia with low pressure and flow produced medial fibrosis in the vein, but no subendothelial intimal proliferative lesions (Table 2). Elevated intravascular pressure alone, however, without disruption of the vasa vasorum produced intimal lesions without evidence of medial fibrosis. The combination of both ele-

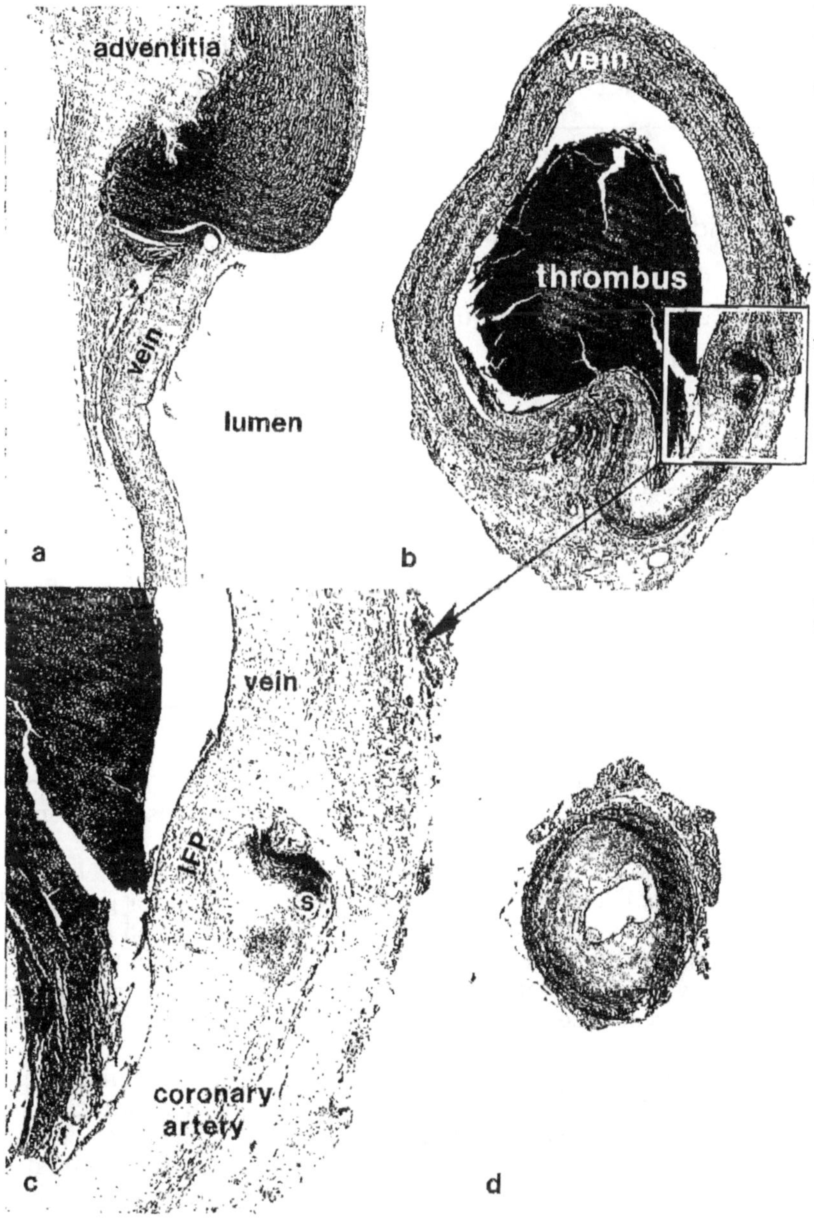

Figure 11. Graft thrombosis and intimal fibrous proliferation (IFP) extending into the coronary artery at the site of vein graft anastomosis in a man (PHWT A73 – 28) who died suddenly 34 days after bypass grafting to the right coronary artery. (a) Anastomosis of vein graft to aortic wall, showing intimal proliferation of the vein and adventitial fibrosis extending from the aorta over the exterior of the graft. (b) Section taken at the veno-coronary anastomosis showing antemortem thrombosis of the vein graft extending into the coronary artery. (c) Higher power view of area enclosed by box (in b) showing moderate IFP of the vein with extension across the suture line(s) into the coronary artery. (d) Section of the coronary artery distal to the anastomosis of the graft showed marked narrowing by plaque and fibrous tissue. Movat stains; reduced 20% from × 13 (a), × 11 (b), × 31 (c), × 12 (d).

TABLE 1
CAUSES AND CONSEQUENCES OF CHANGES IN VEINS USED FOR ARTERIAL CONDUITS

CAUSE	CONSEQUENCE
1. Endothelial damage	Fibrous intimal proliferation
a. Trauma	
b. Elevated transmural pressure	
c. Increased flow	
2. Thrombosis	
3. Intimal damage	
4. Increased wall O_2 tension	
5. Medial ischemia	Medial fibrosis
a. Loss of vasa vasorum	
b. Increased transmural pressure	
6. Adventitial ischemia	

vated intraluminal pressure and flow and medial ischemia resulted in medial and intimal changes similar to the changes seen in human saphenous veins used as aortocoronary conduits.

Several factors unique to aortocoronary bypass grafting make the changes of ischemia and pressure more likely in these grafts than in grafts used for peripheral arterial bypass. While the excised vein is rapidly revascularized when placed in the retroperitoneum and the extremities,[46] the unsupported nature of the grafts in the aortocoronary position makes delay in revascularization of the wall more likely. In addition, flow in the coronary system occurs under diastolic, not systolic, pressure and consequently has lower velocity.[24, 46]

The mechanisms whereby pressure and ischemia cause the intimal and medial changes are unclear (Table 3). Brody and associates[25] suggest that both changes are the result of transformation of medial myocytes in response to injury or to change in their nutritional status (ischemia). It has been postulated that the myocyte response may be mediated by an elevated mural oxygen tension in the vein with resulting direct effects on phospholipid[25, 47] or by the exposure of the smooth muscle cells to plasma factors or blood products as a result of recurrent endothelial damage.[3, 10, 24] The medial myocyte may have two fates: (1) it may be transformed into a fibrocyte[26, 48] and produce medial fibrosis, or (2) it may become a "myointimal cell" and migrate to the intimal layer in response to some unknown stimulus to produce intimal thickening.[26, 48, 49]

The fact that the amount and severity of fibrous intimal proliferation is often variable along the length of a vein graft[7, 29] (Fig. 7) or among separate grafts in the same patient (Fig. 8) suggests that elevated pressure alone does not account for the extent of changes in these conduits. Some anatomic and technical factors, therefore, must modify the effects of pressure and ischemia on the vein graft and the distal coronary artery. These

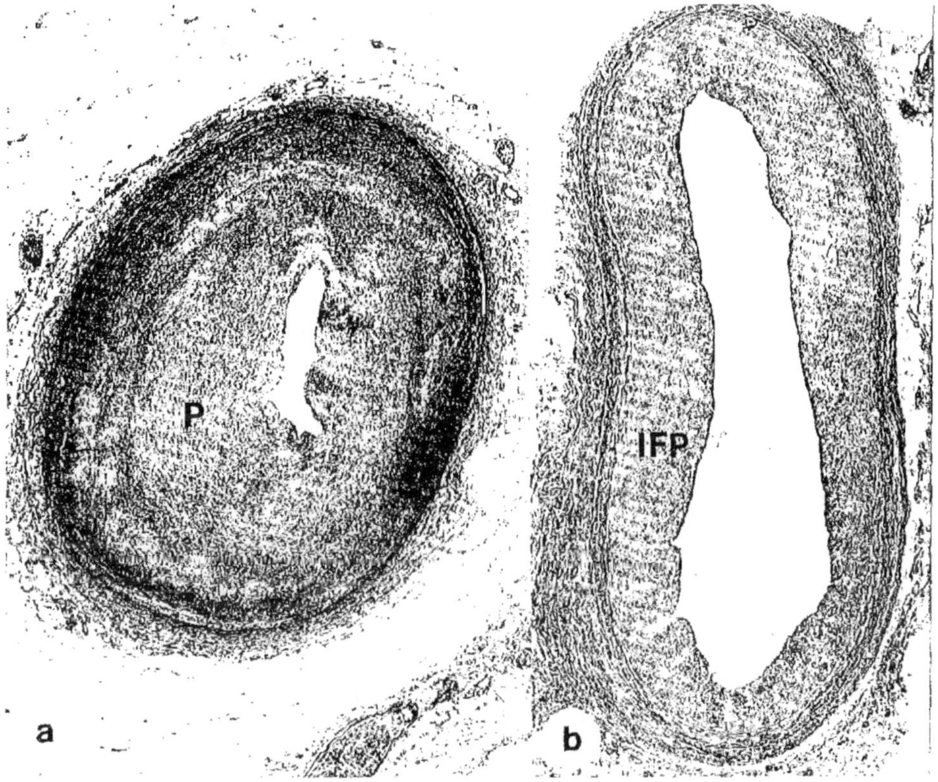

Figure 12. Similarity of atherosclerotic plaque (P) in a coronary artery (a), and the intimal fibrous proliferation (IFP) in a 26-month-old saphenous vein coronary bypass graft (b). Both show intimal thickening by fibrous tissue and loss of medial smooth muscle layers. Movat stains; × 16 (a), × 15 (b).

factors are all related in some fashion to the magnitude or turbulence of flow in the vein graft or the coronary artery into which the graft inserts.

Faulkner and associates[24] studied the effect of flow rate on the development of intimal fibrous proliferative lesions in femoral vein grafts in dogs. Grafts subjected to low flows (30 to 50 ml./min.) showed significantly greater and more generalized intimal proliferation than grafts subjected to high flows (790 ml./min. average). Intimal fibrous proliferation, however, occurred in all grafts just distal to the proximal anastomoses and at the distal anastomoses in both the vein and the native femoral artery, suggesting that turbulence of flow at anastomoses produces augmented vein response, perhaps by causing localized recurrent endothelial damage.[2, 5, 10] It is possible, therefore, that elevated pressure or flow may result in recurrent damage to the endothelial layer. Conversion to intimal lesions by progressive fibrin deposition may then follow. High flow may keep the endothelium "washed" and prevent formation of thrombi, while low flow may encourage thrombi and consequently luminal narrowing.

Studies by Jones and associates[10] support the concept that progressive intimal fibrous proliferation may be the result of progressive organization of subendothelial or mural deposits of fibrin which accumulate as a result of recurrent endothelial damage. Fibrin and platelet thrombi are known to accumulate in response to exposure of collagen, basement membrane, or elastin to the blood[26, 50] and mural thrombi may become incor-

TABLE 2
EFFECTS OF PRESSURE AND ISCHEMIA ON VENOUS CONDUITS*

VASA VASORUM INTACT

Low Pressure (Venous)	High Pressure (Arterial)
↓	↓
Normal Histology	Intimal Proliferation and Fibrosis
Intact Myocytes	Intact Myocytes

VASA VASORUM INTERRUPTED

Low Pressure (Venous)	High Pressure (Arterial)
↓	↓
Medial Fibrosis	Intimal Proliferation and Fibrosis
Loss of Myocytes	Medial Fibrosis
	Loss of Myocytes

*After Brody, *et al.*, *J. Thor. Cardiovasc. Surg.* 64:847, 1972.

TABLE 3
VENOUS CONDUITS FOR AORTOCORONARY BYPASS:
Factors Promoting
Fibrinous or Fibrous Intimal Proliferation With or Without Occlusion

1. Severe narrowing distal to insertion of the graft
2. Insertion of graft in area of plaque
   a. Thrombosis
   b. Hemorrhage
   c. Dissection
3. Hyperacute angle of aortic anastomosis (90° optimal)
4. Tension on grafted vein
   a. Decreases flow
   b. Damages endothelium or intima
   c. Causes tension on anastomoses
5. Previous sclerosis of vein used for conduit
6. Overdistension of vein with saline
   a. Damages endothelium and intima
   b. Possible direct effect on phospholipids of smooth muscle

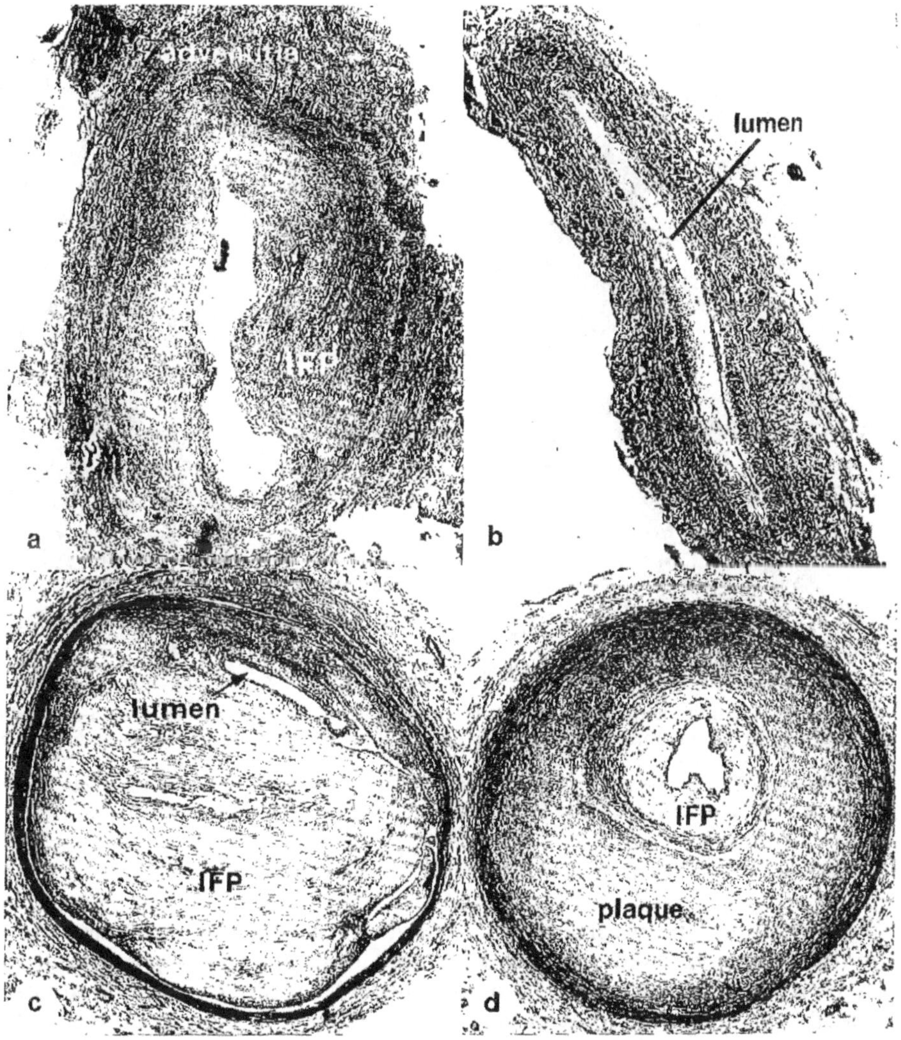

Figure 13 Saphenous vein graft from a 34-year-old man (A75–279) who died seven months after placement of a graft to the left anterior descending (LAD) coronary artery. Endarterectomy was done at the site of the anastomosis to the coronary. He did well for 6.5 months, when angina returned. At reoperation, the vein graft (a) was found to be narrowed proximally by intimal fibrous proliferation (IFP), and flattened and sclerosed distally (b). He died after repeat bypassing of the LAD and placement of vein grafts to the right and posterior descending coronary arteries. (c) Section of LAD immediately distal to the anastomosis of the vein graft at the area of previous endarterectomy showing almost complete occlusion of the vessel by fibrous tissue plaque (IFP). Only a tiny lumen remains. The IFP extended down the LAD for several centimeters, and appeared to be superimposed on preexisting plaque (d), further narrowing the lumen of the vessel. Movat stains; reduced 20% from × 20 (a), × 22 (b), × 34 (c), × 45 (d).

porated into atherosclerotic plaques.[51, 52] Also, fibrous lesions similar to those seen in venous bypass grafts have been observed in native coronary arteries after endothelial damage from perfusion cannulae or after endarterectomy (Fig. 13).[5] Fibrin deposition on venous valves has been suggested as a cause of segmental stenosis of femoropopliteal vein grafts[30] and involvement of the venous valves with intimal proliferation has been observed in aortocoronary vein grafts (Fig. 14). The laminated appearance of

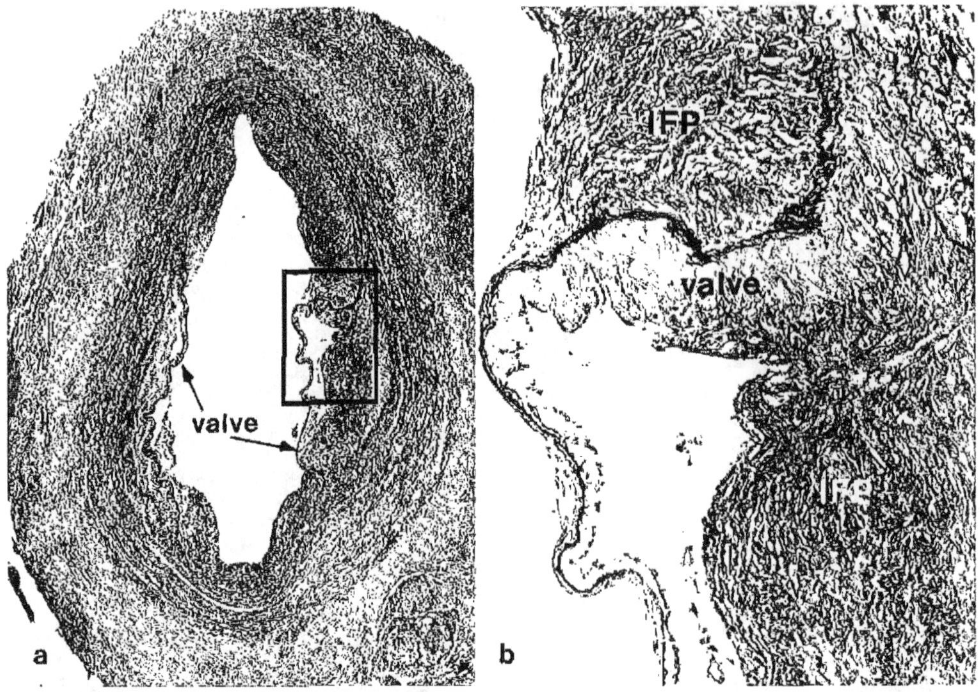

Figure 14. Development of intimal fibrous proliferation (IFP) behind venous valves in a 56-day-old saphenous vein graft (A71–94). (a) Intimal fibrous proliferation lines the vein graft. The valve leaflets are not bound down against the vein wall. Marked adventitial fibrosis also is present. (b) Enlargement of area shown in box (in a), showing IFP above and behind the venous valve. The leaflet remains relatively uninvolved. Movat stains; reduced 20% from × 23 (a), × 130 (b).

some areas of intimal fibrous proliferative lesions in vein bypass grafts and the occasional finding of new vascular channels in the plaques themselves, plus the histologic similarity of recanalized thrombus to intimal fibrous proliferation and demonstrable fibrin deposits in some subendothelial lesions (see Fig. 9), lend support to the concept of continued organization of thrombi as the etiology of these lesions.[12]

The anatomic and technical factors which may cause obstruction to blood flow in saphenous grafts may be divided into two groups: (1) those that affect inflow (refers to the status of the graft itself), and (2) those that affect outflow (refers to the status of the coronary artery and vascular bed into which the graft inserts) (Fig. 15). Each of these factors may affect any single graft and may result in fibrous intimal proliferation or thrombosis of the graft or both.

Dissection of the coronary artery at the vein graft anastomosis and atherosclerotic narrowing of the coronary artery at the site of vein implantation have been observed in some grafts (Figs. 16, 17, and 18).[13] A high percentage of grafts in one study[13] were inserted into coronary arteries which showed significant degrees of obstruction by atherosclerotic plaque in the vessel just *distal* to the site of the graft anastomosis (Figs. 19, 20, and 21).

Some authors[5] have suggested obstruction to coronary graft outflow due to a small distal coronary vessel. Although what constitutes a small coronary artery is somewhat subjective, coronary artery size appears to be slightly smaller in women than in men, even when adjustment is made for differences in myocardial mass.[13] Placement of vein

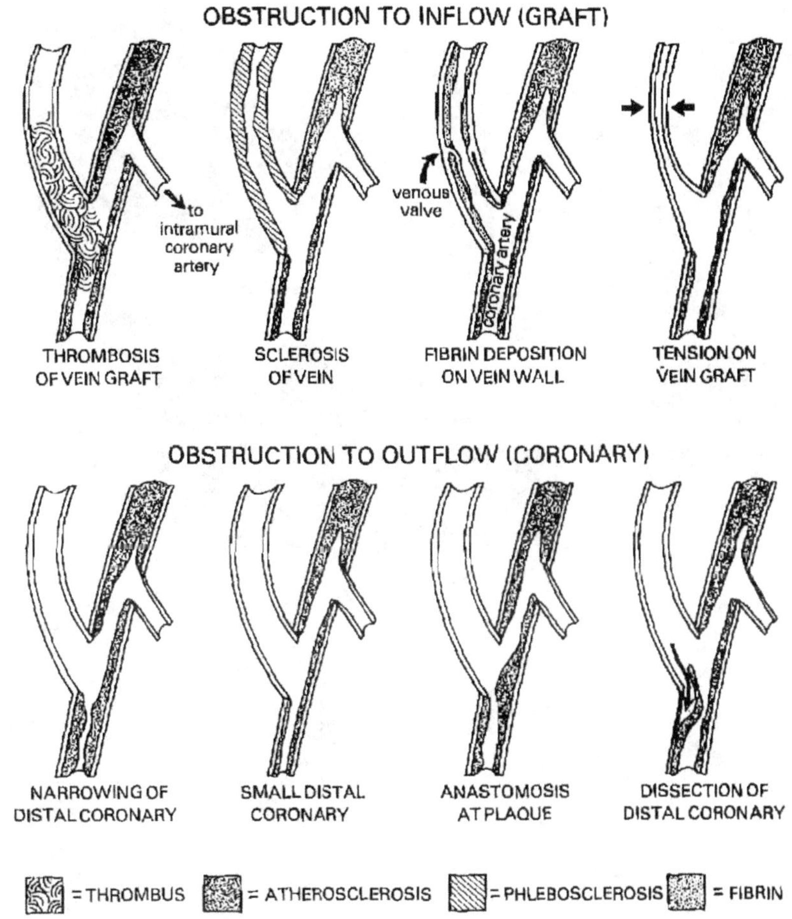

Figure 15. Anatomic and technical factors that affect flow in the coronary arteries following aortocoronary bypass.

grafts too short to allow for the normal distension of the cardiac chambers after discontinuation of cardiopulmonary bypass or the abnormal distension with the development of congestive cardiac failure has been suggested as a possible cause of graft flow obstruction (Fig. 22).[53]

Although some authors have suggested that a 90 degree angle of take-off of the vein graft from the aorta may reduce turbulence of flow,[2, 54] experimental studies have indicated that the effect may be minimal in terms of the overall changes observed in the grafted veins.[12]

The reported frequency of aortocoronary saphenous vein bypass graft occlusion from thrombus or fibrous intimal proliferation may be decreasing.[9, 55, 58] The reasons are unclear but less traumatic handling of the vein before implantation and improvements in surgical techniques may be important. Although probably all veins used as aortocoronary conduits develop some intimal thickening with time, few appear to become totally occluded by this proliferative process. It is probable that this observed variation in the ultimate fate of the vein grafts is related to the relative contributions of

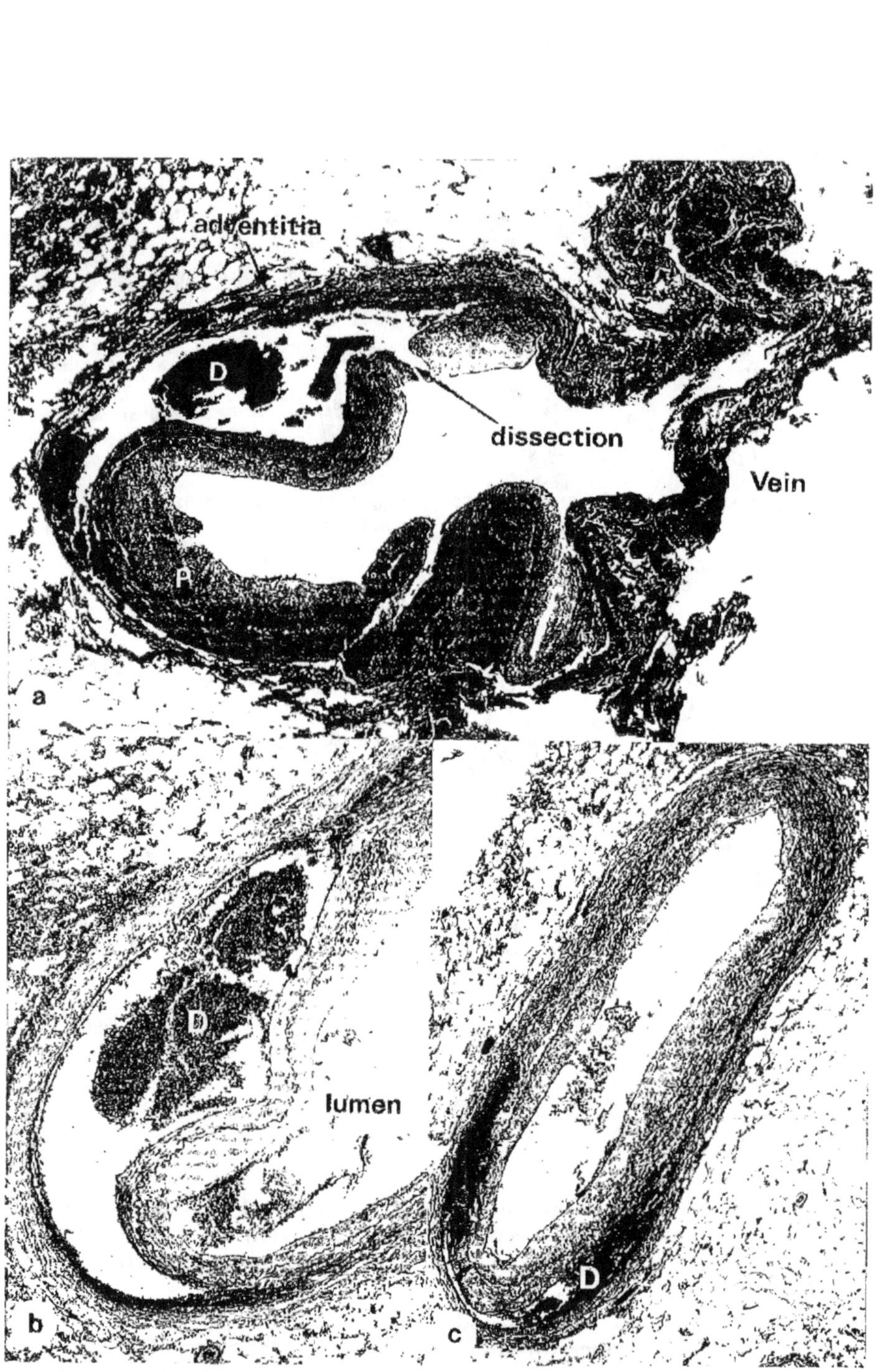

Figure 16. Coronary artery dissection in the left circumflex coronary artery after bypass grafting in a woman who died shortly after operation (A72–209). (a) Anastomosis of the vein graft to the coronary artery showing entrance site of the dissection. The media of the coronary artery and the associated atherosclerotic plaque (p) are separated from the adventitia by the false lumen (D). (b) Circumflex coronary artery distal to insertion of the vein graft. The dissection has progressed distally, causing some narrowing of the lumen. (c) Section of cornary artery proximal to site of venocoronary anastomosis. Mild dissection (D) without luminal narrowing is seen. Movat stains; reduced 20% from × 38 (a), × 44 (b), × 34 (c).

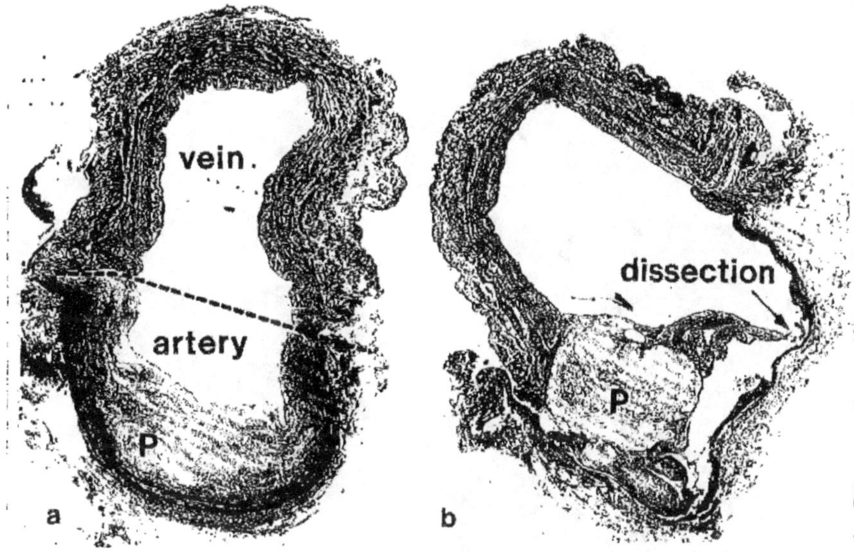

Figure 17. Anastomosis of vein graft at plaque. (a) Anastomosis of vein graft to the proximal right coronary artery in a man (A75–279) who died shortly after operation. Significant narrowing of the coronary artery by plaque (p) at the site of insertion of the graft is seen. (b) Dissection of atherosclerotic plaque from coronary wall at the anastomosis of the vein graft to the posterior descending coronary artery in the same patient. The dissection extended for 2 cm. proximal to the anastomosis. Movat stains; reduced 20% from × 11 (a), × 16 (b).

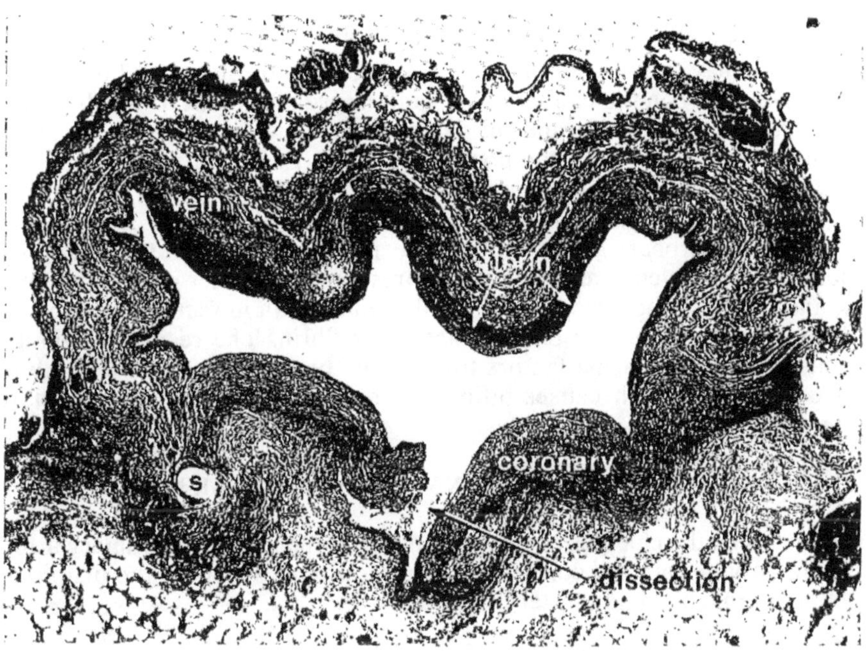

Figure 18. Minimal dissection of the coronary artery immediately beneath the anastomosis in 4-day-old bypass graft. Incision of the posterior wall of the artery at the time of arteriotomy is the most likely cause of this localized dissection. Fibrin deposition on the vein wall is present. S = suture. Phosphotungstic acid–hematoxylin stain; reduced 20% from × 39.

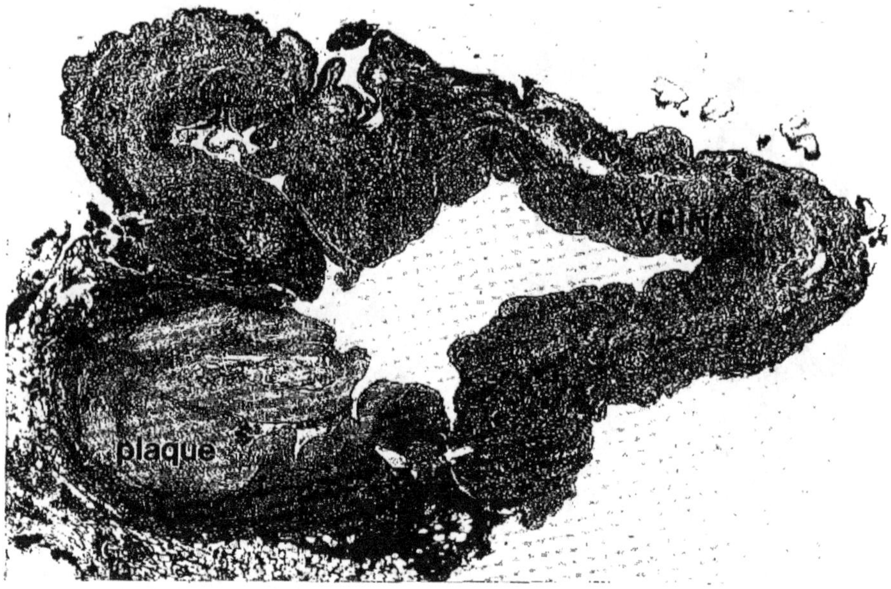

Figure 19. Insertion of vein graft at site of plaque in a 46-year-old man (NA75 – 107) who died 24 hours after insertion of three grafts. The vein graft to the right coronary artery is large in relation to the coronary artery into which it inserts. A large atherosclerotic plaque is present at the anastomosis. Movat stain; reduced 20% from × 22.6.

the various factors which affect graft flow (Fig. 23).[59] Stabilization of the amount of intimal proliferation may occur when the flow becomes less turbulent and damaging to the endothelial layer or when the caliber of the graft approaches that of the distal coronary artery into which it inserts. If transient decreases in flow occur at this stage, progression to complete occlusion by thrombosis may result. Early graft thrombosis might be expected when restrictions to flow are severe.

Although the exact explanations for the development of stenosis or occlusion of saphenous vein aortocoronary grafts remains speculative, a likely factor is progressive or recurrent injury to the vein wall by elevated pressure. The latter is modified by several anatomic and technical factors which affect flow and result in recurrent exposure of the intimal basement membrane to plasma factors or fibrin. The resulting stimulation of smooth muscle cells by plasma factors transforms the myocytes into myointimal cells or fibroblasts which in turn causes intimal fibrous thickening and medial fibrous replacement.

AUTOGENOUS INTERNAL MAMMARY ARTERY

Before discussing the changes observed in autogenous internal mammary arteries utilized as aortocoronary arterial conduits, it is appropriate to discuss the histology of the normal adult internal mammary artery.

Normal Internal Mammary Artery

The internal mammary artery has a musculoelastic wall consisting of an extremely thin intima of ground substance and endothelium overlying a thick internal elastic

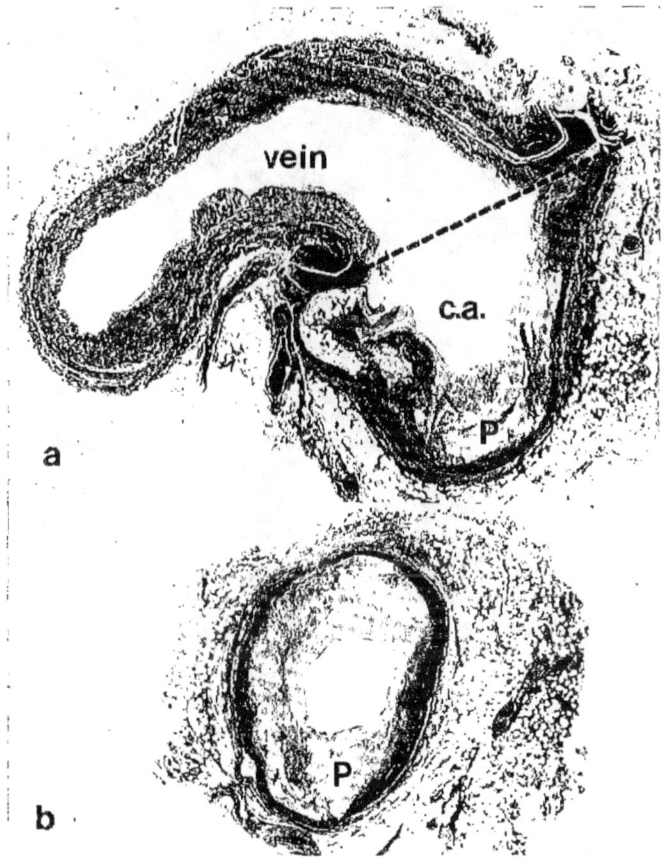

Figure 20. Narrowing of coronary artery distal to insertion of vein graft in a 50-year-old man (MHCMH–4961) who died less than 24 hours after triple vessel bypass grafting. (a) Section of the anastomosis of the vein graft to the left anterior descending coronary artery (c.a.) at the site of considerable narrowing by atherosclerotic plaque (p). (b) Coronary artery section *distal* to the anastomosis showing significant narrowing by plaque. Movat stains; × 11 (a and b).

membrane (Fig. 24). The media is composed of multiple layers of circularly oriented smooth muscle separated by thick elastic fiber layers and collagen. The adventitia is composed of loose alveolar tissue, broad bands of elastic fibers, fibrous tissue, and blood vessels. The blood supply to the media is largely by vasa vasorum which penetrate the wall from the adventitia. As in all arteries, atherosclerotic changes may involve the internal mammary arteries. Thus, these arterial conduits may be involved by the same process as the coronary arteries to which they are anastomosed.

Reported Changes in Internal Mammary Arteries Used as Aortocoronary Implants or Bypass Conduits

Few reports have concerned the histologic fate of internal mammary arteries used in myocardial revascularization procedures.[17, 18, 19, 60, 61] The reports concerned with internal mammary implants into myocardium have demonstrated early thrombotic occlusion of the implants with later recanalization, especially in the segment of the artery

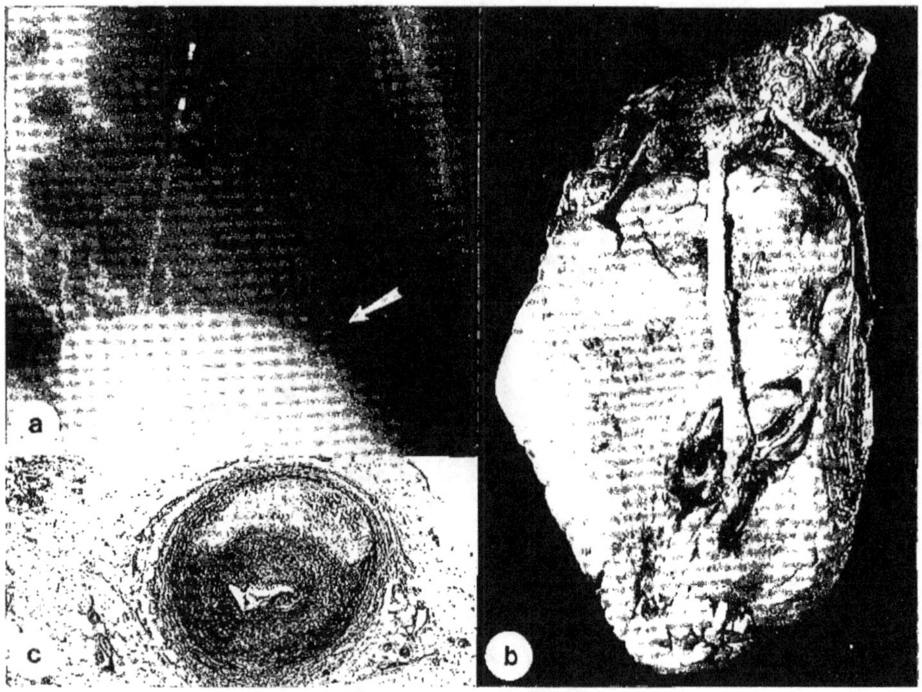

Figure 21. Severe obstruction of coronary artery distal to the site of insertion of a vein bypass graft in a 40-year-old woman (A74–212) who could not be weaned from cardiopulmonary bypass after three-vessel vein grafting. (a) Preoperative coronary angiogram showing total occlusion of the left anterior descending (LAD) coronary artery with reconstitution distally. The distal vessel was interpreted as showing no significant narrowing. (b) Anterior view of heart showing anastomosis of vein graft to the LAD. (c) Section of LAD at approximate area shown by arrow in (a). Severe narrowing of the vessel is present despite a normal appearing angiogram. (c) Movat stain; reduced 20% from × 22.

imbedded in myocardium.[17, 19] The remainder of the artery shows less severe changes of subendothelial intimal thickening by fibroelastic tissue and smooth muscle, loss of medial myocytes, and marked adventitial fibrosis.[17, 18, 19] Experimental studies suggest that devascularization of the wall plays little part in the changes seen, but trauma to the vessel wall increases the amount of subendothelial intimal proliferation.[19]

Histologic studies of internal mammary arteries used as aortocoronary bypass conduits rather than as implants are rare.[18, 19] Most reports have shown little or no structural change of the arterial intima with time.[18, 60, 61] One experimental study showed intimal changes similar to those observed in saphenous veins, but to a much lesser degree.[19] The major change is subendothelial intimal cellular proliferation with associated collagen and mucopolysaccharide deposition.[17, 19] Loss of medial smooth muscle was minimal, but adventitial fibrosis was observed around the arterial pedicle.[19] Thus, the internal mammary artery appears to be relatively resistant to the changes seen in saphenous veins used as aortocoronary bypass grafts. Since the internal mammary artery is taken down with an adventitial pedicle, some medial blood supply may be preserved and revascularization of the wall may occur more quickly than in the unsupported vein grafts. The smaller size and higher velocity of blood flow in the internal mammary arteries may be favorable in terms of prevention of endothelial damage and thrombosis.[61, 62] Significant degrees of subendothelial intimal proliferation, therefore, may be related to

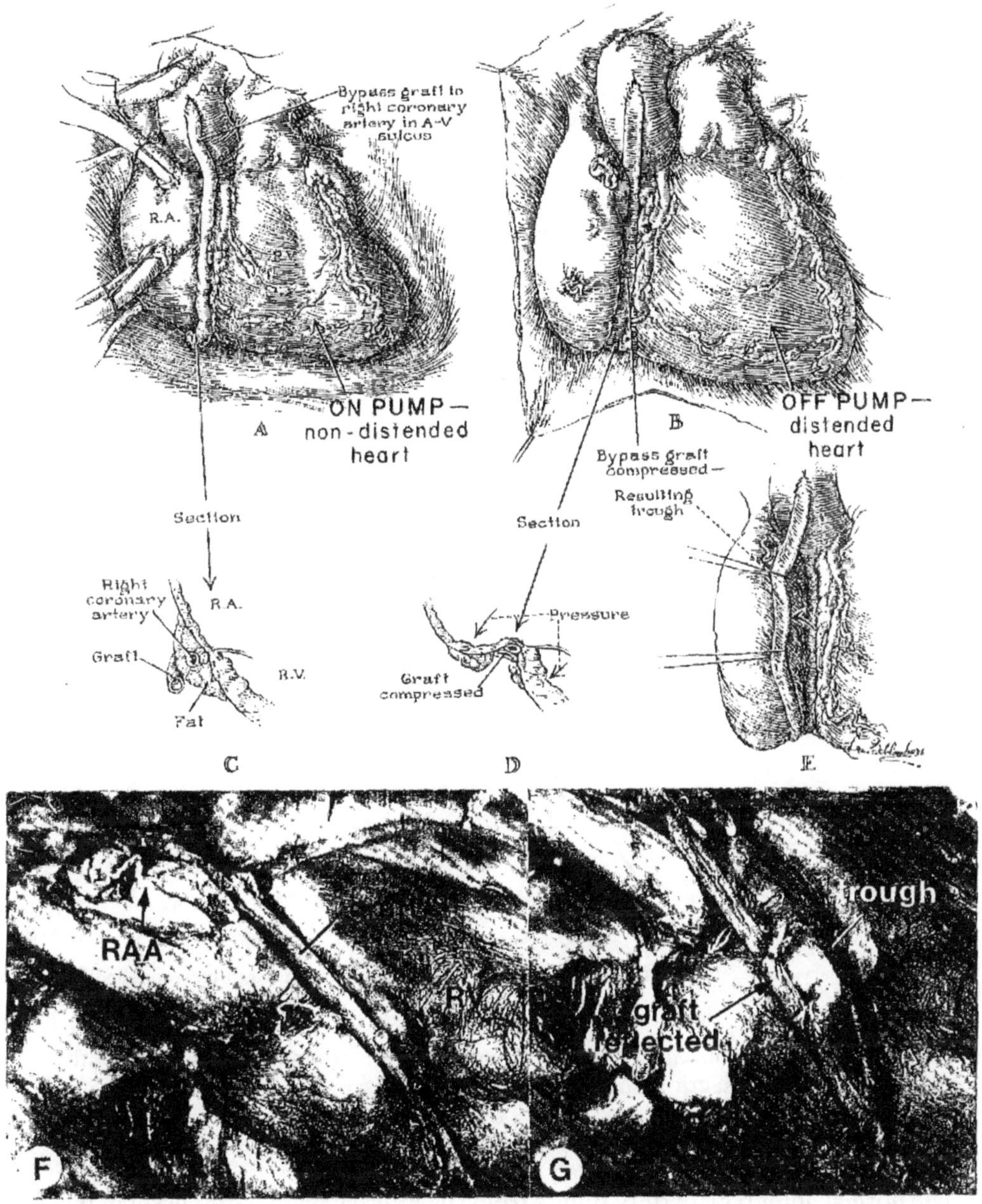

Figure 22. Tension produced on a vein graft to the right coronary artery. *Above:* (A, C) Patient on bypass, heart empty. The vein graft passes along the atrioventricular (AV) sulcus without tension. (B, D) Patient off bypass, heart beating. Distension of the right atrium and ventricle compresses the vein graft in the AV sulcus. (E) Reflection of the vein graft shows the trough which results from excessive tension. R.A. = right atrium, R.V. = right ventricle. *Below:* Saphenous vein aortocoronary bypass graft from the aorta (dashed circle, upper left) to the right posterior descending coronary artery in a 49-year-old man (GT 75A – 107) who died two hours after operation from refractory hypotension. (F) The graft passes along the right atrioventricular sulcus below the ligated right atrial appendage (RAA) and the right atrial body. (G) A view of the graft after it has been reflected. A deep trough is present in the AV sulcus, indicating that the graft was under significant tension. RV = right ventricle.

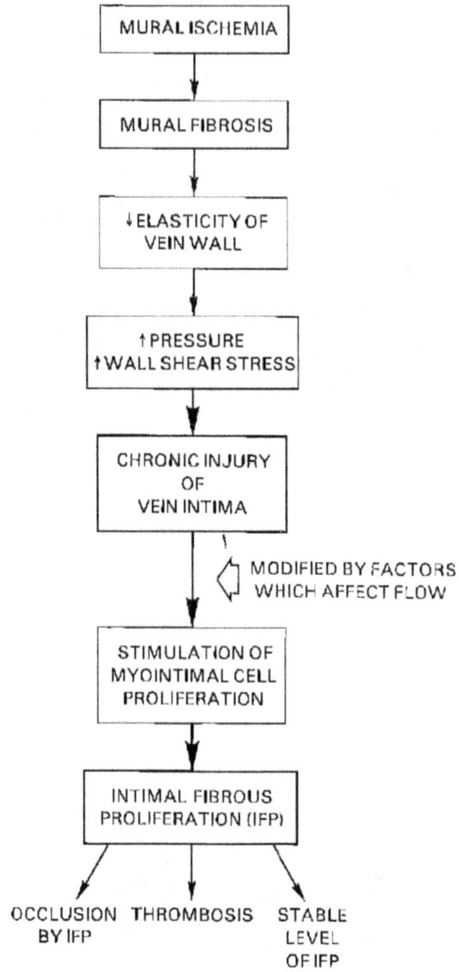

Figure 23. Summary of the relationship of various factors to the development of graft changes and the ultimate fate of the graft.

traumatic handling of the artery or to the presence of other anatomic or technical factors as outlined in the section on saphenous vein grafts.

AUTOGENOUS RADIAL ARTERY

The normal adult radial artery differs from the internal mammary vessel in that it has a muscular, rather than a musculoelastic, media.[21] In this regard, the radial artery is similar to the coronary artery. The muscular media is separated from the thin intima by a well developed internal elastic membrane, and the adventitia is formed by vasa vasorum, collagen bundles, and occasional elastic fibers and smooth muscle.

Reported Changes in Radial Arteries Used as Aortocoronary Bypass Conduits

Early clinical studies have suggested that use of the free radial artery for aortocoronary bypass grafting might prevent the late intimal changes and graft closure observed

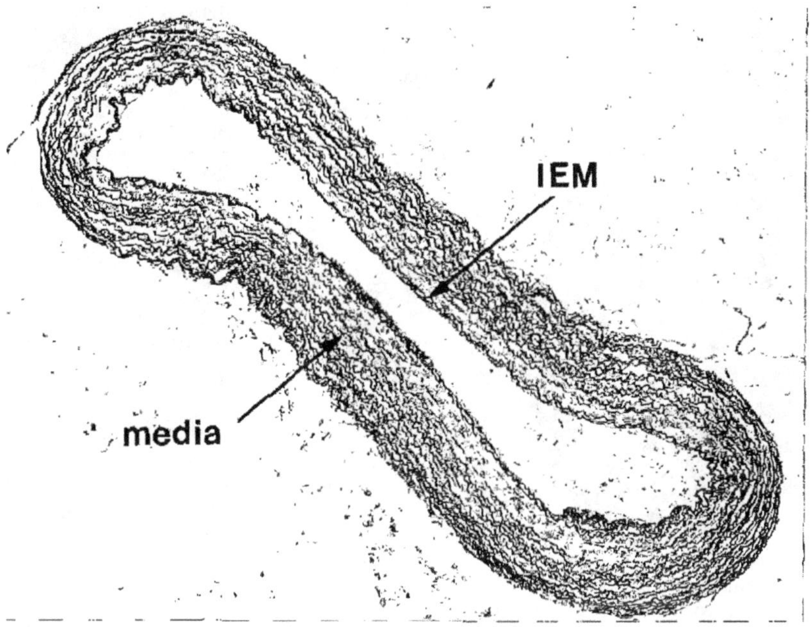

Figure 24. Section of internal mammary artery used as a bypass graft. The thick internal elastic membrane (IEM) and the multiple elastic lamina of the media are shown. Little adventitia is present due to dissection of the artery for use as an aortocoronary bypass conduit. Movat stain; × 40.

in autogenous saphenous veins.[20] Recently, however, later angiographic and histologic studies have documented severe stenosis and graft occlusion in free radial arterial bypass conduits.[21]

The histologic changes in radial artery grafts have been observed as early as eight months after implantation, and consist of severe concentric intimal fibrous thickening and thinning of the medial smooth muscle layers.[21] The internal elastic membrane, however, appears to remain intact.

The causes of the histologic changes observed in radial artery grafts are speculative. Dissection of the adventitia in harvesting the artery and delay in its implantation may result in the medial ischemia and endothelial sloughing seen in saphenous vein grafts. Since the medial smooth muscle layer is thicker in the radial artery than in the saphenous vein a greater degree of medial smooth muscle ischemia and necrosis might be expected.

HETEROGRAFTS AS AORTOCORONARY BYPASS CONDUITS

Only a rare report[63] has described the use of heterograft tissue as aortocoronary bypass conduits. Although great interest and some success[64-68] has surrounded the use of such heterografts as bypass conduits in the peripheral circulation, use of these materials in the aortocoronary position thus far has met with failure.[63]

Histologic observations in sheep carotid arterial grafts fixed in glutaraldehyde and implanted in the aortocoronary position for 30 months have shown extensive infiltration of the entire length of the walls of the vessel by granulomas containing giant cells.[63] In several areas, including both anastomoses, the lumen of the graft was obliterated by fibrous and granulomatous tissue (Figs. 25 and 26).

The cause of the granulomatous reaction and thrombosis and fibrosis of the conduits

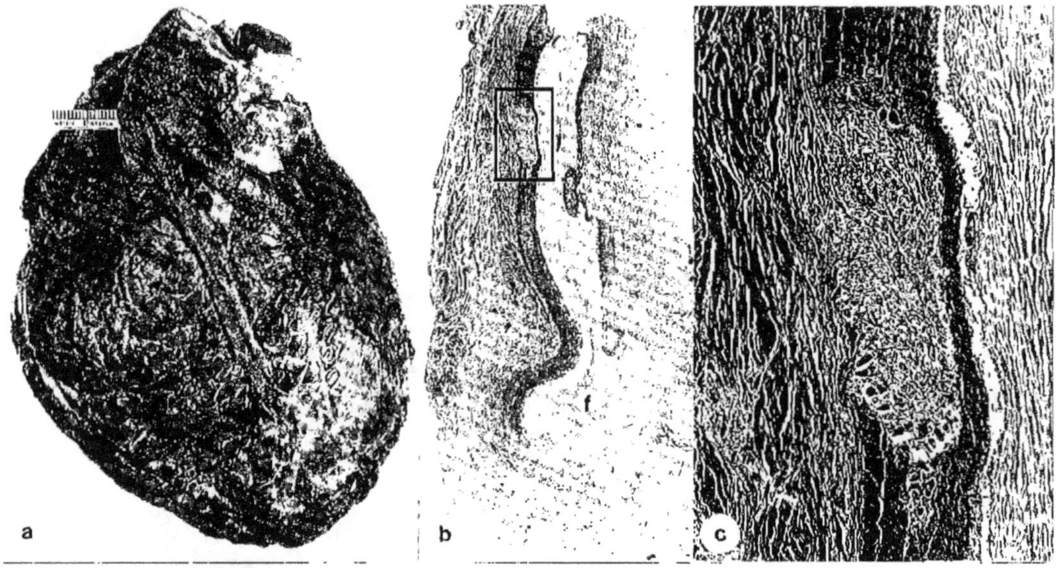

Figure 25. Glutaraldehyde-preserved sheep carotid arterial heterografts used as aortocoronary bypass conduits 30 months before death in a 45-year-old man. (a) The heart at necropsy, showing heterograft conduits to the left anterior descending (LAD) and circumflex coronary arteries. (b) Histologic section of the distal portion of the LAD graft showing adventitial fibrosis, fibrous tissue occlusion of the graft (f), and invasion and fibrous replacement of the walls of the graft. (c) Higher power view of area enclosed by box in (b) showing granulomatous reaction in the heterograft vessel wall. Hematoxylin-eosin stains; reduced 35% from × 14 (b), × 90 (c).

is uncertain; however, a foreign body type reaction to a fixed, and therefore possibly nonantigenic, tube or an active rejection response to the fixed tissue are the most likely possibilities. The severity of the cellular reaction and the structural changes observed when heterografts are implanted in the coronary position and the size differential between heterograft tissue of 4 to 8 mm. diameter and the coronary arteries suggest that heterografts are presently unsatisfactory for use as aortocoronary bypass conduits.

COMMENTS

As already discussed, morphologic changes occur in all biologic materials used as aortocoronary bypass conduits. With the saphenous vein and the internal mammary artery, most changes observed are normal responses to injury and repair and do not affect the function of the graft. Progression of these normal or expected changes, however, may occur and result in "graft failure". Means of predicting which grafts may be expected to fail on the basis of structural changes are not available, except for the observed early thrombosis rate of grafts which carry low flows (<40 to 50 ml./min.) at the time of operation.[69-71] This observation suggests that *maintenance of graft patency in the face of normal or expected structural responses to increased pressure and flow is dependent, as in grafts in the peripheral circulation, upon good run-off from the graft.* As outlined above, many factors may contribute to the status of the run-off of a coronary graft system.

Unlike the saphenous vein and internal mammary coronary bypass grafts, the free radial artery and heterologous tissue grafts develop severe structural changes which make them unsuitable for use as aortocoronary conduits. The normal or expected structural changes in these grafts appear to be too severe to maintain patency of the graft.

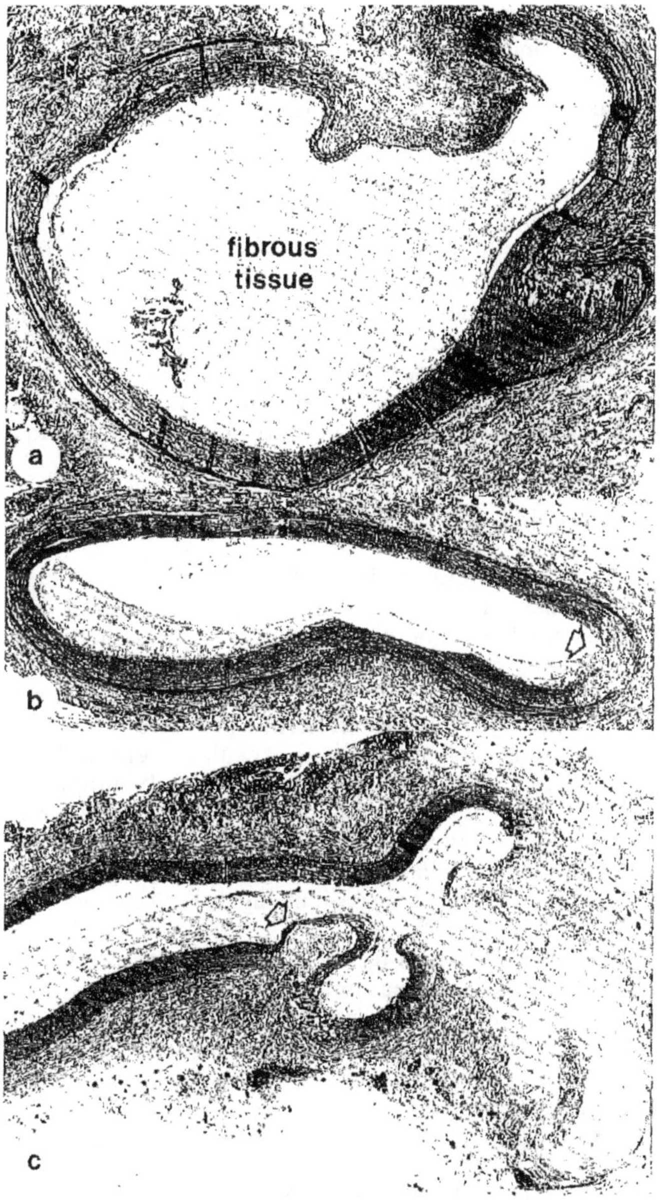

Figure 26. Sheep carotid heterograft aortocoronary conduit from same patient as Figure 25. (a) Proximal portion of graft to the left anterior descending (LAD) coronary artery showing occlusion of the conduit by fibrous tissue. (b) Mid-portion of graft showing focal transmural replacement of the wall with granulomatous and fibrous tissue and a layer of fibrous tissue on the luminal surface of the graft. (c) Distal anastomosis of the heterograft. Severe granulomatous reaction (arrow) and fibrosis is present with occlusion of the vessel. Movat stains; reduced 20% from × 16 (a), × 13.5 (b), × 14 (c).

Again, the failure of these materials probably is related to inadequate run-off to maintain patency in the presence of normal structural alterations, since larger grafts of these materials have been successful when used in the peripheral circulation.[64-68]

There are advantages and disadvantages to the use of all presently available biologic conduits. Use of autogenous saphenous vein has the advantages of (1) ready availability; (2) accessibility; (3) appropriate size and length; (4) thin wall; (5) observed high patency rate; and (6) rare aneurysm formation. Disadvantages include (1) production of venous stasis at the time of its excision with resulting risk of embolism; (2) possibly higher rate of atherosclerosis and occlusion than internal mammary grafts;[18] (3) lack of availability in some patients who have had vein stripping procedures, and (4) phlebosclerotic thickening.

The internal mammary artery has the advantages of (1) the absence of an aortic anastomosis; (2) lack of turbulent flow due to venous valves and higher velocity of flow; (3) better size match with some small coronary arteries, and (4) lack of significant structural changes in most. Disadvantages are[18] (1) the difficulty with which it is dissected via a median sternotomy; (2) the rapidity with which it tapers to inadequate size; (3) its involvement by preexisting atherosclerosis; (4) its size and location, which makes it most useful only for bypassing left coronary arteries; (5) its low flows which, despite patency, may be inadequate to provide satisfactory myocardial revascularization,[72] and (6) its excision leaves a raw tissue bed which may predispose to chostochondral infection.[73]

SUMMARY

This report describes morphologic observations in autogenous saphenous veins, autogenous internal mammary arteries, radial arteries and arterial heterografts used as aortocoronary bypass conduits. The normal or expected changes and the abnormal or unexpected changes observed in each type of bypass conduit is discussed. The three major changes seen in saphenous vein grafts in the aortocoronary position are: (1) medial fibrous replacement; (2) adventitial fibrous proliferation; and (3) intimal fibrous proliferation. Medial fibrous replacement is the result of vein wall ischemia and necrosis and ultimately replacement of smooth muscle cells; adventitial fibrosis is the result of organization of fibrin and red cell clot and repair of ischemic damage. The cause of intimal fibrous proliferation is unclear but appears to be the result of chronic repair of injured intima and endothelium. That the severity of the changes varies along the length of one graft or among grafts in the same patient suggests that other factors contribute to the development of the changes observed.

Although some structural changes have been observed, internal mammary arteries are relatively resistant to the changes seen in saphenous veins. Radial arterial grafts have shown severe structural changes with time, to a degree greater than that seen in the saphenous vein grafts. Heterograft conduits so far have been unsuccessful in the aortocoronary position in humans. The severe changes seen in radial artery and heterograft conduits indicate that they are inadequate for use as substitutes for saphenous vein and mammary artery as bypass conduits from aorta to coronary artery.

ACKNOWLEDGMENT

Technical assistance was provided by Filippina Giacometti, Carol L. Schurtz, Monica J. Clark, and Barbara E. Winterrowd. Secretarial assistance was provided by Zulienne F. Moyer and Carole C. Kreider.

REFERENCES

1. Johnson, W. D., Auer, J. E., and Tector, A. J.: *Late changes in coronary vein grafts*. Am. J. Cardiol. 26:640, 1970.

2. Kennedy, J. H., Wieting, D. W., Hwang, N. H., et al.: *Hydraulic and morphologic study of fibrous intimal hyperplasia in autogenous saphenous vein bypass grafts*. J. Thorac. Cardiovasc. Surg. 67:805, 1974.

3. UNNI, K. K., KOTTKE, B. A., TITUS, J. L., ET AL.: *Pathologic changes in saphenous vein aorto-coronary bypass grafts.* Am. J. Cardiol. 34:526, 1974.

4. HAMAKER, W. R., DOYLE, W. F., O'CONNELL, T. J., ET AL.: *Subintimal obliterative proliferation in saphenous vein grafts.* Ann. Thorac. Surg. 13:488, 1972.

5. VLODAVER, Z., AND EDWARDS, J. E.: *Pathologic analysis in fatal cases following saphenous vein coronary arterial bypass.* Chest 64:555, 1973.

6. VLODAVER, Z., AND EDWARDS, J. E.: *Pathologic changes in aortic-coronary arterial saphenous vein grafts.* Circulation 44:719, 1971.

7. MARTI, M. C., BOUCHARDY, B., AND COX, J. N.: *Aorto-coronary bypass with autogenous saphenous vein grafts: Histopathologic aspects.* Virchows Arch. (Pathol. Anat.) 352:255, 1971.

8. KERN, W. H., DERMER, G. B., AND LINDESMITH, G. G.: *The intimal proliferation in aorto-coronary saphenous vein grafts: Light and electron microscopic studies.* Am. Heart J. 84:771, 1972.

9. CAMPEAU, L., CROCHET, D., LESPERANÇE, J., ET AL.: *Postoperative changes in aortocoronary vein grafts revisited: Angiographic studies at two weeks and at one year in two series of consecutive patients.* Circulation 52:369, 1975.

10. JONES, M., CONKLE, D. M., FERRANS, V. J., ET AL.: *Lesions observed in arterial autogenous vein grafts. Light and electron microscopic evaluation.* Circulation 47 & 48:III–198, 1973.

11. BARBORIAK, J. J., BATAYIAS, G. E., PINTAR, K., ET AL.: *Pathologic changes in surgically removed aorto-coronary vein grafts.* Ann. Thorac. Surg. 21:524, 1976.

12. BREYER, R. H., SPRAY, T. L., KASTL, D. G., ET AL.: *Histologic changes in saphenous vein aorto-coronary bypass grafts: The effect of the angle of the aortic anastomosis.* J. Thorac. Cardiovasc. Surg. 72: (in press).

13. SPRAY, T. L., AND ROBERTS, W. C.: *Status of native coronary arteries proximal and distal to coronary anastomotic sites of aorto-coronary bypass grafts.* Circulation April, 1977.

14. SPRAY, T. L., AND ROBERTS, W. C.: *Changes in saphenous veins used as aortocoronary bypass grafts.* Am. Heart J. (in press).

15. BARBORIAK, J. J., PINTAR, K., AND KORNS, M. E.: *Atherosclerosis in aortocoronary vein grafts.* Lancet 2:621, 1974.

16. RIAHI, M., VASU, C. M., TOMATIS, L. A., ET AL.: *Aneurysm of saphenous vein bypass graft to coronary artery.* J. Thorac. Cardiovasc. Surg. 70:358, 1975.

17. YARBROUGH, J. W., ROBERTS, W. C., ABEL, R. M., ET AL.: *The cause of luminal narrowing in internal mammary arteries implanted into canine myocardium.* Am. Heart J. 84:507, 1972.

18. ROSSITER, S. J., BRODY, W. R., KOSEK, J. C., ET AL.: *Internal mammary artery versus autogenous vein for coronary artery bypass graft.* Circulation 50:1236, 1974.

19. MULLERWORTH, M. H., DANIEL, F. J., AND LIE, J. T.: *The fate of internal mammary arterial implants and bypass conduits for myocardial revascularization. Experimental angiographic, histologic, and ultrastructural observations.* J. Thorac. Cardiovasc. Surg. 70:89, 1975.

20. CARPENTIER, A., GUERMONPREZ, J. L., DELOCHE, A., ET AL.: *The aorto-to-coronary radial artery bypass graft. A technique avoiding pathological changes in grafts.* Ann. Thorac. Surg. 16:111, 1973.

21. CURTIS, J. J., STONEY, W. S., ALFORD, W. C., JR., ET AL.: *Intimal hyperplasia: A cause of radial artery aortocoronary bypass graft failure.* Ann. Thorac. Surg. 20:628, 1975.

22. CHEANVECHAI, C., EFFLER, D. B., HOOPER, J. R., ET AL.: *The structural study of the saphenous vein.* Ann. Thorac. Surg. 20:636, 1975.

23. DEDOMENICO, M., SAMEH, A. A., BERGER, K., ET AL.: *Experimental coronary artery surgery. Long-term follow-up, bypass venous autografts, longitudinal arteriotomies, and end-to-end anastomoses.* J. Thorac. Cardiovasc. Surg. 56:617, 1968.

24. FAULKNER, S. L., FISHER, R. D., CONKLE, D. M., ET AL.: *The effect of blood flow rate on subendothelial proliferation in venous autografts used as arterial substitutes.* Circulation 51 & 52:I–163, 1975.

25. BRODY, W. R., KOSEK, J. C., AND ANGELL, W. W.: *Changes in vein grafts following aorto-coronary bypass induced by pressure and ischemia.* J. Thorac. Cardiovasc. Surg. 64:847, 1972.

26. BRODY, W. R., ANGELL, W. W., AND KOSEK, J. C.: *Histologic fate of the venous coronary artery bypass in dogs.* Am. J. Pathol. 66:111, 1972.

27. NUNN, D. B., CHUN, B., WHELAN, T. J., JR., ET AL.: *Autogenous veins as arterial substitutes: A study of their histologic fate with special attention to endothelium.* Ann. Surg. 160:14, 1964.

28. MCCABE, M., AND CUNNINGHAM, G. J.: *Histological and histochemical examination of autogenous vein grafts.* Br. J. Surg. 54:147, 1967.

29. MCNAMARA, J. J., DARLING, R. C., AND LINTON, R. R.: *Segmental stenosis of saphenous vein autografts.* N. Engl. J. Med. 277:290, 1967.

30. Barner, H. B., Judd, D. R., Kaiser, G. C., et al.: *Late failure of arterialized in situ saphenous vein.* Arch. Surg. 99:781, 1969.

31. Stein, A. A., Rosenblum, J., and Leather, R.: *Intimal sclerosis in human veins.* Arch. Pathol. 81: 548, 1966.

32. Anderson, W. A. D.: *Pathology,* ed. 6. C. V. Mosby Co., St. Louis, 1971.

33. Esterly, J. A., Glagov, S., and Ferguson, D. J.: *Morphogenesis of intimal obliterative hyperplasia of small arteries in experimental pulmonary hypertension.* Am. J. Pathol. 52:325, 1968.

34. Heath, D., and Edwards, J. E.: *Pathology of hypertensive pulmonary vascular disease: description of six grades of structural changes in the pulmonary artery with special reference to congenital cardiac septal defects.* Circulation 18:533, 1958.

35. Stuart, M., and Magarey, F. R.: *Great veins in venous hypertension.* J. Pathol. Bacteriol. 79:319, 1960.

36. Geiringer, E.: *Venous atheromata.* Arch. Pathol. 48:410, 1949.

37. McGee, W. G., and Ashworth, G. F.: *Fine structure of chronic hypertensive arteriopathy in the human kidney.* Am. J. Pathol. 43:273, 1963.

38. Vlodaver, Z., and Neufeld, H. N.: *The musculo-elastic layer in the coronary arteries: A histological and hemodynamic concept.* Vasc. Dis. 4:136, 1967.

39. Gresham, G. A., Howard, A. N., and King, A. J.: *Comparative histopathological study of the early atherosclerotic lesion.* Br. J. Exp. Pathol. 43:21, 1962.

40. Vlodaver, Z., and Edwards, J. E.: *Pathology of coronary atherosclerosis.* Prog. Cardiovasc. Dis. 14: 256, 1971.

41. Haust, M. D., More, R. H., and Movat, H. Z.: *Role of smooth muscle cells in the fibrogenesis of arteriosclerosis.* Am. J. Pathol. 37:377, 1960.

42. Geer, J. C., McGill, N. C., Jr., and Strong, J. P.: *Fine structure of the human atherosclerotic lesions.* Am. J. Pathol. 38:263, 1961.

43. Geer, J. C.: *Fine structure of human aortic intimal thickening and fatty streaks.* Lab. Invest. 14:1764, 1965.

44. Caro, C. G., Fitz-Gerald, J. M., J. M., and Schroter, R. C.: *Arterial wall shear and distribution of early atheroma in man.* Nature 223:1159, 1969.

45. Flaherty, J. T., Pierce, J. E., Ferrans, V. J., et al.: *Endothelial nuclear patterns in the canine arterial tree with particular reference to hemodynamic events.* Circ. Res. 30:23, 1972.

46. Szilagyi, D. E., Elliot, J. P., Hagenman, J. H., et al.: *Biologic fate of autogenous vein implants as arterial substitutes. Clinical, angiographic and histopathologic observations in femoropopliteal operations for atherosclerosis.* Ann. Surg. 178:232, 1973.

47. Cohn, L. H., Kosek, J. C., and Angell, W. W.: *Pulmonary arteriosclerosis produced by hyperoxemic normotensive perfusion.* Surgery 70:723, 1971.

48. Murray, M., Schrodt, G. R., and Berg, H. F.: *Role of smooth muscle cells in healing of injured arteries.* Arch. Pathol. 82:138, 1966.

49. Wissler, R. W.: *The arterial medial cell smooth muscle, or multifunctional mesenchyma?* Circulation 36:1, 1967.

50. Ts'ao, C. H., and Glagov, S.: *Platelet adhesion to subendothelial components in experimental aortic injury: Role of fine fibrils and basement membrane.* Br. J. Exp. Pathol. 51:423, 1970.

51. Duguid, J. B.: *Thrombosis as a factor in the pathogenesis of aortic atherosclerosis.* J. Pathol. Bacteriol. 60:57, 1948.

52. Roberts, W. C., and Buja, L. M.: *Frequency and significance of coronary arterial thrombi and other observations in fatal acute myocardial infarction: A study of 107 necropsy patients.* Am. J. Med. 52:425, 1972.

53. Spray, T. L., and Roberts, W. C.: *Tension on coronary bypass conduits: A neglected cause of real or potential obstruction of saphenous vein grafts.* J. Thorac. Cardiovasc. Surg. 72:282, 1976.

54. Bond, M. G., Hostetler, J. R., Karayannacos, P. E., et al.: *Intimal changes in arteriovenous bypass grafts: Effects of varying the angle of implantaion at the proximal anastomosis and of producing stenosis in the distal runoff artery.* J. Thorac. Cardiovasc. Surg. 71:907, 1976.

55. Hall, R. J., Garcia, E., Wukasch, D. C., et al.: *Aortocoronary bypass (CAB): Long-term follow-up.* Circulation 51 & 52:11–90, 1975.

56. Grondin, C. M., Castonguay, Y. R., Lesperance, J., et al.: *Attrition rate of aorto-to-coronary artery saphenous vein grafts after one year.* Ann. Thorac. Surg. 14:223, 1972.

57. Flemma, R. J., Johnson, W. D., Lepley, D., Jr., et al.: *Late results of saphenous vein bypass grafting for myocardial revascularization.* Ann. Thorac. Surg. 14:232, 1972.

58. GRONDIN, C. M., MEERE, C., CASTONGUAY, Y., ET AL.: *Progressive and late obstruction of an aorto-coronary venous bypass graft.* Circulation 43:698, 1971.

59. BOURASSA, M. G., LESPERANCE, J., CAMPEAU, L., ET AL.: *Factors influencing patency of aortocoronary vein grafts.* Circulation 45 & 46:I–79, 1971.

60. BARNER, H. B., KAISER, G. C., JELINEK, M., ET AL.: *Aortocoronary vein graft and internal mammary-coronary anastomosis.* Arch. Surg. 105:908, 1972.

61. HIROSE, T., AND MARSHALL, D.: *A comparataive study of the direct internal mammary-to-coronary artery anastomosis and the aortocoronary vein bypass graft.* Ann. Thorac. Surg. 16:471, 1973.

62. GRONDIN, C. M., LESPÉRANCE, J., BOURASSA, M. G., ET AL.: *Coronary artery grafting with the saphenous vein or internal mammary artery.* Ann. Thorac. Surg. 20:605, 1975.

63. BULKLEY, B. H., AND ROBERTS, W. C.: *Heterografts as aortocoronary bypass conduits in human beings.* Am. J. Cardiol. 36:823, 1975.

64. ROSENBERG, N.: *The modified bovine arterial graft.* Arch. Surg. 105:547, 1972.

65. ROSENBERG, N., MARTINEZ, A., SAWYER, P. N., ET AL.: *Tanned collagen arterial prostheses of bovine carotid origin in man.* Ann. Surg. 164:247, 1966.

66. DALE, W. A., AND LEWIS, M. R.: *Modified bovine heterografts for arterial replacement.* Ann. Surg. 169: 927, 1969.

67. DILLON, M. L., SCOTT, S. M., VASQUEZ, M. D., ET AL.: *Tissue response to an arterial substitute of bovine origin.* Arch. Surg. 105:577, 1972.

68. ROSENBERG, N., LORD, G. H., HENDERSON, J., ET AL.: *Collagen arterial graft of bovine origin: seven-year observations in the dog.* Surgery 67:951, 1970.

69. GRONDIN, C. M., LEPAGE, G., CASTONGUAY, Y. R., ET AL.: *Aortocoronary bypass grafts: Initial blood flow through the graft and early postoperative patency.* Circulation 44:815, 1971.

70. WALKER, J. A., FRIEDBERG, H. D., FLEMMA, R. J., ET AL.: *Determinants of the angiographic patency of aortocoronary bypass grafts.* Circulation 45 & 46:I–86, 1972.

71. STINSON, E. B., OLINGER, G. N., AND GLANCY, D. L.: *Anatomical and physiological determinants of blood flow through aortocoronary vein bypass grafts.* Surgery 74:390, 1973.

72. FLEMMA, R. J., SINGH, H. M., TECTOR, A. J., ET AL.: *Comparative hemodynamic properties of vein and mammary artery in coronary bypass operations.* Ann. Thorac. Surg. 20:619, 1975.

73. CULLIFORD, A. T., CUNNINGHAM, J. N., JR., ZEFF, R. H., ET AL.: *Sternal and costrochondral infections following open-heart surgery: A review of 2,594 cases.* J. Thorac. Cardiovasc. Surg. 72:714, 1976.

Changes in saphenous veins used as aortocoronary bypass grafts

Thomas L. Spray, M.D.*
William C. Roberts, M.D.**
Bethesda, Md.

The widespread use of reversed autogenous saphenous veins to bypass obstructed coronary arteries has stimulated interest in the long-term morphologic and functional fate of the grafts. Stenosis or complete occlusion of the graft is now recognized as an all too frequent complication of its use as an aortocoronary conduit.[1-13] While all grafts develop some morphologic changes, the degree and the functional significance of the changes may be related to several factors, including intraluminal pressure, graft-wall ischemia, thrombosis or fibrin deposition, and repair of damaged endothelium and intima, either from ischemia or trauma or both.[8-11, 14-23] This paper describes structural changes observed in saphenous veins used as aortocoronary conduits and discusses the relative contribution of the above factors to these changes.

Normal saphenous vein

The normal human saphenous vein contains a thin *intima* consisting of relatively acellular fibrous tissue covered by a single layer of endothelial cells and separated from the media by a rudimentary internal elastic membrane (Fig. 1). The *media* consists of multiple layers of smooth muscle cells, separated by bundles of collagen, ground substance, and occasional short elastic fibers. The majority of medial smooth muscle layers have a circular orientation; in areas near the venous valves, however, the middle circular layers have a more longitudinal arrangement. Frequently, longitudinally oriented smooth muscle fasicles make up the innermost layers of the media. The *adventitia* is composed of bundles of collagen with scattered fasicles of longitudinally oriented smooth muscle cells. Broad loose bands of elastic fibers are present in abundance. Vasa vasorum are present and may extend into the outermost portion of the media.

Reported changes in saphenous vein grafts used as arterial conduits

Seven changes have been described in veins implanted in the arterial circulation:[18] (1) endothelial damage, (2) medial hypertrophy, (3) medial necrosis, (4) graft-wall fibrosis (media and adventitia), (5) intimal fibrous thickening, (6) intimal lipid deposition, and (7) aneurysmal dilatation.

In 1906, Carrel and Guthrie[24] described intimal thickening in veins implanted in dogs, and concluded that veins placed in the arterial circulation had a strong tendency to assume the character of an artery. In further vein transplantation experiments in 1908, Carrel[25] described four characteristic changes in veins used as arteries in the *peripheral* circulation: (1) intimal thickening, (2) adventitial thickening (from fibrosis), (3) loss of the inner one-third of the media, and (4) loss of elasticity producing a fibrous tube. In addition, medial hypertrophy was observed in some grafts. The development of vascular surgery utilizing saphenous veins for femoropopliteal bypass and aortocoronary bypass brought renewed interest in the long-term fate of these grafts.

In early studies of the use of veins as conduits

From the Pathology Branch, National Heart, Lung, and Blood Institute, National Institutes of Health, Bethesda, Md.

Received for publication Aug. 25, 1976.

Reprint requests: William C. Roberts, M.D., Chief, Pathology Branch, National Heart, Lung, and Blood Institute, NIH, Bethesda, Md. 20014.

*Staff Associate, Pathology Branch, National Heart, Lung and Blood Institute, National Institutes of Health, Bethesda, Md.

**Chief, Pathology Branch, National Heart, Lung and Blood Institute, National Institutes of Health, Bethesda, Md., and Clinical Professor of Pathology and Medicine (Cardiology), Georgetown University, Washington, D. C.

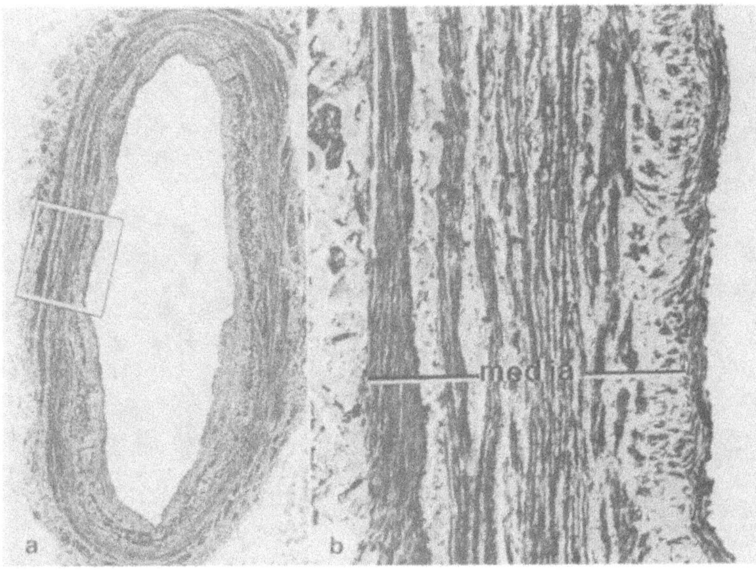

Fig. 1. Normal saphenous vein. *a*, Low power view showing medial circular and longitudinal smooth muscle layers. *b*, High power view of area enclosed in box in *a*. Multiple layers of circular smooth muscle separated by layers of fibrous tissue make up the media. Occasional longitudinal smooth muscle fascicles are present near the lumen. (Movat Stain; original magnifications ×20 *(a)*, ×130 *(b)*.)

in the *aortocoronary* position, Dedomenico and associates[26] described changes up to 2.5 years after implantation in canine jugular veins and in saphenous veins. A marked increase in both fibrous tissue and smooth muscle was noted in the media. Up to a threefold dilatation of vessel caliber occurred in the jugular vein grafts. Johnson and associates[5] noted considerable thickening of the subendothelial portion of saphenous veins used as aortocoronary vein grafts in three patients, and this thickening has been observed to be extensive enough to result in severe luminal narrowing or total obstruction of the bypass graft.[2, 9, 10] Grondin and colleagues,[2] in addition to the intimal fibrosis, described fibrotic changes involving the entire vein wall in a patient who died 114 days after bypass grafting.

Vlodaver and Edwards[10] noted changes in each of eight saphenous vein grafts used as aortocoronary bypass conduits in place for more than 100 days: fibrous subendothelial thickening with severe luminal narrowing occurred in six and thrombosis occurred in two. No changes were observed by these authors in venous grafts in place for less than one month.

Marti and associates[11] examined eight grafts at necropsy which were in place up to 300 days and noted wall thickening with intimal hyperplasia and transient medial muscular hypertrophy, followed by atrophy and loss of some medial myocytes. Kern and co-workers[12] examined 16 grafts from age 2 days to 29 months, both with light and electron microscopy. Intimal fibrosis was present in the nine patients in whom the grafts had been in place for over two months. Ultrastructural study of the intimal lesions showed proliferation of "fibroblasts" and smooth muscle cells and developing capillaries. Unni and associates[7] studied 62 grafts from 40 patients at various times up to 28 months after operation. The earliest changes were infusion of blood elements into the intima and migration of leukocytes into the media and intima, presumably in response to endothelial damage. The major change after one month was intimal fibrous proliferation, resulting in graft occlusion in three patients.

Lipid deposition and atherosclerotic change has been a rare finding in vein grafts in the peripheral circulation[27-29] and has been reported infrequently in aortocoronary vein grafts.[6, 30, 31] In addition, aneurysmal dilatation, which has been observed in canine jugular veins used as aortocoronary grafts,[26] is exceedingly rare when saphenous veins are used as aortocoronary conduits. Aneurysm formation in a saphenous vein aortocoronary bypass graft has been reported in only one patient.[32]

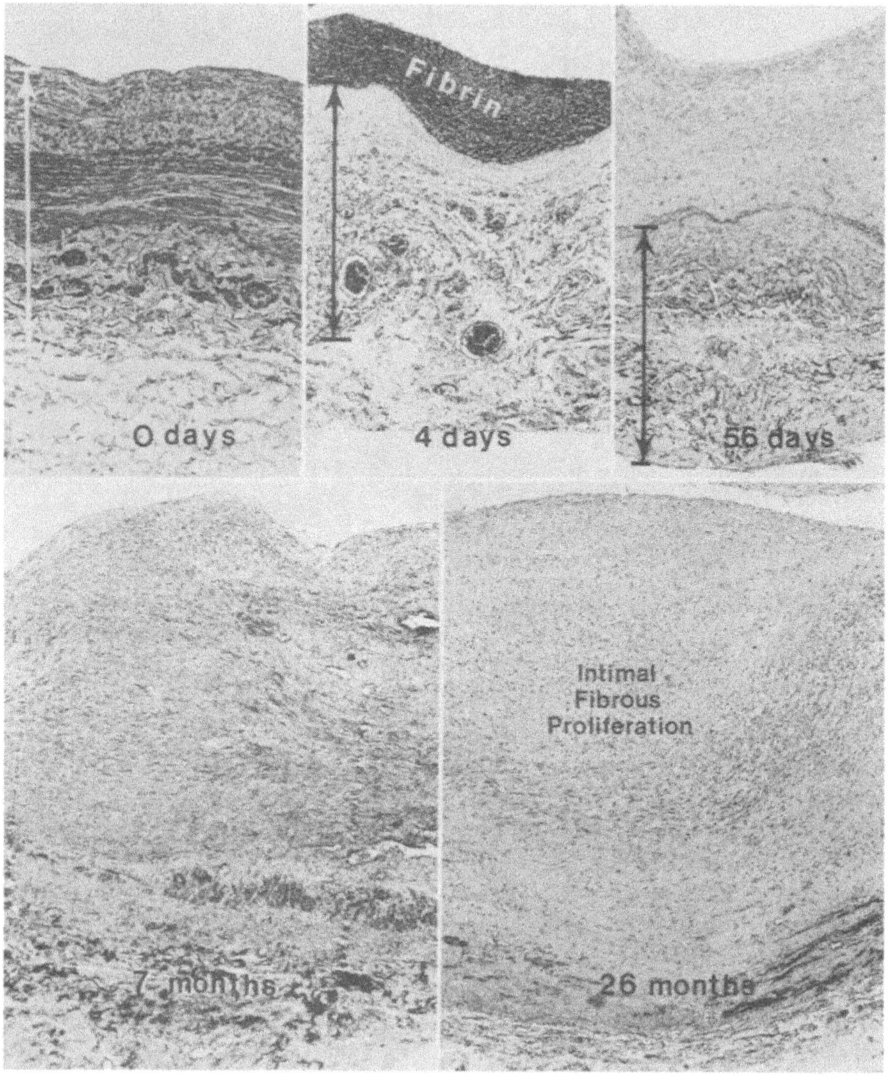

Fig. 2. Composite of changes seen in saphenous vein aortocoronary grafts from 0 days (normal vein) to 26 months after implantation *at the same magnification* (×54). Arrows indicate normal wall thickness (media + adventitia). *0 days* = intima thin, marked medial smooth muscle layers in both circular and longitudinal directions, loose adventitial tissue. *4 days* = Large deposit of fibrin over slightly thickened intima. Marked loss of medial smooth muscle with cellular infiltration. *56 days* = Thickened vein wall with marked intimal fibrous proliferation. The media and adventitia show loss of muscle cells and fibrosis. *7 months* = Severe intimal fibrous proliferation is present, containing some neovascular channels. Marked loss of medial smooth muscle and replacement fibrosis is present. *26 months* = The vein wall has become almost completely replaced by fibrous tissue and intimal proliferation, creating a fibrous tube. Only small areas of medial smooth muscle cells remain. (All Movat stains.)

Brody and associates[17] performed experimental studies of the progression of graft changes in dogs. During the first week after implantation, they noted endothelial cell damage, fibrin deposition, subendothelial edema, and necrosis and inflammatory cell infiltration of medial smooth muscle. In later grafts, the medial smooth muscle either hypertrophied, died, or underwent fibroblastic transformation with resulting medial and intimal fibrosis.

Further delineation of the time course of changes in aortocoronary grafts came from Jones and associates[18] in dogs. During the first two weeks after implantation the grafts showed focal endothelial disruption, mural fibrin deposition, medial edema, and inflammatory infiltration into

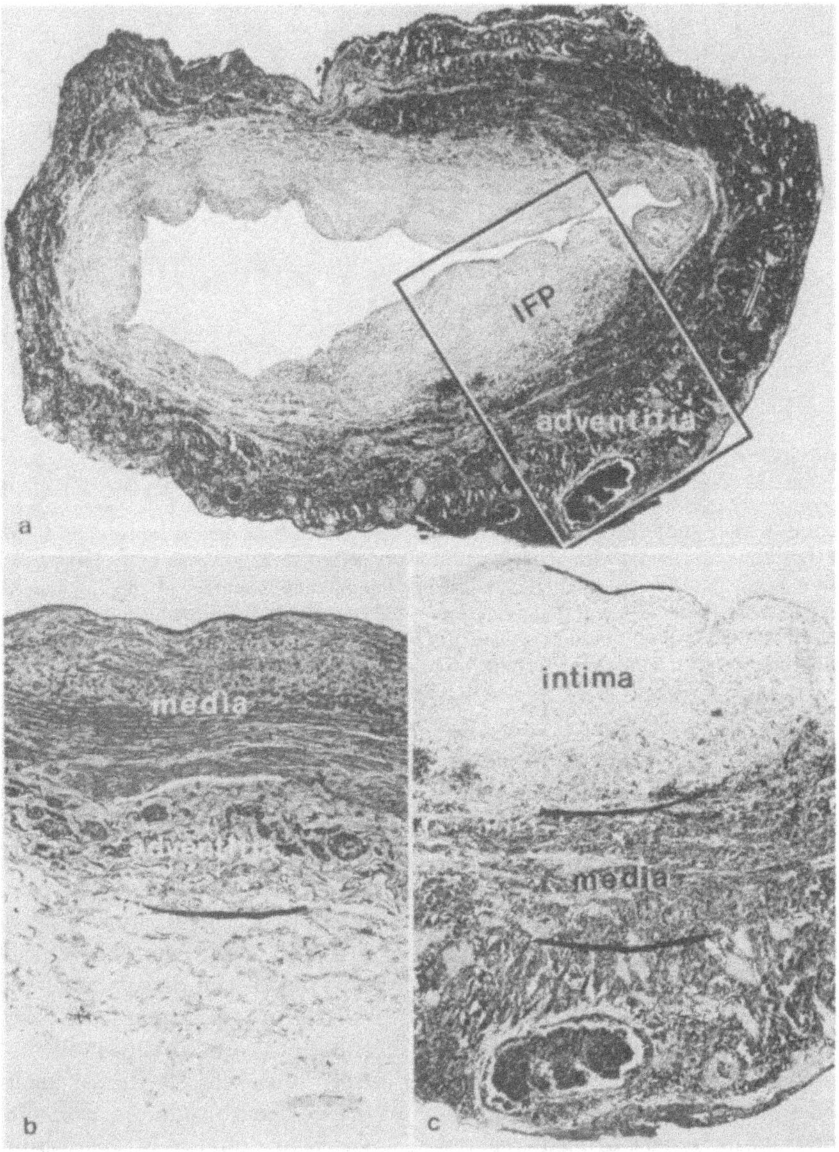

Fig. 3. Phlebosclerosis in a saphenous vein used for aortocoronary bypass grafting (N-A75-171). *a*, Section of a saphenous vein segment left over after use of the major segment for bypass grafting. Phlebosclerosis is present, creating intimal thickening histologically identical to intimal fibrous proliferation (IFP). *b*, Normal saphenous vein for comparison. *c*, Higher power view of area enclosed in box in *a*, showing intimal thickening, loss of some medial smooth muscle and adventitial hemorrhage. (Movat stains; original magnification ×28 *(a)*, ×54 *(b)*, ×54 *(c)*.)

the vein wall. These changes were followed by loss of smooth muscle cells and the appearance of focal subendothelial proliferative lesions and fibrin deposits. By three months, diffuse subendothelial fibrous deposits had developed, and these became extensive by six to 12 months after grafting.

The endothelial changes in grafted autogenous veins have been debated, largely because normal histologic and other morphologic studies involve techniques that may produce artifactual losses of endothelial layers. Ramos and associates[33] recently described the course and extent of endothelial damage in experimental studies in dogs. Progressive changes were seen in all layers of the vein walls, including intimal fibrous proliferation.

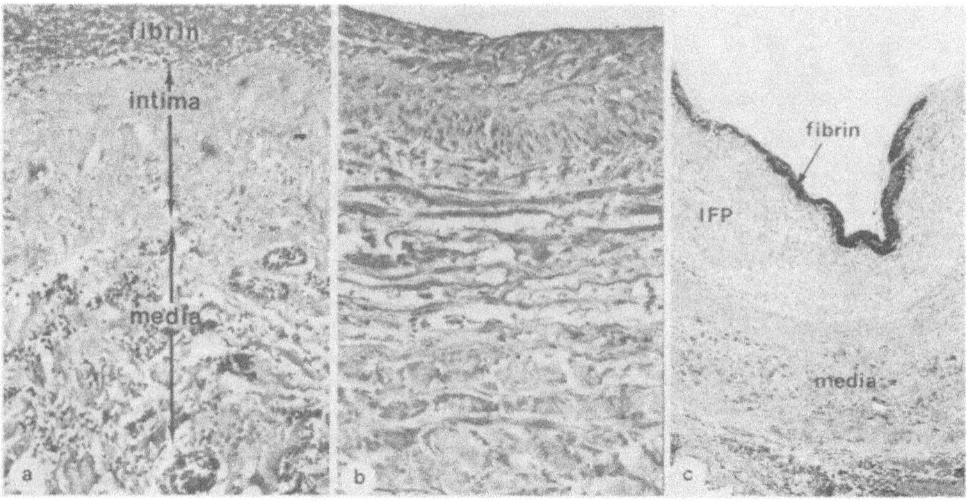

Fig. 4. *a*, Wall of a vein graft taken 4 days after implantation. Fibrin deposition on the intimal surface and infiltration of the intima and media with acute inflammatory cells is seen. Necrosis of medial smooth muscle also is present. *b*, Vein graft implanted for 18 days showing edema and necrosis of medial smooth muscle cells. (Hematoxylin and eosin stains; original magnification ×220 [*a* and *b*]). *c*, Subendothelial fibrin in a 2-month-old vein bypass graft. Marked intimal fibrous proliferation *(IFP)* is present and loss of smooth muscle in the media is noted. (Phosphotungstic acid-hematoxylin stain; original magnification ×54.)

Endothelial cell layers were sloughed but re-endothelialization occurred in all grafts. In veins distended with saline before implantation, the changes occurred earlier (two to four weeks) and were more severe than in nondistended veins. Distention with blood tended to cause less endothelial damage but ultimately no difference in the degree of fibrotic changes in the vein walls.

Personally studied saphenous veins used as aortocoronary bypass conduits in humans

We have examined at necropsy 65 saphenous vein grafts from 38 patients who died up to 72 months after aortocoronary bypass procedures. A composite of the histologic changes in these grafts from day zero (normal unused vein) to 26 months after operation is shown in Fig. 2. Vein grafts from patients who died intraoperatively showed minimal medial edema and disruption of the adventitia due to dissection and excision of the vein before grafting. In several patients (Fig. 3) marked intimal thickening was present in grafts which had been in place for only a few hours. Preexisting phlebosclerosis is considered the etiology of the intimal changes in these grafts.

By two weeks mural edema was more pronounced, some medial smooth muscle cells were necrotic, and inflammatory infiltrates were present. The edema was evidenced by the presence of clear spaces between the layers of smooth muscle (Fig. 4). The endothelium often appeared disrupted and the intimal surface usually was covered, either partially or completely, by fibrin.

By three weeks cells with characteristics of smooth muscle appeared in the subendothelial portion of the intima. The cells generally were oriented such that their longest diameter was parallel to the direction of blood flow (Fig. 2).

In grafts in place from two to 72 months, the subendothelial intimal lesions were more generalized and less cellular, ground substance was present in abundance, and short elastic fibers and vascular channels occasionally were present. Deposits of fibrin also often were present both on the luminal surface and in the subendothelial lesions themselves (Fig. 4). The smooth muscle fibers of the media now were markedly diminished in numbers and they were replaced, in part or in whole, by fibrous tissue and collagen. In the adventitia there was a marked increase in fibrous tissue with severe disruption or complete replacement of elastic fibers. Organizing fibrin on the external surface of the grafts contributed to the adventitial fibrosis (Fig. 5*c*). Vasa vasorum were infrequent, but capillary channels were present and extended into the fibrotic media in several patients. Thus, the saphenous vein used as an artery became a stiff, fibrous–tissue conduit.

The subendothelial proliferation of fibrous

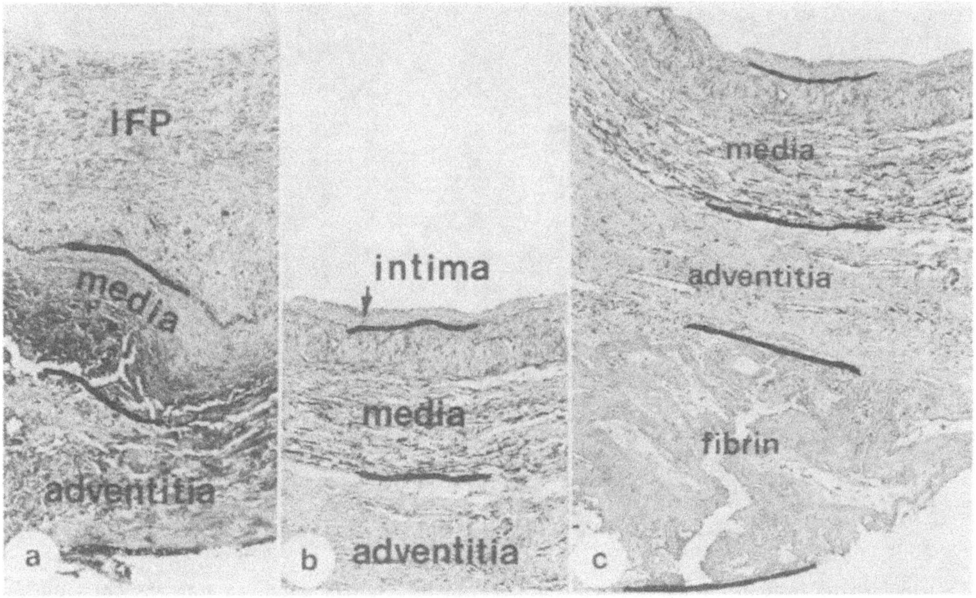

Fig. 5. Variable intimal fibrous proliferation *(IFP)* in a 56-day-old saphenous vein graft from a 46-year-old man (A71-94) who died of renal failure after aortic and mitral valve replacements and vein grafting to the right and left anterior descending coronary arteries. *a*, Proximal vessel. There is marked IFP and smooth muscle loss in the media. *b*, Distal vessel. Minimal IFP is present. *c*, Adventitial fibrosis and organizing fibrin in same area of graft as *b*. (Movat stains; original magnification of each ×54.)

tissue was quite variable in magnitude and location and infrequently was extensive enough to cause severe narrowing. Occasionally, it was seen to involve the base of venous valves (Fig. 6). Two grafts (7 months, and 56 months) did show complete occlusion from intimal fibrous proliferation, yet the occlusions were only within 2 cm. of the proximal (aortic) anastomosis and the intima of the distal portion of the grafts appeared minimally changed. A later graft (26 months) showed changes similar to a 2-month-old graft in which luminal narrowing of about 50 per cent was seen. In one 19-month-old graft, very little intimal thickening was present, but large collections of subendothelial cells resembling smooth muscle cells were seen (Fig. 7). In addition, this graft showed extensive subendothelial fibrin deposition. Thus, the intimal fibrous proliferation appeared to progress at varying rates and locations and often stabilized at some ill-defined degree of luminal narrowing.

Table I. Causes and consequences of changes in veins used for arterial conduits

Cause	*Consequence*
1. Endothelial damage a. Trauma b. Elevated transmural pressure 2. Thrombosis 3. Intimal damage 4. Increased wall O_2 tension	Intimal fibrous proliferation
5. Medial ischemia a. Loss of vasa vasorum b. Increased transmural pressure	Medial fibrous replacement
6. Adventitial ischemia	Adventitial fibrous proliferation

Causes of morphologic changes in saphenous veins used as aortocoronary conduits

Although the causes of the above-described changes in saphenous vein grafts are unclear, several possible mechanisms have been proposed[8-11, 15-23] (Table I). Similar subendothelial proliferation of smooth muscle cells is seen in several situations in the vascular system. The phlebosclerotic lesions in venous varicosities are presumably the response of the vein to increases in hydrostatic pressure.[34] Arteriovenous shunts of any origin (congenital, traumatic, or iatrogenic) show intimal thickening, presumably the result of

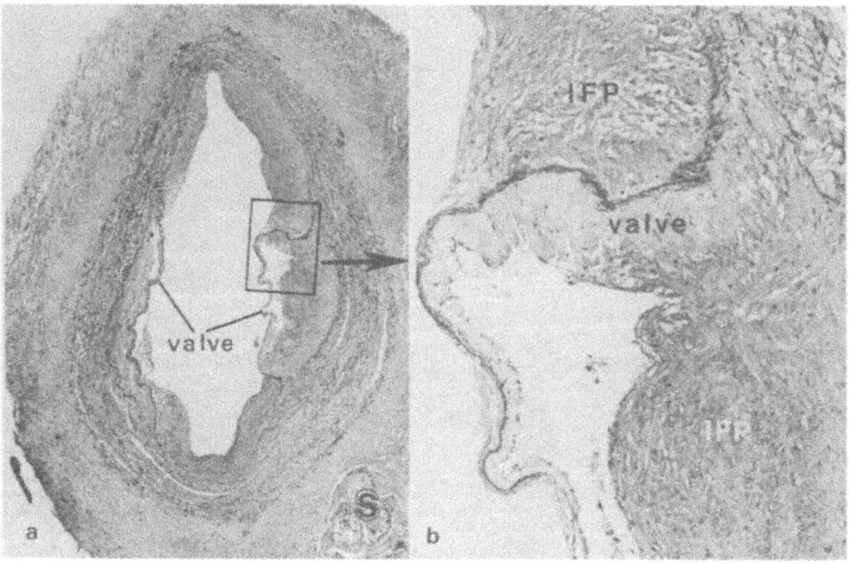

Fig. 6. Development of intimal fibrous proliferation *(IFP)* behind venous valves in a 56-day-old saphenous vein graft (A71-94). *a*, Intimal fibrous proliferation lines the vein graft. The valve leaflets are not bound down against the vein wall. Marked adventitial fibrosis also is present. *S* = suture. *b*, Enlargement of area shown in box in *a*, showing *IFP* above and behind the venous valve. The leaflet remains relatively uninvolved. (Movat stains; original magnification ×23 *(a)*, and ×130 *(b)*.)

Table II. Effects of pressure and ischemia on venous conduits*

Vasa vasorum intact	
Low pressure (venous)	High pressure (arterial)
↓	↓
Normal histology	Intimal proliferation and fibrosis
Intact myocytes	Intact myocytes
Vasa vasorum interrupted	
Low pressure (venous)	High pressure (arterial)
↓	↓
Medial fibrosis	Intimal proliferation and fibrosis
Loss of myocytes	Medial fibrosis Loss of myocytes

*Modified from Brody, *et al.*, J. Thor. Cardiovasc. Surg. **64**:847, 1972.

increased pressure and flow.[12, 35] Subendothelial proliferative lesions also occur in the small pulmonary arteries of patients with pulmonary hypertension,[36, 37] in vena cava and portal veins in patients with chronic right-sided congestive cardiac failure or portal hypertension,[38, 39] and in peripheral arteries of some patients with systemic hypertension.[40] In addition, the subendothelial intimal lesions resemble the fibrous and musculoelastic plaques of atherosclerosis[41-46] (Fig. 8).

The common denominator in each of the above examples appears to be an elevation of intravascular pressure or magnitude of flow or both, or a decreased velocity of flow, with resulting increased shear stress on the vascular walls.[6, 15, 47, 48] Brody and colleagues[17] attempted to differentiate the effects of pressure and ischemia on femoral vein grafts in dogs. Vein segments were either left intact or dissected free from their adventitia, thereby severing the vasa vasora and producing medial ischemia. Next, the vein segments were either left in the venous system or were arterialized by creation of an arteriovenous fistula. The presence of medial ischemia in the absence of elevated pressure and flow produced medial fibrosis in the vein without subendothelial intimal proliferative lesions (Table II). Elevated intravascular pressure alone, however, without alterations in blood supply to the media by the vasa vasorum produced intimal lesions without evidence of medial fibrosis. The combination of both elevated intraluminal pressure and medial ischemia resulted in medial and intimal changes similar to the changes seen in human saphenous veins used as aortocoronary conduits.

Several factors unique to aortocoronary bypass grafting make the changes of ischemia and pressure more likely in these grafts than in grafts used

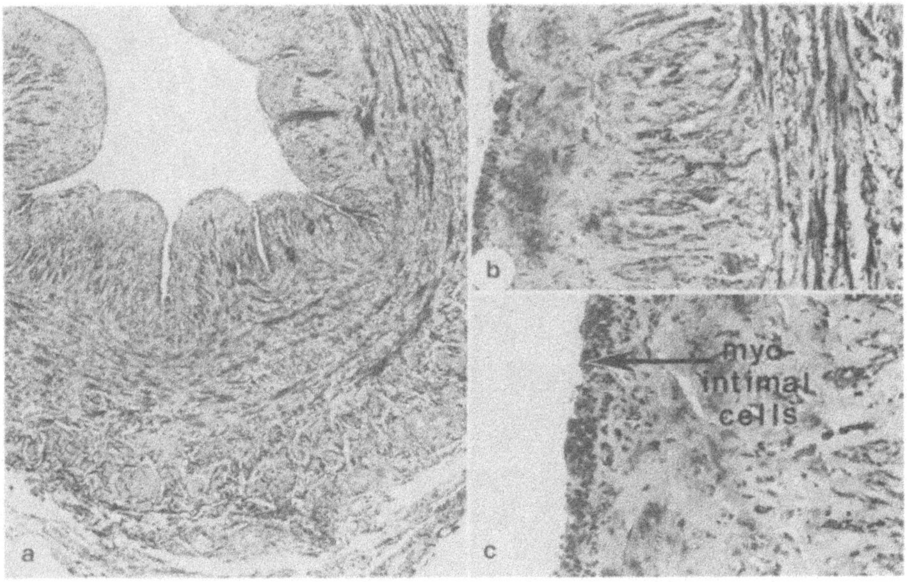

Fig. 7. Subendothelial myointimal cell accumulation in a 19-month-old graft to the circumflex coronary artery from a 52-year-old man (GT 75A-69) who died at reoperation for replacement of an occluded graft to the left anterior descending coronary artery. *a*, Marked medial and subendothelial cellularity is noted. *b*, Higher power view showing subendothelial collections of cells, intimal thickening and increased cellularity of the media. *c*, Myointimal cells are seen immediately under the endothelial layer. Beneath these cells is proliferative intimal tissue. (Movat stains; original magnification ×54 *(a)*, ×130 *(b)*, ×220 *(c)*.)

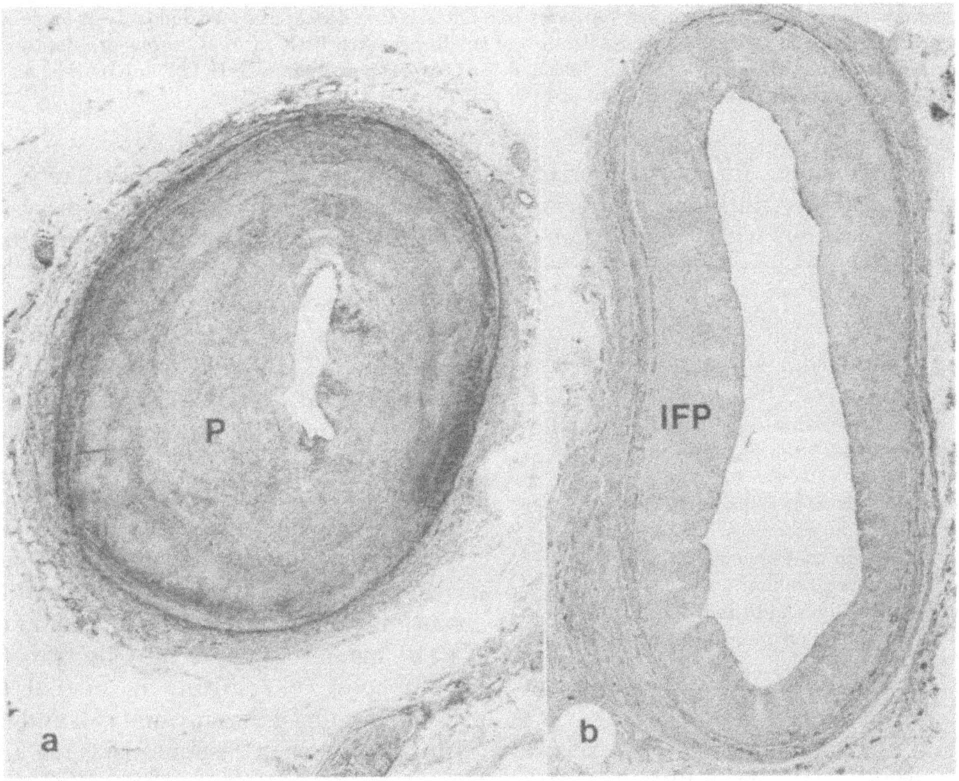

Fig. 8. Similarity of atherosclerotic plaque *(P)* in a coronary artery *(a)*, and the intimal fibrous proliferation *(IFP)* in a 26-month-old saphenous vein coronary bypass graft (*b*). Both show intimal thickening by fibrous tissue and loss of medial smooth muscle layers. (Movat stains, original magnification ×16 *(a)*, and ×15 *(b)*.)

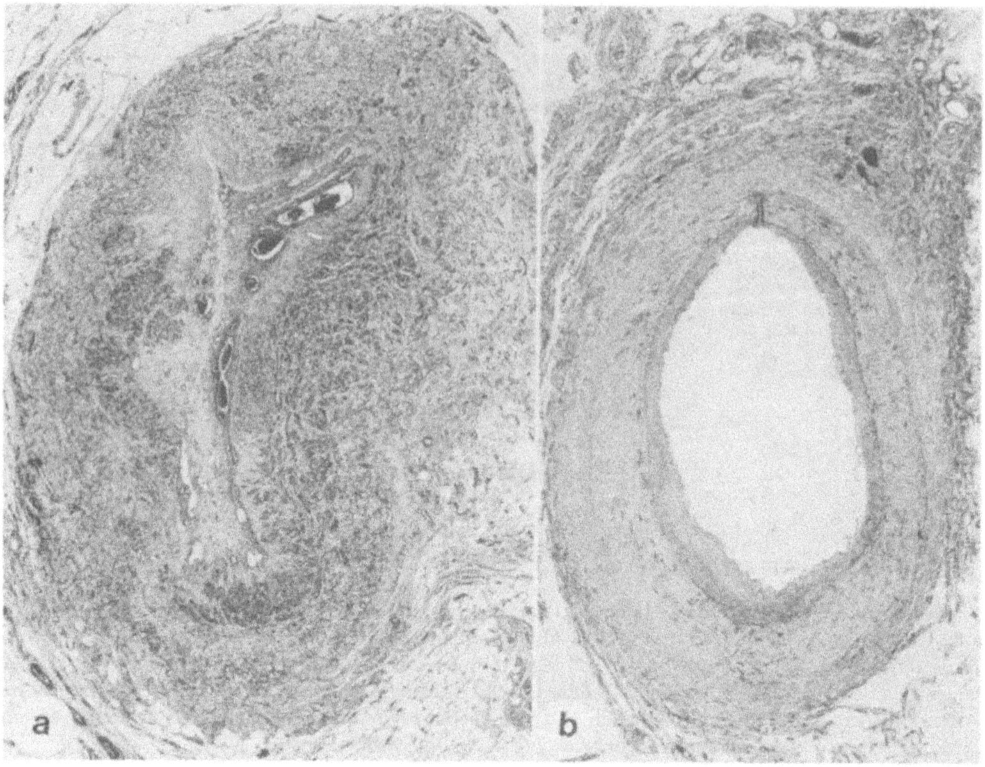

Fig. 9. Saphenous vein bypass grafts from a 44-year-old woman (7983) who underwent grafting to the right *(a)*, and left anterior descending (LAD) *(b)*, coronary arteries 26 months before death. She died suddenly at home. *a*, Right coronary graft showing occlusion and recanalization of the lumen with little intimal fibrous proliferation (IFP). Thrombus was the probable cause of graft occlusion. *b*, LAD graft showing moderate IFP and marked adventitial fibrosis. (Movat stains; original magnification of each ×27.)

Table III. Venous conduits for aortocoronary bypass: Factors promoting fibrinous or fibrous intimal proliferation with or without occlusion

1. Severe narrowing distal to insertion of the graft
2. Insertion of graft in area of plaque
    a. Thrombosis
    b. Hemorrhage
    c. Dissection
3. Hyperacute angle of aortic anastomosis (90° optimal)
4. Tension on grafted vein
    a. Decreases flow
    b. Damages endothelium or intima
    c. Causes tension on anastomoses
5. Previous sclerosis of vein used for conduit
6. Overdistension of vein with saline
    a. Damages endothelium and intima
    b. Possible direct effect on phospholipids of smooth muscle

in the peripheral circulation. While the excised vein is revascularized early when placed in the highly vascular tissue beds in the extremities,[49] the unsupported nature of the grafts in the aortocoronary position make delay in revascularization of the media more likely. Furthermore, flow occurs under diastolic, not systolic, pressure in the coronary system and flow consequently is slower.[15, 49]

The mechanisms whereby pressure and ischemia cause the intimal and medial changes are unclear (Table III). Brody and associates[16] suggest that both the intimal and medial changes are produced by the transformation of medial myocytes in response to injury or to change in their nutritional status. The myocyte response may be mediated by elevated wall oxygen tension with resulting effects on phospholipid[16, 50] or by the presence of plasma factors or blood products as a result of recurrent endothelial damage.[7, 15, 18] The medial myocyte may be transformed into a fibrocyte[17, 51] resulting in medial fibrosis, or it may become a myointimal cell and migrate to the intimal layer in response to some unknown stimulus to produce intimal thickening.[17, 51, 52]

That the degree of fibrous intimal proliferation is often variable along the length of a vein graft[11, 21] (Fig. 5) or between two grafts in the

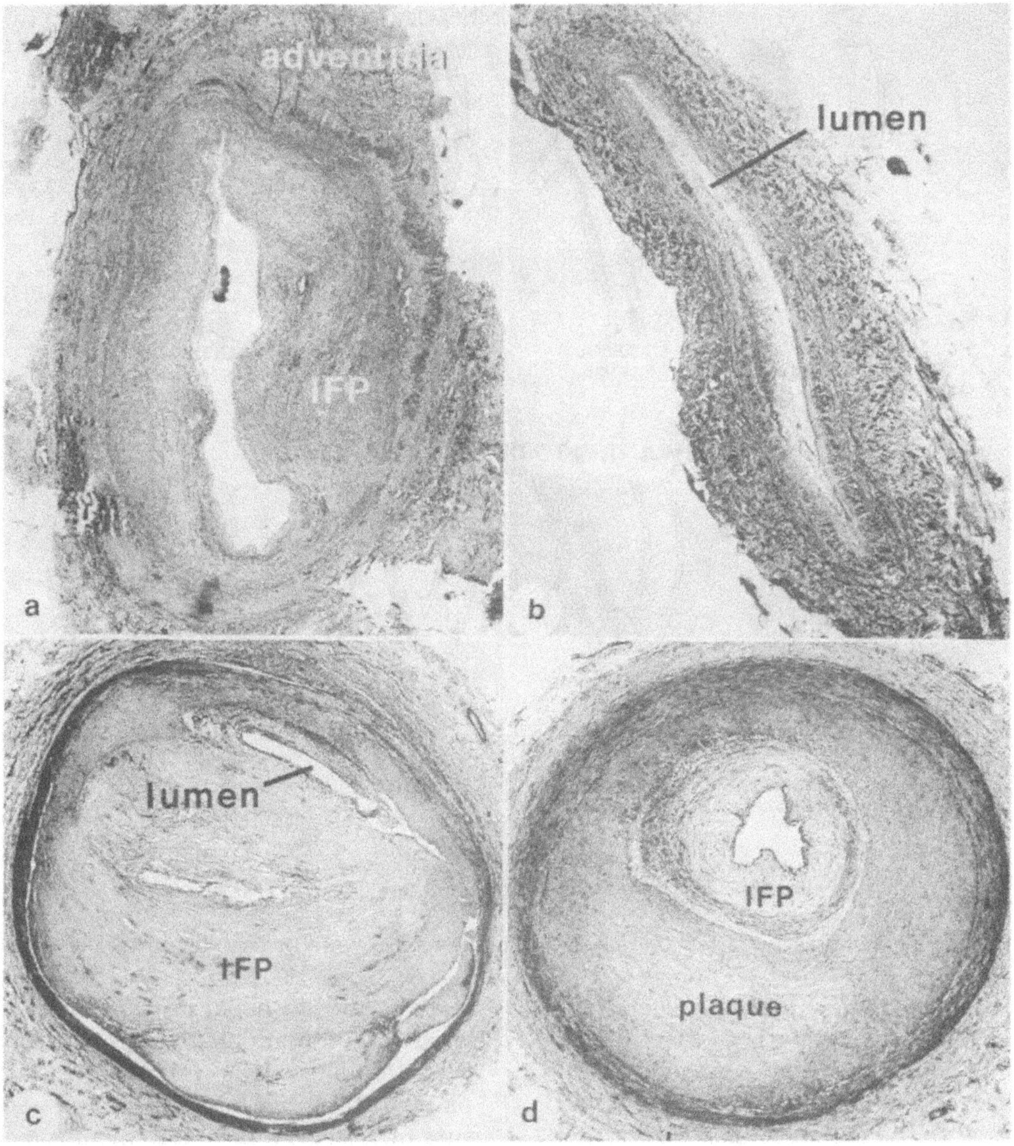

Fig. 10. Saphenous vein graft from a 34-year-old man (A75-279) who died 7 months after placement of a graft to the left anterior descending (LAD) coronary artery. Endarterectomy was done at the site of the anastomosis to the coronary. He did well for 6.5 months, when angina returned. At reoperation, the vein graft *(a)* was found to be narrowed proximally by intimal fibrous proliferation *(IFP)*, and flattened and sclerosed distally *(b)*. He died after repeat bypassing of the LAD and placement of vein grafts to the right and posterior descending coronary arteries. *c*, Section of LAD immediately distal to the anastomosis of the vein graft at the area of previous endarterectomy showing almost complete occlusion of the vessel by fibrous tissue plaque *(IFP)*. Only a tiny lumen remains. The IFP extended down the LAD for several centimeters, and appeared to be superimposed on preexisting plaque *(d)*, further narrowing the lumen of the vessel. (Movat stains; original magnification ×20 *(a)*, ×22 *(b)*, ×34 *(c)*, ×45 *(d)*.)

same patient (Fig. 9) indicates that elevated pressure alone does not account for the extent of changes in these conduits. Some anatomic and technical factors, therefore, must modify the effects of pressure and ischemia on the grafted vein and the distal coronary artery. These factors, which are listed in Table III, are all related in some fashion to the amount of flow or to the velocity or turbulence of flow in the graft or the coronary artery into which the graft inserts.

Faulkner and associates[15] studied the effect of flow rate on the development of subendothelial proliferative lesions in femoral vein grafts in dogs. Grafts subjected to low flows (30 to 50 ml./min.)

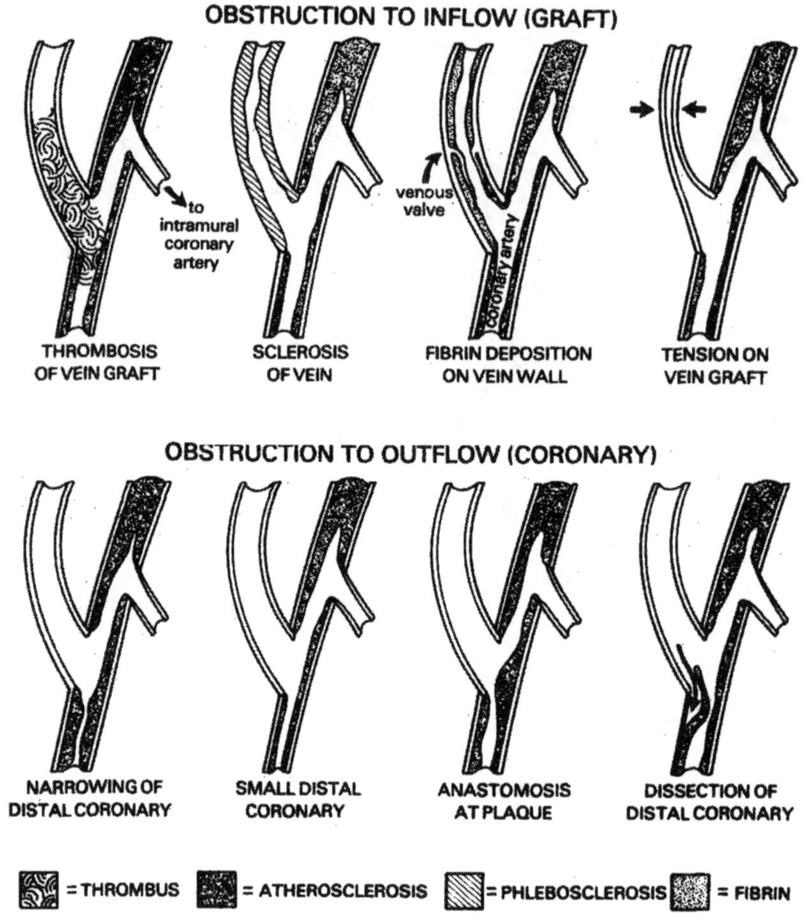

Fig. 11. Anatomic and technical factors that affect flow in the coronary arteries following aortocoronary bypass.

showed significantly greater and more generalized intimal proliferation than grafts subjected to high flows (790 ml./min. average). Subendothelial intimal proliferation, however, occurred in all grafts just distal to the proximal anastomosis and at the distal anastomosis in both the vein and the native artery, indicating that turbulence of flow caused by the anastomosis produces augmented vein response, perhaps by causing localized recurrent endothelial disruption.[6, 9, 18] Elevations in pressure, therefore, may result in recurrent endothelial damage which is then converted to intimal lesions by progressive fibrin deposition. High flow states may keep the endothelium "washed" of thrombi, while low flow may encourage such thrombi and result in significant luminal narrowing.

Jones and associates[18] offer support for the concept that progressive intimal fibrous proliferation may be the result of progressive organization of subendothelial or mural deposits of fibrin which accumulate as a result of recurrent endothelial damage. It is well known that fibrin and platelet thrombi accumulate in response to exposure of collagen, basement membrane, or elastin to the blood,[17, 53] and that mural thrombi may become incorporated into plaques.[54, 55] In addition, fibrous lesions similar to those seen in bypass grafts occur in native coronary arteries after endothelial damage from perfusion cannulae or after endarterectomy (Fig. 10).[9] Fibrin deposition on venous valves has been implicated in causing stenoses of femoropopliteal vein grafts.[23] The laminated appearance of some areas of subendothelial intimal proliferative lesions in vein bypass grafts and the new vascular channels in the plaques themselves, plus the histologically demonstrable fibrin deposits in some subendothelial lesions (Fig. 4), lend support to the concept of continued organization of thrombi as the etiology

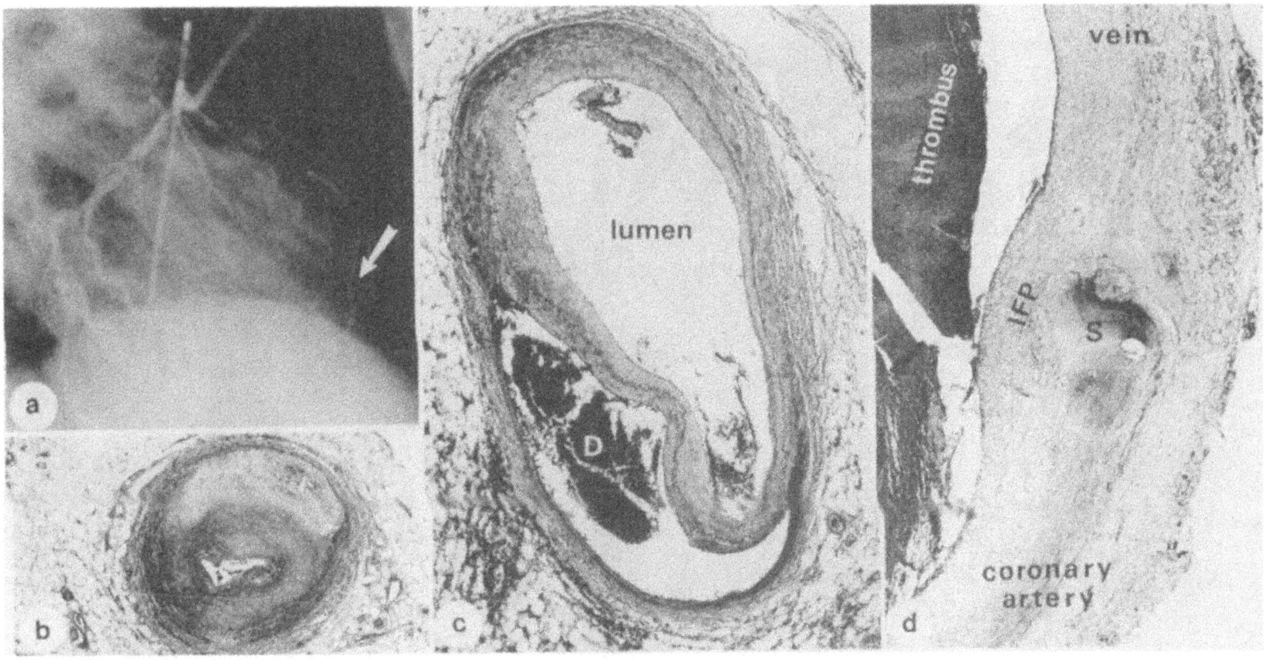

Fig. 12. *a*, and *b*, Severe obstruction of coronary artery distal to the site of insertion of a vein bypass graft in a 40-year-old woman (A74-212) who could not be weaned from cardiopulmonary bypass after 3 vessel vein grafting. *a*, Preoperative coronary angiogram showing total occlusion of the left anterior descending (LAD) coronary with reconstitution distally. The distal vessel was interpreted as showing no significant narrowing. *b*, Section of LAD vessel at approximate area shown by *arrow* in *a*. Severe narrowing of the vessel is seen despite a normal-appearing angiogram. *c*, Coronary artery dissection in the left circumflex coronary artery after bypass grafting (A72-209). The dissection *(D)* has progressed distally, narrowing the lumen of the vessel. *d*, Intimal fibrous proliferation *(IFP)* extending into the coronary artery at the site of vein graft anastomosis in a patient (PHWT A73-28) who died suddenly at home 34 days after bypass grafting to the right coronary artery. Section taken at the venocoronary anastomosis showing antemortem thrombosis of the vein graft extending into the coronary artery (CA), and moderate intimal fibrous proliferation *(IFP)* of the vein with extension across the suture line *(S)* into the coronary artery. (Movat stains; original magnification ×22 *b*, ×38 *c*, ×31 *d*.)

of these lesions. In addition, the histologic similarity of recanalized thrombus to intimal fibrous proliferation has been described in grafts in dogs.[56]

The anatomic and technical factors which may alter blood flow in saphenous grafts may be divided into two groups: (1) those that limit inflow (refers to the status of the graft itself), and (2) those that limit outflow (refers to the status of the coronary artery into which the graft inserts) (Fig. 11). Any of these factors may result in fibrous subendothelial intimal proliferation or thrombosis of the graft or both.

Studies of the coronary bypass grafts (37 saphenous veins) and native coronary arteries in 20 patients who died early (< 2 months) after aortocoronary procedures were carried out to evaluate the frequency of the presence of any anatomic or technical factors that might lead to decreased graft flow.[57] Two of the 37 grafts were occluded by thrombus, but the remaining 35 were free of occluding thrombus. Fibrin deposits (usually small) were present on the walls of 27 per cent of the grafts (Fig. 2) and 29 per cent of the coronary arteries at or near the site of the anastomosis. Fibrin also was present proximal to the anastomosis in some patients, and occasionally the proximal artery was thrombosed, probably due to the "watershed effect" of a subtotal proximal obstruction.[58]

In 38 graft systems (graft plus the entire coronary artery into which the graft inserted), sections of the anastomosis were adequate to estimate degrees of luminal narrowing. In one graft the lumen of the coronary artery was > 75 per cent narrowed at the anastomosis itself, while in seven it was 51 to 75 per cent narrowed by atherosclerotic plaque at this point. Significant

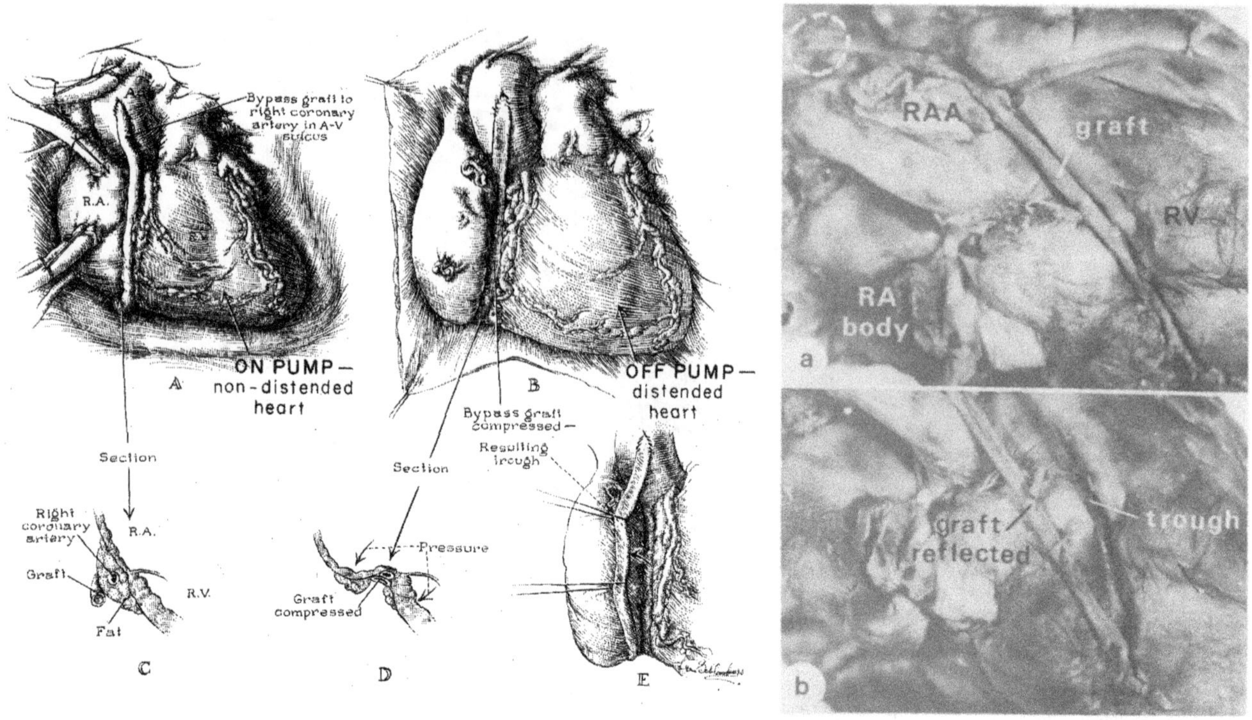

Fig. 13. Tension produced on a vein graft to the right coronary artery. *Left: A,* and *C,* Patient on bypass, heart empty. The vein graft passes along the atrioventricular (AV) sulcus without tension. *B,* and *D,* Patient off bypass, heart beating. Distension of the right atrium and ventricle compresses the vein graft in the AV sulcus. *E,* Reflection of the vein graft shows the trough which results from excessive tension. *R.A.* = right atrium; *R.V.* = right ventricle. ***Right:*** Saphenous vein aortocoronary bypass graft from the aorta *(dashed circle)* to the right posterior descending coronary artery (RCA) in a 49-year-old man (GT 75A-107) who died 2 hours after operation from refractory hypotension. *a,* The graft passes along the right atrioventricular (A-V) sulcus below the ligated right atrial appendage *(RAA)* and the right atrial body. *b,* A view of the graft after it has been reflected. A deep trough is present in the A-V sulcus, indicating that the graft was under significant tension. *RV* = right ventricle.

obstruction to graft flow might be expected in these patients. In some grafts intimal proliferation extended from the vein graft across the anastomosis and into the distal artery (Fig. 12*d*).

Dissection of the coronary artery at or near the anastomosis, due primarily to separation of atherosclerotic plaque, occurred in seven (19 per cent) graft systems studied (Fig. 12*b*).

Atherosclerotic narrowing of the coronary artery distal to the anastomosis of the aortocoronary bypass graft often was pronounced. Significant (> 75 per cent) cross-sectional narrowing in this segment occurred in 16 (44 per cent) of the graft systems examined (Fig. 12*a, b*). Narrowing of 51 per cent to 75 per cent occurred in an additional 31 per cent. Thus, residual severe atherosclerosis in the native coronary artery distal to the graft anastomosis is the most frequent cause of poor graft run-off.

Small caliber of the coronary artery distal to the vein graft anastomosis also has been suggested as a factor which may decrease flow through the graft. While estimates of what constitutes a "small" distal artery are debated, measurements of *relative* vessel size in men versus women after bypass grafting indicates that vessel size in women is smaller than in men even when rough correction is made for variations in cardiac weight.[57, 59-61] Luminal areas, however, are similar when correction is made for myocardial mass, suggesting that less atherosclerotic narrowing is necessary to produce a given limitation to blood flow in women than in men. While coronary size *per se* may not be important in terms of over-all blood flow, the smaller coronary arteries in women may make creation of the venocoronary anastomosis more difficult technically. This feature may contribute to the higher (2 times) early mortality rate in women than in men after saphenous vein aortocoronary bypass operation.[62, 63]

A possible but neglected cause of obstruction to graft flow is tension on the graft caused by underestimation of graft length at operation or by excessive cardiac distention postoperatively[64] (Fig. 13). In a study of 41 saphenous vein aortocoronary grafts from 21 patients at necropsy, abnormal graft tension (as indicated by grooving of the right atrial wall or right atrioventricular sulcus [Fig. 13] or by fattening of a graft passing in front of the pulmonary trunk) was present in six grafts (15 per cent) from five patients (24 per cent). The abnormal graft tension was observed in five (33 per cent) of 15 grafts to the distal right or posterior descending coronary artery but in only one (3 per cent) of 26 grafts to left coronary arteries. Graft tension appeared to result from placement of a graft of inadequate length to accommodate normal or abnormal distention of the right atrium and right ventricle or of the pulmonary trunk after discontinuation of cardiopulmonary bypass or development of congestive cardiac failure. Localized graft occlusion also may occur as a result of local hematoma formation and tamponade.

The hydraulics of the angle of take-off of the graft from the aorta may influence graft flow and, therefore, may predispose to graft occlusion by thrombosis or intimal fibrous proliferation.[6] The optimal angle for maximal flow and minimal turbulence has been calculated to be 90 degrees.[6] Among eight patients studied by Kennedy and associates,[6] the angle of the aortic anastomosis ranged from 30 to 80 degrees (average 45 degrees). Even when the graft initially is placed at an angle of 90 degrees to the aorta, shortening later may cause this angle to become more acute.[65] Although experimental studies of vein grafts in the peripheral circulation indicate that greater intimal fibrous proliferation occurs in grafts placed at an acute angle,[66] examination of aortocoronary bypass grafts in 13 dogs with either acute, obtuse, or perpendicular take-off of the aortic anastomosis showed no effect of the angle of the aortic anastomosis on the location or severity of the intimal changes.[56]

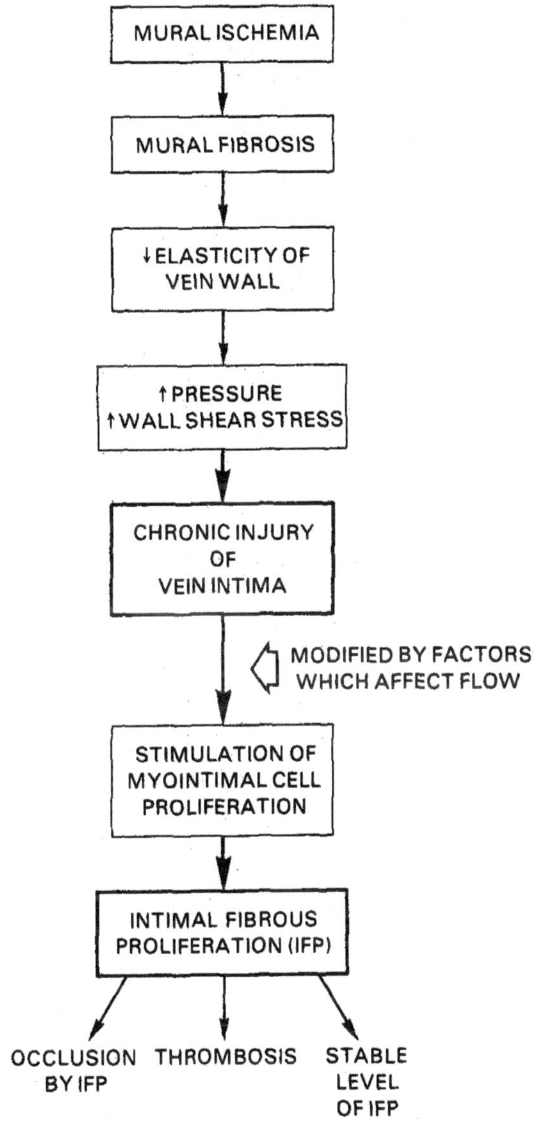

Fig. 14. Summary of the relationship of various factors to the development of graft changes and the ultimate fate of the graft.

The frequency of aortocoronary saphenous vein bypass graft occlusion from thrombus or fibrous intimal proliferation appears to be decreasing.[13] The reasons for this decrease are not known, but less traumatic handling of the vein before implantation and changes in the population of patients considered for bypass procedures may be large contributing factors. Although probably all vein grafts develop some intimal thickening with time, relatively few become totally occluded by this proliferative process. It is likely that this variation in the ultimate fate of grafts is related to the relative contributions of the various factors affecting graft flow. These are described above and outlined in Fig. 14. Perhaps stabilization of the degree of intimal proliferation occurs when flow has been modified to become less turbulent and damaging to the endothelial layer or when the caliber of the graft approaches that of the distal coronary artery into which it inserts. If severe alterations in flow occur at this stage, progression to complete occlusion by thrombosis may result. Early graft thrombosis would be expected in situations where restrictions to flow were severe soon after operation.

Although the explanation for the development of occlusion or stenosis of saphenous vein aortocoronary grafts remains speculative, we believe that progressive injury to the vein by elevated pressure and modified by several anatomic and technical factors which affect flow results in progressive exposure of collagen to plasma factors or fibrin deposition with resulting stimulation of smooth muscle cells. Further study of the relative contributions of the various influencing factors may permit alterations in surgical technique or patient selection to minimize both early and late graft failures.

Summary

This report describes morphologic changes in saphenous veins used as aortocoronary bypass conduits, and discusses the relative contribution of various factors to these changes. The three primary changes are: (1) *medial fibrous replacement,* (2) *adventitial fibrous proliferation,* and (3) *intimal fibrous proliferation.* Medial fibrous replacement is caused by vein wall ischemia with loss of smooth muscle cells; adventitial fibrous proliferation is the result of organization of fibrin deposits and repair of ischemic injury; and intimal fibrous proliferation results from some stimulus, probably fibrin deposition on injured intima, which causes stimulation of smooth muscle cells to become fibroblasts or "myointimal cells." Although all grafts show some changes, the degree and severity of these three changes is variable along the length of the grafts and among separate grafts in the same patient.

REFERENCES

1. Flemma, R.J., Johnson, W.D., Lepley, D., Jr., et al.: Late results of saphenous vein bypass grafting for myocardial revascularization. Ann. Thorac. Surg. **14**:232, 1972.
2. Grondin, C.M., Meere, C., Castonguay, Y., et al.: Progressive and late obstruction of an aortocoronary venous bypass graft, Circulation **43**:698, 1971.
3. Grondin, C.M., Castonguay, Y.R., Lesperance, J., et al.: Attrition rate of aorta-to-coronary artery saphenous vein grafts after one year, Ann. Thorac. Surg. **14**:223, 1972.
4. Grondin, C.M., Dyrda, I., Pasternac, A., et al.: Discrepancies between cineangiographic and postmortem findings in patients with coronary artery disease and recent myocardial revascularization, Circulation **49**:703, 1974.
5. Johnson, W.D., Auer, J.E., and Tector, A.J.: Late changes in coronary vein graft, Am. J. Cardiol. **26**:640, 1970.
6. Kennedy, J.H., Wieting, D.W., Hwang, N.H., et al.: Hydraulic and morphologic study of fibrous intimal hyperplasia in autogenous saphenous vein bypass grafts, J. Thorac. Cardiovasc. Surg. **67**:805, 1974.
7. Unni, K.K., Kottke, B.A., Titus, J.L., et al.: Pathologic changes in aortocoronary saphenous vein grafts, Am. J. Cardiol. **34**:526, 1974.
8. Hamaker, W.R., Doyle, W.F., O'Connell, T.J., et al.: Subintimal obliterative proliferation in saphenous vein grafts, Ann. Thorac. Surg. **13**:488, 1972.
9. Vlodaver, Z., and Edwards, J.E.: Pathologic analysis in fatal cases following saphenous vein coronary arterial bypass, Chest **64**:555, 1973.
10. Vlodaver, Z., and Edwards, J.E.: Pathologic changes in aortic-coronary arterial saphenous vein grafts, Circulation **44**:719, 1971.
11. Marti, M.C., Bouchardy, B., and Cox, J.N.: Aortocoronary bypass with autogenous saphenous vein grafts: Histopathologic aspects, Virchows Arch. (Pathol Anat.) **352**:255, 1971.
12. Kern, W.H., Dermer, G.B., and Lindesmith, G.G.: The intimal proliferation in aortocoronary saphenous vein grafts: Light and electron microscopic studies, AM. HEART J. **84**:771, 1972.
13. Campeau, L., Crochet, D., Lesperance, J., et al.: Postoperative changes in aortocoronary vein grafts revisited: Angiographic studies at 2 weeks and at one year in two series of consecutive patients, Circulation **52**:369, 1975.
14. Bourassa, M.G., Lesperance, J., Campeau, L., et al.: Factors influencing patency of aortocoronary vein grafts, Circulation **45** and **46** (Suppl. I):I-79, 1971.
15. Faulkner, S.L., Fisher, R.D., Conkle, D.M., et al.: The effect of blood flow rate on subendothelial proliferation in venous autografts used as arterial substitutes, Circulation **51** and **52** (Suppl. I):I-163, 1975.
16. Brody, W.R., Kosek, J.C., and Angell, W.W.: Changes in vein grafts following aortocoronary bypass induced by pressure and ischemia, J. Thorac. Cardiovasc. Surg. **64**:847, 1972.
17. Brody, W.R., Angell, W.W., and Kosek, J.C.: Histologic fate of the venous coronary artery bypass in dogs, Am. J. Pathol. **66**:111, 1972.
18. Jones, M., Conkle, D.M., Ferrans, V.J., et al.: Lesions observed in arterial autogenous vein grafts. Light and electron microscopic evaluation, Circulation **47** and **48** (Suppl. III):III-198, 1973.
19. Nunn, D.B., Chun, B., Whelan, T.J., Jr., et al.: Autogenous veins as arterial substitutes: A study of their histological fate with special attention to endothelium, Ann. Surg. **160**:14, 1964.
20. McCabe, M., and Cunningham, G.J.: Histological and

histochemical examination of autogenous vein grafts, Br. J. Surg. **54**:147, 1967.

21. McNamara, J.J., Darling, R.C., and Linton, R.R.: Segmental stenosis of saphenous vein autografts, N. Engl. J. Med. **277**:290, 1967.
22. Mullerworth, M.H., Daniel, F.J., and Lie, J.T.: The fate of internal mammary arterial implants and bypass conduits for myocardial revascularization. Experimental angiographic, histologic, and ultrastructural observations, J. Thorac. Cardiovasc. Surg. **70**:89, 1975.
23. Barner, H.B., Judd, D.R., Kaiser, G.C., et al.: Late failure of arterialized in situ saphenous vein, Arch. Surg. **99**:781, 1969.
24. Carrel, A., and Guthrie, C.C.: Results of biterminal transplantation of veins, Am. J. Med. Sci. **132**:415, 1906.
25. Carrel, A.: Results of transplantation of blood vessels, organs, and limbs, J.A.M.A. **51**:1662, 1908.
26. Dedomenico, M., Sameh, A.A., Berger, K., et al.: Experimental coronary artery surgery: Long-term follow-up, bypass venous autografts, longitudinal arteriotomies, and end-to-end anastomoses, J. Thorac. Cardiovasc. Surg. **56**:617, 1968.
27. Ejrup, B., Hiertonn, T., and Moberg, A.: Atheromatous changes in autogenous venous grafts, Acta Chir. Scand. **121**:211, 1961.
28. Beebe, H.G., Clark, W.F., and DeWeese, J.A.: Atherosclerotic change occuring in an autogenous venous arterial graft, Arch. Surg. (Chicago) **101**:85, 1970.
29. Penn, I., Schenk, E., Rob, C., DeWeese, J., et al.: Evaluation of the development of athero-arteriosclerosis in autogenous venous grafts inserted into the peripheral arterial system, *in* Simeone, F.A., ed.: Cardiovascular surgery, American Heart Association Monograph 11, Circulation **31** and **32** (Suppl. I):I-192, 1965.
30. Barboriak, J.J., Pintar, K., and Korns, M.E.: Atherosclerosis in aortocoronary vein grafts, Lancet **2**:621, 1974.
31. Barboriak, J.J., Batayias, G.E., Pintar, K., et al.: Pathological changes in surgically removed aortocoronary vein grafts, Ann. Thorac. Surg. **21**:524, 1976.
32. Riahi, M., Vasu, C.M., Tomatis, L.A., et al.: Aneurysm of saphenous vein bypass graft to coronary artery, J. Thorac. Cardiovasc. Surg. **70**:358, 1975.
33. Ramos, J.R., Berger, K., and Mansfield, P.B.: Histologic fate and endothelial changes of distended and nondistended vein grafts, Ann. Surg. **183**:205, 1976.
34. Stein, A.A., Rosenblum, J., and Leather, R.: Intimal sclerosis in human veins, Arch. Pathol. **81**:548, 1966.
35. Anderson, W.A.D.: Pathology, 6th ed, St. Louis, 1971, The C.V. Mosby Company, pp. 126, 127, 755.
36. Esterly, J.A., Glagov, S., and Ferguson, D.J.: Morphogenesis of intimal obliterative hyperplasia of small arteries in experimental pulmonary hypertension, Am. J. Pathol. **52**:325, 1968.
37. Heath, D., and Edwards, J.E.: Pathology of hypertensive pulmonary vascular disease: Description of six grades of structural changes in the pulmonary artery with special reference to congenital cardiac septal defects, Circulation **18**:533, 1958.
38. Stuart, M., and Magarey, F.R.: Great veins in venous hypertension, J. Pathol. Bacteriol. **79**:319, 1960.
39. Geiringer, E.: Venous atheromata, Arch. Pathol. **48**:410, 1949.
40. McGee, W.G., and Ashworth, G.F.: Fine structure of chronic hypertensive arteriopathy in the human kidney, Am. J. Pathol. **43**:273, 1963.
41. Vlodaver, Z, and Neufeld, H.N.: The musculo-elastic layer in the coronary arteries: A histological and hemodynamic concept, Vasc. Dis. **4**:136, 1967.
42. Gresham, G.A., Howard, A.N., and King, A.J.: Comparative histopathological study of the early atherosclerotic lesion, Br. J. Exp. Pathol. **43**:21, 1962.
43. Vlodaver, Z., and Edwards, J.E.: Pathology of coronary atherosclerosis, Progr. Cardiovasc. Dis. **14**:256, 1971.
44. Haust, M.D., More, R.H., and Movat, H.Z.: Role of smooth muscle cells in the fibrogenesis of arteriosclerosis, Am. J. Pathol. **37**:377, 1960.
45. Geer, J.C., McGill, N.C., Jr., and Strong, J.P.: Fine structure of the human atherosclerotic lesions, Am. J. Pathol. **38**:263, 1961.
46. Geer, J.C.: Fine structure of human aortic intimal thickening and fatty streaks, Lab. Invest. **14**:1764, 1965.
47. Caro, C.G., Fitz-Gerald, J.M., and Schroter, R.C.: Arterial wall shear and distribution of early atheroma in man, Nature **223**:1159, 1969.
48. Flaherty, J.T., Pierce, J.E., Ferrans, V.J., et al.: Endothelial nuclear patterns in the canine arterial tree with particular reference to hemodynamic events, Circ. Res. **30**:23, 1972.
49. Szilagyi, D.E., Elliot, J.P., Hagenman, J.H., et al.: Biologic fate of autogenous vein implants as arterial substitutes: clinical, angiographic and histopathologic observations in femoropopliteal operations for atherosclerosis, Ann. Surg. **178**:232, 1973.
50. Cohn, L.H., Kosek, J.C., and Angell, W.W.: Pulmonary arteriosclerosis produced by hyperoxemic normotensive perfusion, Surgery **70**:723, 1971.
51. Murray, M., Schrodt, G.R., and Berg, H.F.: Role of smooth muscle cells in healing of injured arteries, Arch. Pathol. **82**:138, 1966.
52. Wissler, R.W.: The arterial medial cell, smooth muscle or multifunctional mesenchyma? Circulation **36**:1, 1967.
53. Ts'ao, C.H., and Glagov, S.: Platelet adhesion to subendothelial components in experimental aortic injury: Role of fine fibrils and basement membrane, Br. J. Exp. Pathol. **51**:423, 1970.
54. Duguid, J.B.: Thrombosis as a factor in the pathogenesis of aortic atherosclerosis, J. Pathol. Bacteriol. **60**:57, 1948.
55. Roberts, W.C., and Buja, L.M.: Frequency and significance of coronary arterial thrombi and other observations in fatal acute myocardial infarction: A study of 107 necropsy patients, Am. J. Med. **52**:425, 1972.
56. Breyer, R.H., Spray, T.L., Kastl, D.G., et al.: Histologic changes in saphenous vein aortocoronary bypass grafts: The effect of the angle of the aortic anastomosis, J. Thorac. Cardiovasc. Surg. **72**:916, 1976.
57. Spray, T.L., and Roberts, W.C.: Status of native coronary arteries proximal and distal to coronary anastomotic sites of aortocoronary bypass grafts, Circulation (In press April, 1977)
58. Rees, S.: The watershed: A factor in coronary vein graft occlusion, Br. Heart J. **38**:197, 1976.
59. Lewis, B.S., and Gotsman, M.S.: Relation between coronary artery size and left ventricular wall mass, Br. Heart J. **35**:1150, 1973.
60. Wilens, S.L., Plair, C.M., and Henderson, D.: Size of the major epicardial coronary arteries at necropsy, J.A.M.A. **198**:1325, 1966.
61. Milles, G., and Dalessandro, W.: The relationship of the weight of the heart and the circumference of the coronary arteries to myocardial infarction and myocardial failure, Am. J. Pathol. **30**:31, 1954.
62. Bolooki, H., Vargas, A., Green, R., et al.: Results of direct

coronary artery surgery in women, J. Thorac. Cardiovasc. Surg. **69**:271, 1975.

63. Hall, R.J., Garçia, E., Wukasch, D.C., et al.: Aortocoronary bypass (CAB): Long-term follow-up (Abstr.), Circulation **51** and **52** (Suppl. II):II-90, 1975.
64. Spray, T.L., and Roberts, W.C.: Tension on coronary bypass conduits: A neglected cause of real or potential obstruction of saphenous vein grafts, J. Thorac. Cardiovasc. Surg. **72**:282, 1976.
65. Cody, M.C., Smith, H.C., Frye, R.L., et al.: Long-term followup of flow and dimension changes in saphenous vein bypass grafts to the coronary arteries (Abstr.), Circulation **49** and **50** (Suppl. III):III-132, 1974.
66. Bond, M.G., Hostetler, J.R., Karayannacos, P.E., et al.: Intimal changes in arteriovenous bypass grafts: Effects of varying the angle of implantation at the proximal anastomosis and of producing stenosis in the distal runoff artery, J. Thorac. Cardiovasc. Surg. **71**:907, 1976.

Twisting of an aorta-coronary bypass conduit

A complication of coronary surgery

Twisting of an aorta-coronary bypass conduit was observed at necropsy in each of three patients. Three twists (540 degrees) just distal to the aortic anastomosis caused total obstruction of the bypass conduit to the left anterior descending coronary artery in one patient. A single twist (180 degrees) occurred in a bypass conduit in each of the other two patients. Obviously, prevention of graft twisting is essential for successful bypass grafting.

William C. Roberts, M.D., Anthony S. Lachman, M.D., and Renu Virmani, M.D.,
Bethesda, Md.

There are many causes of occlusion of a saphenous vein graft used as a conduit between the aorta and coronary arteries. The most common is severe narrowing of the native coronary artery at, or distal to, the coronary anastomosis so that there is poor run-off of blood from the graft.[1] Other causes include tension on the bypass graft owing to shortening or to abnormal or even normal expansion of an underlying cardiac chamber or pulmonary trunk,[2] hypotension from any cause,[3, 4] dissection of the coronary artery at the site of, or distal to, a coronary anastomosis,[5] prior phlebosclerosis of the saphenous vein used as the bypass graft,[4] abnormal clotting factors,[4] atherosclerosis of the graft itself,[5] occlusion of the aortic anastomotic site by an atherosclerotic process in the aorta,[4] and technically poor anastomoses.[6] Another cause of the graft occlusion is *twisting* of the bypass conduit. To our knowledge this complication has not been described previously, but such was the case in three patients to be described in the report which follows.

Patients studied

Certain clinical and morphologic observations in the three patients are summarized in Table I and features of the twisted grafts are illustrated in Figs. 1 to 3. Each patient underwent coronary bypass grafting primarily because of severe angina pectoris. Each had greater than 75 percent narrowing on cross section of the lumen of the native right, left anterior descending, and left circumflex coronary arteries. In Patient 1 (Table I), three twists were observed in the graft just past its aortic anastomosis (Fig. 1). These three twists resulted in virtually total occlusion of this conduit at the site of the twists (Fig. 1). In Patients 2 and 3, only a single twist was observed in the twisted bypass conduit (Figs. 2 and 3). The twisted graft in two patients was anastomosed to the left anterior descending coronary artery (Figs. 1 and 2) and, in the third patient, to the distal right coronary artery (Fig. 3). Patients 1 and 3 died in the operating room; neither could be weaned from cardiopulmonary bypass. Patient 2 died about 6 hours after entering the recovery room from the operating room.

From the Pathology Branch, National Heart, Lung, and Blood Institute, National Institutes of Health, Bethesda, Md. 20014.

Received for publication Oct. 31, 1977.

Accepted for publieation Nov. 15, 1977.

Address for reprints: William C. Roberts, M.D., Building 10-A, Room 3E30, National Institutes of Health, Bethesda, Md. 20014.

Comment

A twisted conduit is not an ideal conduit. A single (180 degree) twist occurred in two of the three patients described herein; it is unlikely, however, that a twist of this degree would lead to significant luminal obstruction by itself. A twist of this order, however, could be a cause of altered blood flow which in turn might accelerate the process of intimal fibrous proliferation.[3, 4, 7] Three twists (540 degrees) within 1 cm., however, occurred in one bypass conduit of Patient 1; this degree of twisting caused virtually complete occlusion of this bypass conduit and therefore was equivalent to no conduit at all.

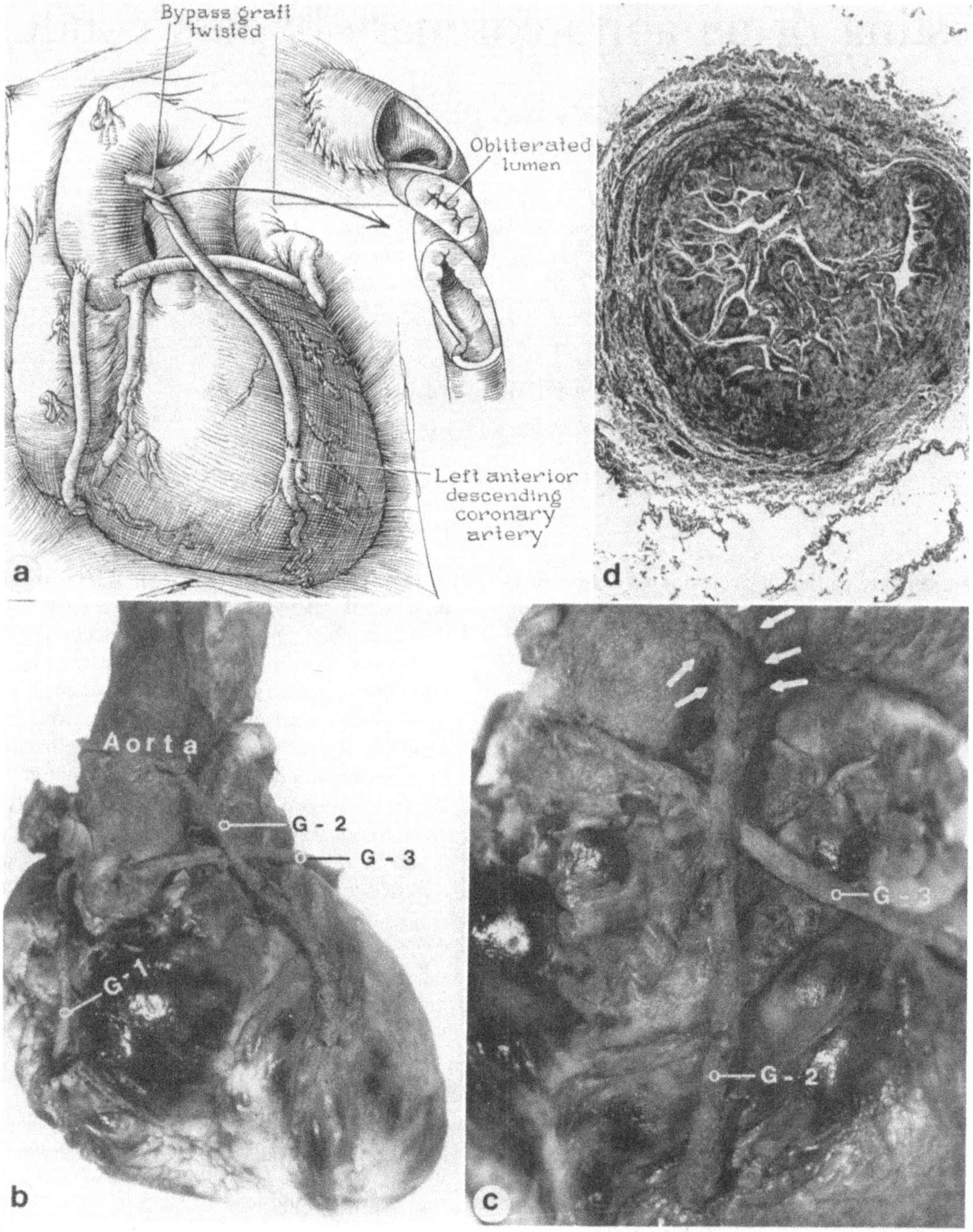

Fig. 1. Patient 1 (Table I). *a,* Drawing showing the twisted (540 degrees) saphenous vein bypass conduit. *b,* Exterior view of the heart showing saphenous vein bypass conduits to the right *(G-1),* left anterior descending *(G-2),* and left circumflex *(G-3)* coronary arteries. *c,* Close-up view showing the twists *(arrows)* in graft *(G-2)* to the proximal portion of the left anterior descending coronary artery. *d,* Photomicrograph of cross-section at the site of the twists in the bypass conduit. (Movat stain: Original magnification ×25.)

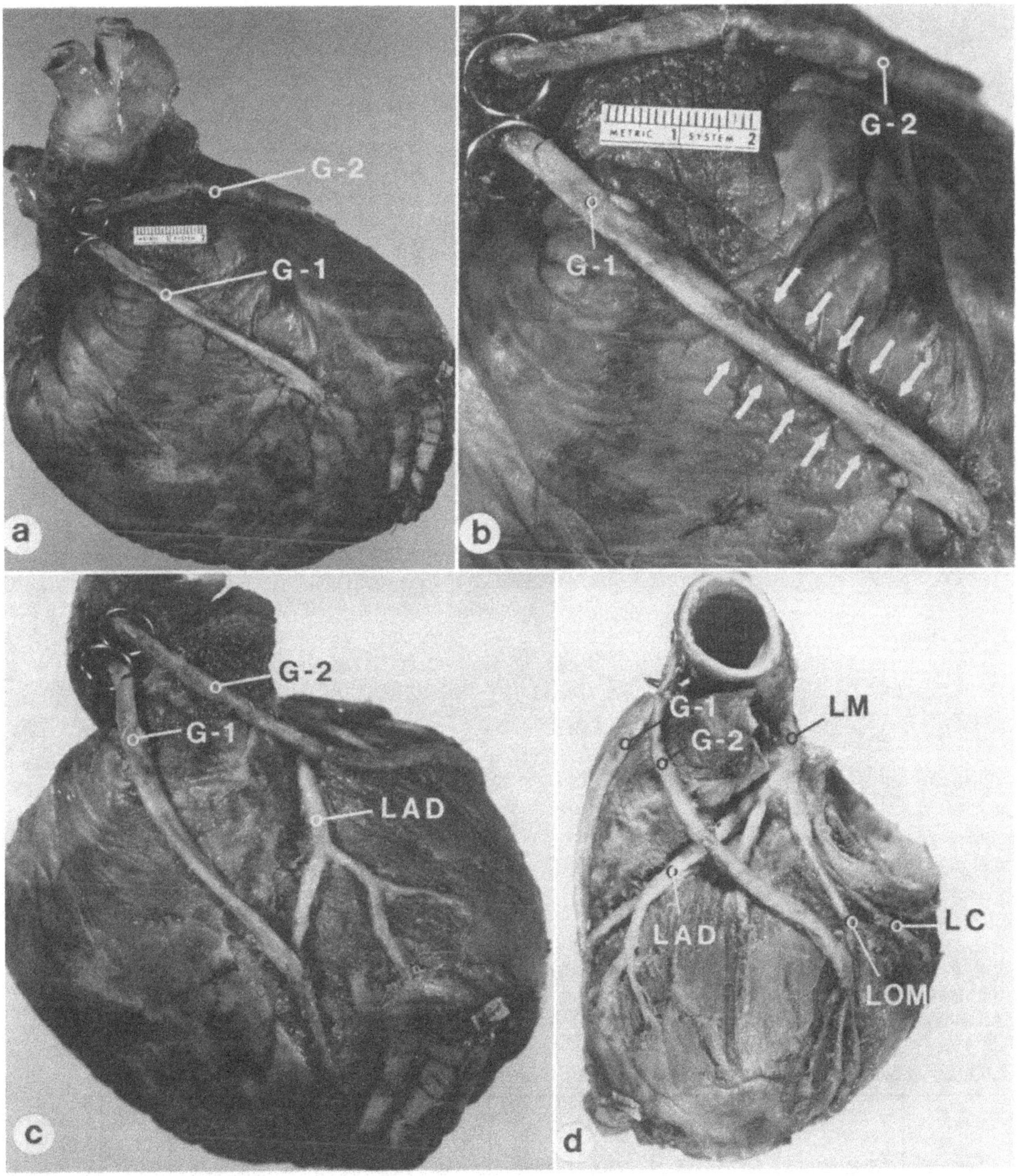

Fig. 2. Patient 2 (Table I). *a,* Exterior view of heart showing saphenous vein bypass grafts *(G-1* and *G-2)* to the left anterior descending and left obtuse marginal coronary arteries. *b,* Close-up view showing a 180 degree twist *(arrows)* of the bypass conduit *(G-1)* to the left anterior descending coronary artery. *c,* Exterior view of heart after dissecting out the native left coronary arteries. *LAD,* Left anterior descending. *d,* Lateral view showing the untwisted graft to the left obtuse marginal *(LOM)* and the twisted graft *(G-1)* to the left anterior descending *(LAD)* coronary artery. *LC,* Left circumflex. *LM,* Left main coronary artery.

The frequency of twisting of coronary bypass conduits is unknown. This complication was observed in our three patients within a 6 month period. This complication is not simply a matter of inexperience of the surgeon with the coronary bypass procedure. Each of our three patients underwent coronary operation in 1976 or 1977, each by a different surgeon at different institutions. However, each surgeon was quite experienced with this procedure.

Careful attention to proper alignment of a bypass

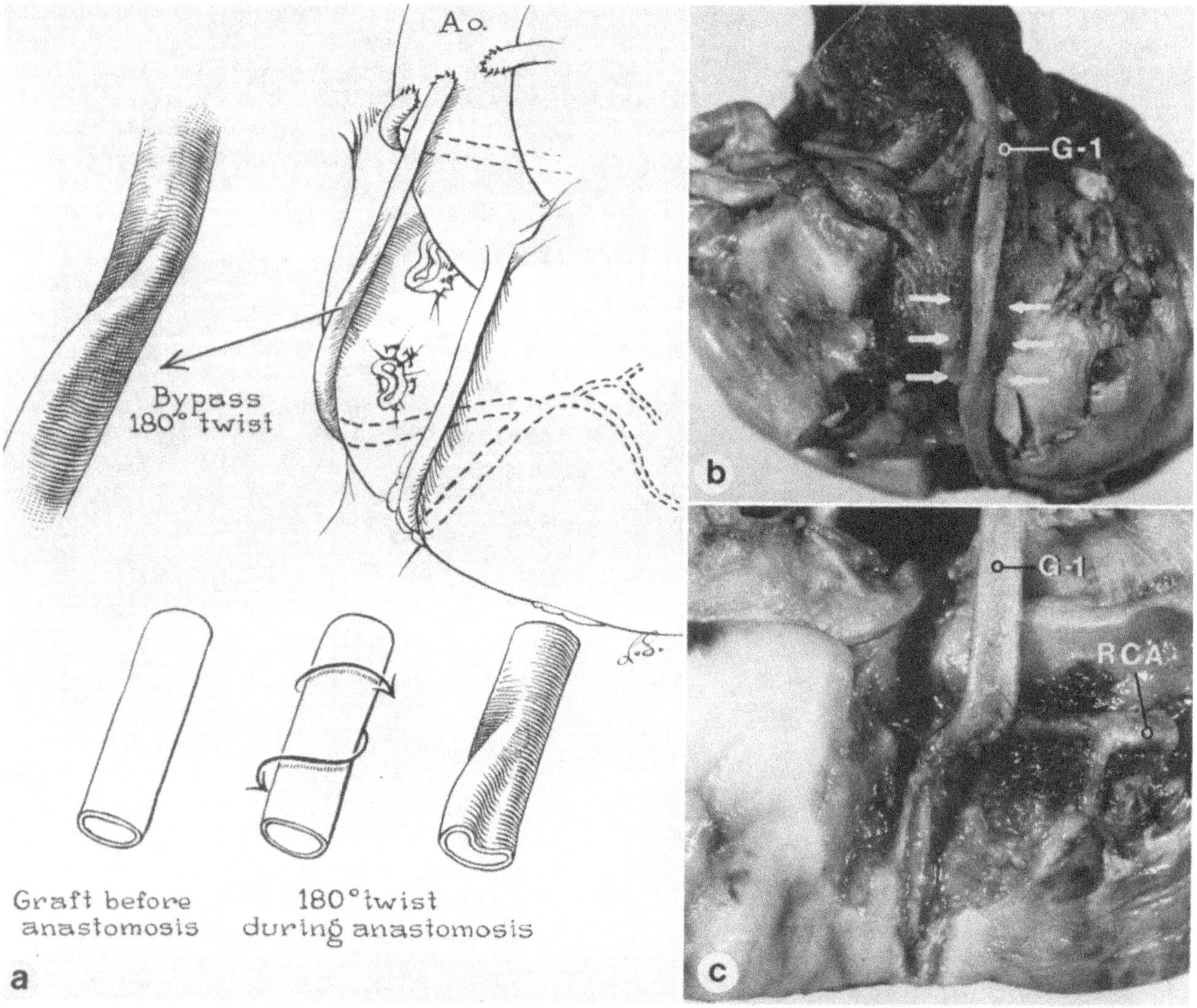

Fig. 3. Patient 3 (Table I). *a,* Drawing showing the 180 degree twist of the bypass conduit to the distal portion of the right coronary artery. *b,* Exterior view of heart showing a 180 degree twist *(arrows)* of the graft *(G-1). c,* Anastomosis of the graft *(G-1)* to the right coronary artery *(RCA).*

Table I. *Observations in each of three patients with twisting of one aorta-coronary bypass conduit*

Pt.	*Number*	*Age (yr.)*	*Sex*	*AP*	*HMI*	*CHF*	*Coronary artery receiving graft*					*Interval: Op → death (hr.)*
							LAD	*LOM*	*LC*	*Right*	*LD*	
1	76A-211	72	M	+	+	0	+*	0	+	+	0	0
2	A77-137	63	M	+	0	+	+*	+	0	0	0	6
3	N77-80	50	M	+	0	0	+	0	0	+*	+	0

Legend: AP, Angina pectoris. HMI, Healed myocardial infarct. CHF, Congestive heart failure. LAD, Left anterior descending. LOM, Left obtuse marginal. LC, Left circumflex. LD, Left diagonal. Op, Operation.
*Graft to this artery was twisted.

graft between the aorta and coronary artery should prevent graft twisting.

REFERENCES

1 Spray TL, Roberts WC: Status of the grafts and the native coronary arteries proximal and distal to coronary anastomotic sites of aortocoronary bypass grafts. Circulation **55**:741-749, 1977

2 Spray TL, Roberts WC: Tension on coronary bypass conduits. A neglected cause of real or potential obstruction of saphenous vein grafts. J THORAC CARDIOVASC SURG **72**:282-287, 1976

3 Vlodaver Z, Edwards JE: Pathologic analysis in fatal cases following saphenous vein coronary arterial bypass. Chest **64:**555-563, 1973

4 Spray TL, Roberts WC: Changes in saphenous veins used as aortocoronary bypass grafts. Am Heart J **94:**500-516, 1977

5 Bulkley BH, Roberts WC: Isolated coronary arterial dissection. A complication of cardiac operations. J THORAC CARDIOVASC SURG **67:**148-151, 1974

6 Breyer RH, Spray TL, Kastl DG, Roberts WC: Histologic changes in saphenous vein aorto-coronary bypass grafts. The effect of the angle of the aortic anastomosis. J THORAC CARDIOVASC SURG **72:**916-924, 1976

7 Jones M, Conkle DM, Ferrans VJ, Roberts WC, Levine FH, Melvin DB, Stinson EB: Lesions observed in arterial autogenous vein grafts. Light and electron microscopic evaluation. Circulation **48,49:**Suppl 3:198-210, 1973

Amount of Narrowing by Atherosclerotic Plaque in 44 Nonbypassed and 52 Bypassed Major Epicardial Coronary Arteries in 32 Necropsy Patients Who Died Within 1 Month of Aortocoronary Bypass Grafting

BRUCE F. WALLER, MD
WILLIAM C. ROBERTS, MD, FACC

Bethesda, Maryland

In 32 necropsy patients who died within 30 days of an aortocoronary bypass operation performed for relief of angina pectoris, the lumens in 42 (95 percent) of 44 nonbypassed and in 52 (100 percent) of 52 bypassed arteries were narrowed 76 to 100 percent in cross-sectional area by atherosclerotic plaque. Of 616 five mm segments of the 44 nonbypassed arteries examined histologically, 292 (47 percent) were narrowed 76 to 100 percent in cross-sectional area by atherosclerotic plaque; of 728 segments examined in the 52 bypassed arteries, 375 (52 percent) were similarly narrowed. Thirty-two (73 percent) of the 44 nonbypassed coronary arteries (in 23 patients) had been judged to be narrowed 50 percent or less in diameter on preoperative coronary angiography, but at necropsy 31 (97 percent) of these arteries were narrowed 76 to 100 percent in cross-sectional area and the other artery was narrowed 51 to 75 percent. Thus, significant amounts of atherosclerotic plaque tend to be present at necropsy in all three major coronary systems of patients with angina pectoris who die early after an aortocoronary bypass operation.

In patients undergoing aortocoronary bypass operations, one, two or three or more bypass conduits are inserted. The decision to bypass one major coronary artery and not another is usually determined by the degree and location of the narrowing or the size of the coronary artery on preoperative angiography. The accuracy of angiographic judgment or the status of the nonbypassed coronary artery has, to our knowledge, not been evaluated at necropsy in patients who died early after aortocoronary bypass operations. Thus, 44 nonbypassed coronary arteries were examined in 32 necropsy patients who died within 30 days of an aortocoronary bypass operation carried out for relief of angina pectoris, and the observations on the nonbypassed arteries were compared with those on the bypassed arteries.

Methods

Study patients: In the Pathology Branch of the National Heart, Lung, and Blood Institute, from 1972 through July 1979, we examined at necropsy the hearts of 117 patients who died after aortocoronary bypass procedures; 75 patients (64 percent) died within 60 days of the operation and 42 (36 percent) died later. Of the 75 patients who died within 60 days of operation, 43 (57 percent) had three or more aortocoronary bypass conduits inserted. The remaining 32 patients, all of whom died within 30 days of the bypass operation, had one (13 patients) or two (19 patients) bypass conduits inserted. This paper concerns only the latter 32 patients, whose ages ranged from 34 to 70 years (mean 55); 22 were men and 10 were women. All 32 patients had angina pectoris preoperatively, which was stable in 6 (19 percent) and unstable in 26 (81 percent). (Unstable angina pectoris was defined as anterior thoracic pain of recent onset [less than 1 month before clinical evaluation] or a recent change in the pattern of the pain

From the Pathology Branch, National Heart, Lung, and Blood Institute, National Institutes of Health, Bethesda, Maryland. Manuscript received November 26, 1979; revised manuscript received June 24, 1980, accepted June 27, 1980.

Address for reprints: William C. Roberts, MD, Building 10A, Room 3E30, National Heart, Lung, and Blood Institute, National Institutes of Health, Bethesda, Maryland 20205.

in terms of frequency, severity, intensity and ease of provocation. Nocturnal angina or angina at rest or prolonged angina within 3 months of death was considered unstable.)

In addition to coronary heart disease, six patients (all with stable angina pectoris) also had valvular heart disease: isolated aortic-valve stenosis in two, isolated mitral stenosis in one, pure mitral regurgitation secondary to papillary muscle dysfunction in one and combined aortic and mitral stenosis in two. These six patients also had replacement of the mitral or aortic valve, or both, with a prosthesis in addition to the aortocoronary bypass procedure. In these six patients with associated valvular heart disease, 12 of the 18 major coronary arteries received a bypass conduit, or one major coronary artery was not bypassed in each. Excluding the 6 patients with associated valvular heart disease, none of the other 26 patients had had clinical evidence of congestive cardiac failure and none of the total 32 patients had had a clinical event compatible with acute myocardial infarction. However, at necropsy 4 of the 32 patients had one or more transmural left ventricular scars, and 7 other patients had relatively small subendocardial foci of left ventricular necrosis.

Eighteen of the 32 patients died in the operating room because of inability to be separated from cardiopulmonary bypass. The remaining 14 patients died after varying periods of shock (low cardiac output syndrome). The interval from the end of the operation to death in these 14 patients ranged from 2 hours to 24 days; in 4 patients, 12 hours or less; in 3 patients, from 16 to 24 hours; in 4 patients, from 2 to 4 days; and in 3 patients, from 6, 14 and 24 days, respectively. None of the 18 patients who died in the operating room had left ventricular myocardial necrosis detected histologically at necropsy. Of the remaining 14 patients who died later, 4 had one or more foci of left ventricular myocardial necrosis (that is, acute myocardial infarction) at necropsy.

Examination of coronary arteries: This report focuses on the status of the 44 major nonbypassed and the 52 bypassed epicardial coronary arteries in the 32 patients. The major arteries analyzed were the right, left anterior descending and left circumflex (Table I). However, if a conduit had been

TABLE I

Summary of Coronary Arterial Findings in 32 Patients With Angina Pectoris Who Died Within 30 Days of Aortocoronary Bypass

Nonbypassed coronary arteries		
Left anterior descending (LAD) only	1	20 patients (single artery)
Left circumflex (LCx) only	9	
Right (RCA) only	10	
LAD and LCx	2	12 patients (two arteries)
LAD and RCA	1	
LCx and RCA	9	
Nonbypassed coronary arteries and (number of arteries) narrowed more than 75% in cross-sectional area by atherosclerotic plaque		
LAD	4 (4)	44 arteries (42 > 75%)
LCx	20 (19)	
RCA	20 (19)	
Number of 5 mm segments in 44 nonbypassed coronary arteries and (number of arteries) [%] narrowed more than 75% in cross-sectional area by atherosclerotic plaque	616 (292) [47%]	
Bypassed coronary arteries		
LAD only	9	12 patients (single artery)
LCx only	1	
RCA only	2	
LAD and LCx	10	20 patients (two arteries)
LAD and RCA	9	
LCx and RCA	1	
Bypassed coronary artery and number of arteries narrowed more than 75% in cross-sectional area by atherosclerotic plaque		
LAD	28 (28)	52 arteries (52 > 75%)
LCx	12 (12)	
RCA	12 (12)	
Total number of 5 mm segments in 52 bypassed coronary arteries and (number of arteries) [%] narrowed more than 75% in cross-sectional area by atherosclerotic plaque	728 (375) [52%]	

TABLE II

Angiographic and Histologic Comparison of Amount of Coronary Arterial Narrowing by Atherosclerotic Plaque in 32 of 44 Nonbypassed Major Epicardial Coronary Arteries With Less Than 50 percent Diameter Reduction on Preoperative Angiography

Histologic Finding at Necropsy	Preoperative Angiographic Narrowing (diameter reduction)		
	0–30%	31–50%	Total
LAD			
Number of arteries	1	2	3
Number narrowed >75%*	1	2	3
Number of 5 mm segments	14	29	43
Number (%) narrowed >75%*	6 (43)	13 (45)	19(44)
LCx			
Number of arteries	1	14	15
Number narrowed >75%*	1	14	15
Number of 5 mm segments	5	133	138
Number (%) narrowed >75%*	1 (20)	65 (49)	66 (48)
RCA			
Number of arteries	2	12	14
Number narrowed >75%*	2	11	13
Number of 5 mm segments	46	216	262
Number (%) narrowed >75%*	20 (43)	106 (49)	126 (48)
Totals			
Number of arteries	4	28	32
Number (%) narrowed >75%*	4 (100)	27 (96)	31 (97)
Number of 5 mm segments	65	378	443
Number (%) narrowed >75%*	27 (42)	184 (49)	211 (48)

* Cross-sectional area.

placed to the left obtuse marginal coronary artery, the left circumflex system then was considered to have been bypassed. If neither the left obtuse marginal nor the left circumflex coronary artery had been bypassed, only the status of the left circumflex artery was included in our analysis. Of the 44 nonbypassed coronary arteries, preoperative coronary angiograms showed some degree of narrowing in 43: diameter reduction 10 to 30 percent in 3 arteries, 31 to 50 percent in 28 arteries, 51 to 75 percent in 1 artery and 76 to 100 percent in 11 arteries (Table II). In the latter 12 arteries, either coronary bypass grafting had not been planned (six cases) or at operation the artery was not found or was deemed too small to bypass (six cases). In all 52 bypassed coronary arteries, preoperative selective angiograms disclosed greater than 50 percent narrowing in diameter.

The nonbypassed and bypassed coronary arteries were examined at necropsy in similar fashion. Each artery was excised intact from the heart and subjected to X-ray examination. If calcific deposits were present radiographically the artery was decalcified. The arteries were then cut transversely to the longitudinal axes into 5 mm long segments. The 5 mm segments were labeled, dehydrated and embedded in paraffin; several histologic sections were cut and one was stained by the Movat method and examined. All determinations of luminal narrowing were based on examination of the Movat-stained sections because this stain clearly outlines the artery's internal elastic membrane. The degree of narrowing was based on histologic examination of each cross section magnified 25 to 50 times. The judgment regarding the degree of luminal narrowing of each 5 mm segment was based on the degree of luminal obliteration within the luminal circle bordered by the internal elastic membrane. This method has been demonstrated[1] to be almost as accurate as videoplanimetry and the intra- and interobserver errors to be less than 5 percent. The percent cross-sectional area luminal narrowing by atherosclerotic plaque in each 5 mm segment was determined as follows: 0 to 25, 26 to 50, 51 to 75, 76 to 95 and 96 to 100. In arteries with eccentric lumens and walls indented artifactually into them, the judgment of degrees of narrowing at necropsy was determined only after visual expansion of the collapsed portion of wall.

Results

Nonbypassed versus bypassed coronary arteries: At necropsy, the lumens in 42 (95 percent) of the 44 nonbypassed coronary arteries and the lumens in all 52 bypassed coronary arteries were narrowed 76 to 100 percent in cross-sectional area by atherosclerotic plaques (Table I). (A 75 percent narrowing of cross-sectional area [necropsy] is equivalent to a 50 percent reduction in diameter [angiogram].[2]) The results of the examination of each 5 mm long segment of the 44 nonbypassed and the 52 bypassed coronary arteries are summarized in Table III and in Figure 1. Of the 616 five mm segments in the 44 nonbypassed arteries, 292 (47 percent) were narrowed 76 to 100 percent in cross-sectional area by atherosclerotic plaque; 143 (23 percent) were narrowed, 51 to 75 percent; 109 (18 percent) were narrowed 26 to 50 percent; and 72 (12 percent) were narrowed 0 to 25 percent. Of the 728 five mm segments in the 52 bypassed arteries 375 (52 percent) were narrowed 76 to 100 percent in cross-sectional area by atherosclerotic plaques; 215 (29 percent) were narrowed 51 to 75 percent; 123 (17 percent) were narrowed 26 to 50 percent, and 15 (2 percent) were narrowed 0 to 25 percent. The amount of severe (more than 75 percent cross-sectional area) narrowing by atherosclerotic plaques in the proximal and distal halves of the nonbypassed and bypassed left anterior descending and right coronary arteries was similar (Fig. 2). The proximal half of the nonbypassed left circumflex coronary artery had a higher proportion of 5 mm segments narrowed 76 to 100 percent than did the distal half of this

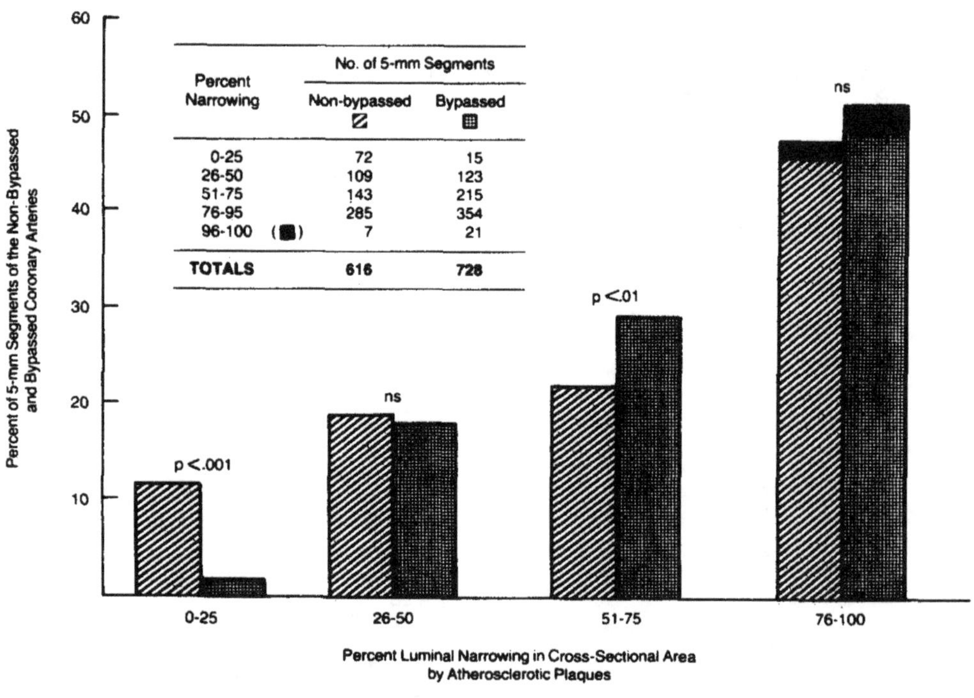

FIGURE 1. Bar graph showing percent of 5 mm segments of 44 nonbypassed and 52 bypassed major epicardial coronary arteries narrowed to various degrees in 32 necropsy patients with angina pectoris who died within 30 days of an aortocoronary bypass operation.

TABLE III

Number and Percent of 5 mm Segments of 44 Nonbypassed (N) and 52 Bypassed (B) Major Epicardial Coronary Arteries and Grade of Cross-Sectional Area Luminal Narrowing

Coronary Artery	Percent Cross-Sectional Area Luminal Narrowing											
	0–25		26–50		51–75		76–95		96–100		Total	
	N	B	N	B	N	B	N	B	N	B	N	B
LAD												
n	6	12	6	72	16	117	25	195	2	8	55	404
%	(11)	(3)	(11)	(18)	(29)	(29)	(45)	(48)	(4)	(2)	(100)	(100)
LCx												
n	28	2	34	28	41	40	95	63	2	4	200	137
%	(14)	(2)	(17)	(20)	(21)	(29)	(47)	(46)	(1)	(3)	(100)	(100)
RCA												
n	38	1	69	23	86	58	165	96	3	9	361	187
%	(11)	(1)	(18)	(12)	(24)	(31)	(46)	(51)	(2)	(5)	(100)	(100)
Total	72	15	109	123	143	215	285	354	7	21	616	728
	(12)†	(2)†	(18)	(17)	(23)*	(29)*	(46)	(49)	(1)	(3)	(100)	(100)

* $p < 0.01$. † $p < 0.001$.
LAD = left anterior descending, LCx = left circumflex, RCA = right coronary artery.

artery but the proportions were similar in the bypassed artery.

Preoperative coronary angiographic versus autopsy findings: Of the 32 nonbypassed coronary arteries (in 23 patients) judged to have a diameter reduction of 50 percent or less on preoperative coronary angiography, at necropsy 31 (97 percent) were narrowed 76 to 100 percent in cross-sectional area by atherosclerotic plaque (211 [48 percent] of 443 five mm segments) and 1 (3 percent) was narrowed 51 to 75 percent in cross-sectional area (Table II). Figures 3 and 4 show, respectively, a cross section from each 5 mm segment of the right coronary artery and the angiogram of this artery in 1 of the 23 patients with one or more major coronary arteries that were not bypassed because of insignificant reduction in diameter. Of the 12 nonbypassed coronary arteries (in nine patients) judged to be either "severely narrowed" or "too small to bypass" on preoperative coronary angiography, at necropsy 11 were narrowed 76 to 100 percent in cross-sectional area by atherosclerotic plaque (81 [47 percent] of 173 five mm segments) and 1 was narrowed 51 to 75 percent.

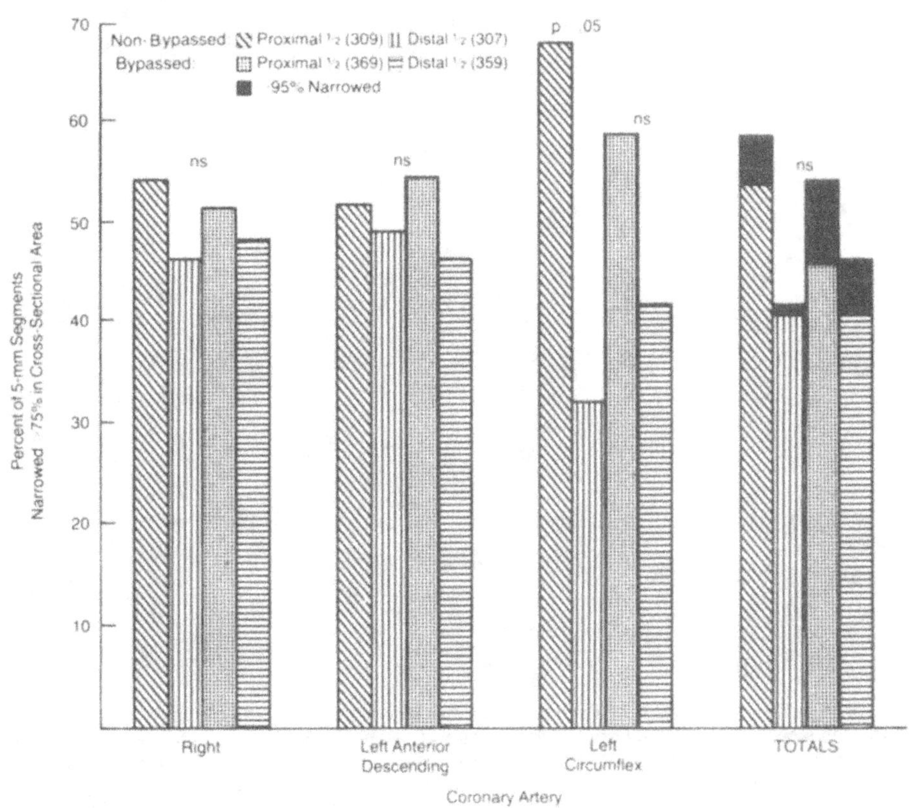

FIGURE 2. Bar graph showing percent of 5 mm segments of the proximal and distal halves of the 44 nonbypassed and 52 bypassed major epicardial coronary arteries narrowed more than 75 percent in cross-sectional area by atherosclerotic plaque in 32 necropsy patients who died within 30 days of aortocoronary bypass grafting.

Comments

Autopsy findings in fatal coronary artery disease: This study demonstrates that our necropsy patients with angina pectoris who died soon after aortocoronary bypass operations had *diffuse* coronary atherosclerosis and that their preoperative angiograms frequently underestimated the severity of the coronary narrowing. Other studies from this laboratory and elsewhere have also shown that among patients with fatal coronary heart disease (irrespective of the type of coronary event), coronary atherosclerosis in the major epicardial coronary arteries is diffuse and severe and that it is unusual to find a normal 5 mm long segment in any of the three major (right, left anterior descending and left

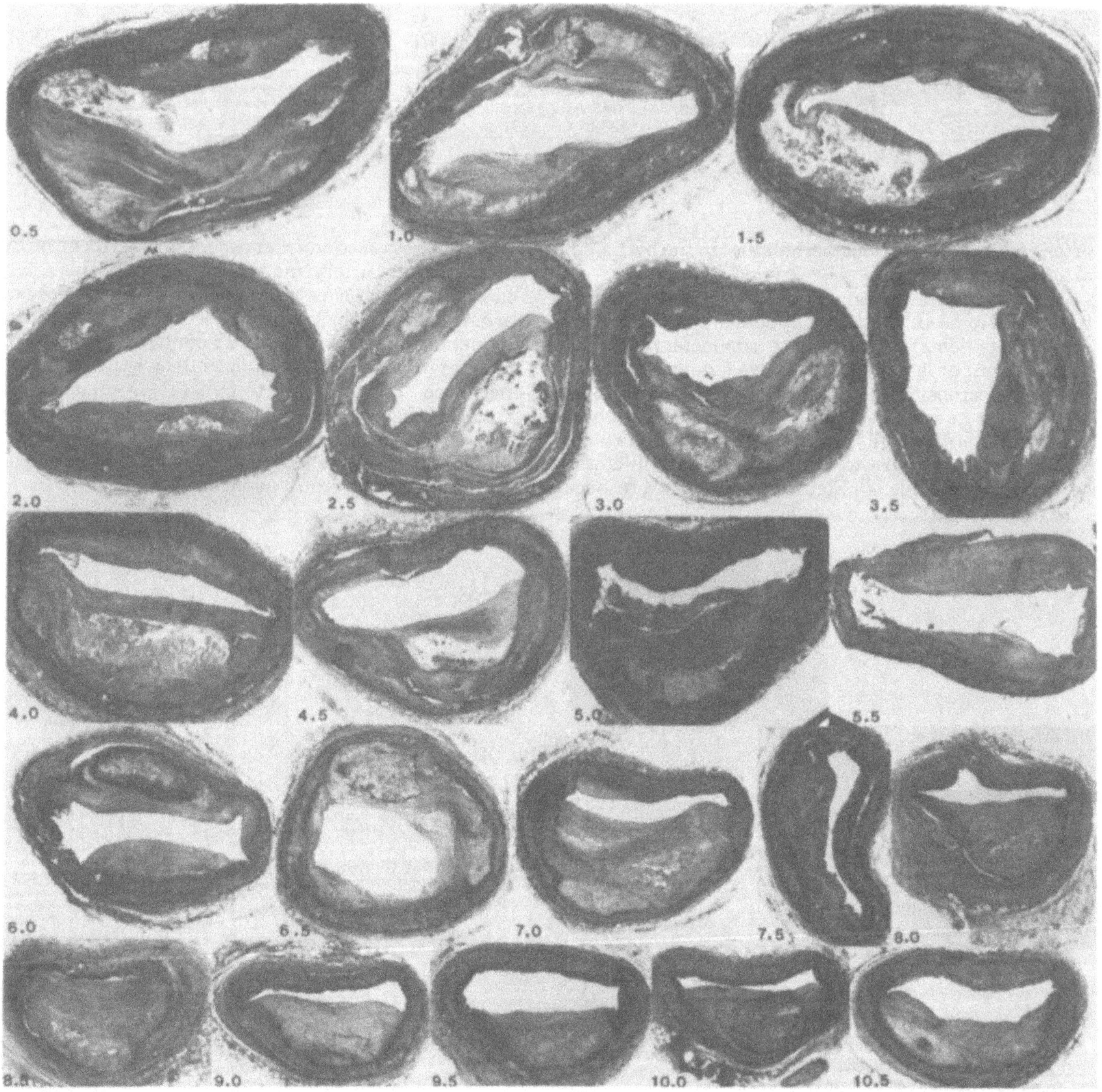

FIGURE 3. Cross-sections from each of 21 five mm segments of the right coronary artery in 1 of the 32 patients in whom one or more major coronary arteries were not bypassed because the preoperative angiogram indicated 50 percent or less diameter reduction. The histologic sections begin with the first 5 mm segment of the right coronary artery (0.5 cm) and extend to the origin of the posterior descending branch (10.5 cm). The amount narrowing of cross-sectional area of the lumen by atherosclerotic plaque (determined with videoplanimetry) in these 21 histologic sections was as follows: 76 to 100 percent in 10 (48 percent), 51 to 75 percent in 6 (28 percent) and 50 percent or less in 5 (24 percent).

circumflex) coronary arteries.[3-8] Among necropsy patients studied in our laboratory with unstable angina pectoris,[4] acute myocardial infarction,[5] sudden coronary death[6] and healed myocardial infarction with either cardiac[7] or noncardiac[8] death, the lumens of at least 30 percent of the three major coronary arteries were narrowed 76 to 100 percent in cross-sectional area by atherosclerotic plaque and about 70 percent of the lengths of these three arteries were narrowed more than 50 percent in cross-sectional area. Additionally, the lumens in only about 10 percent of the lengths of these three arteries were narrowed 25 percent or less in cross-sectional area. Among the 44 nonbypassed coronary arteries in our 32 patients, 292 (47 percent) of 616 five mm segments (an average of 20/artery) of nonbypassed artery were narrowed 76 to 100 percent in cross-sectional area by atherosclerotic plaque and another 23 percent were narrowed 51 to 75 percent. Of the 52 bypassed coronary arteries in our 32 patients, 375 (52 percent) of 728 five mm segments were narrowed 76 to 100 percent in cross-sectional area by atherosclerotic plaque and another 29 percent were narrowed 51 to 75 percent. Furthermore, only 12 percent of the 5 mm long segments of the nonbypassed coronary arteries were narrowed 25 percent or less, and only 2 percent of the bypassed arteries were so narrowed. Thus, the odds appear to favor the view that all three major coronary arteries will be considerably narrowed in necropsy patients with angina pectoris who died early after an aortocoronary bypass operation.

Coronary angiographic versus autopsy findings: Several studies among patients with symptomatic coronary heart disease have emphasized that coronary angiograms tend to underestimate the amount of coronary luminal narrowing. Among 61 coronary arteries examined with angiography during life and subsequently at necropsy in our laboratory,[2] in 17 (40 percent) of the 42 vessels narrowed 76 to 100 percent in cross-sectional area at necropsy, the narrowing was underestimated by two or three angiographers; and in 7 of 8 arteries narrowed 51 to 75 percent in cross-sectional area at necropsy, the narrowing was underestimated by one or more of the three angiographers. Thus, among patients with severe coronary atherosclerosis, coronary angiography tends to underestimate the actual degrees of luminal narrowing. Among 32 (76 percent) of the 44 nonbypassed coronary arteries (from 23 patients) described in this study, preoperative coronary angiography indicated less than 50 percent reduction in diameter in 21 arteries and 50 percent reduction in 11. However, at necropsy 31 of these 32 arteries were narrowed more than 75 percent in cross-sectional area.

Role of coronary bypass grafting: Several clinical studies have demonstrated that the early postoperative mortality rates and the frequency of postoperative acute

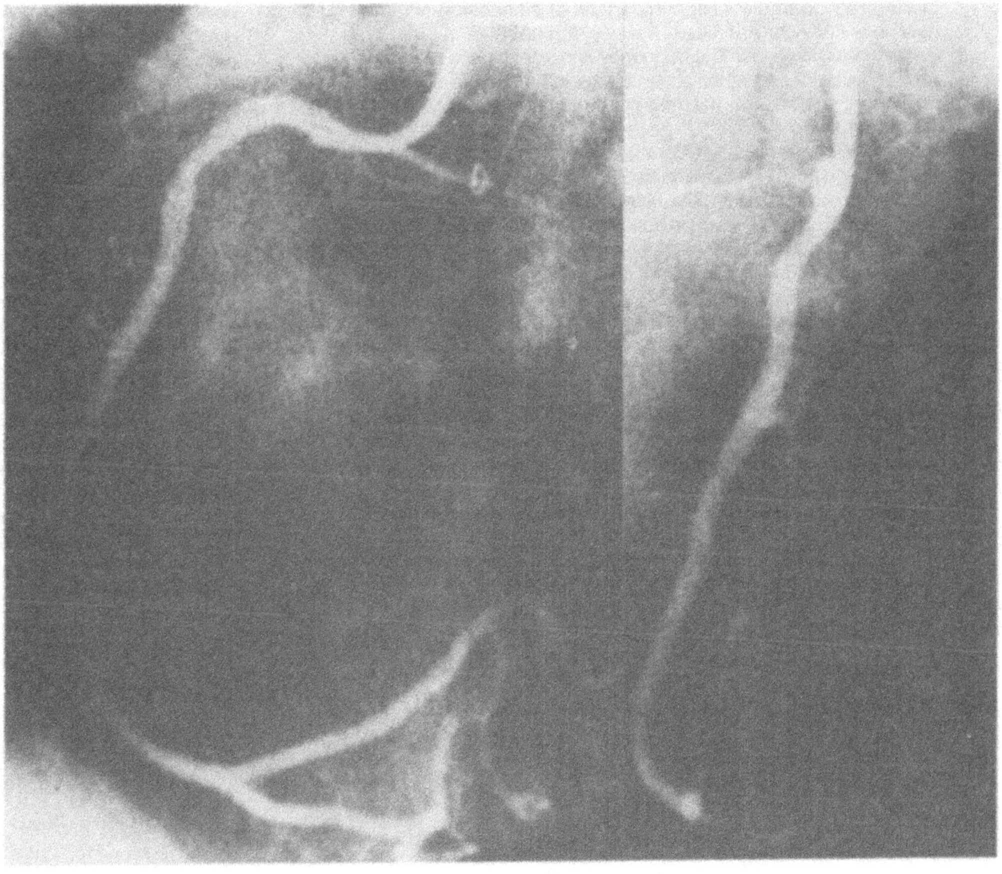

FIGURE 4. Same patient. Two views of the preoperative selective coronary arteriogram of the right coronary artery in the patient whose right coronary artery is shown histologically in Figure 3. The maximal diameter reduction in both right (**right**) and left (**left**) anterior oblique views was judged to be between 40 and 50 percent.

myocardial infarction are lower, and the frequency of disappearance of angina pectoris and improvement in exercise tolerance are greater in patients having three or more aortocoronary grafts than in those with two grafts and less in patients having two grafts than in those having only one. Stiles et al.[9] found the combined immediate and 6 month mortality rate to be 4 percent in 445 patients receiving three grafts, 9 percent in the 416 patients receiving two grafts and 21 percent in the 85 patients receiving a single graft. Sheldon et al.[10] observed clinical evidence of acute myocardial infarction early postoperatively in only 6 (3 percent) of 187 patients having multiple grafts and in 49 (17 percent) of 286 patients having a single graft. Of 58 patients followed up 13 to 36 months by Assad-Morell et al.,[11] 21 (80 percent) of 26 receiving three or more grafts had no angina pectoris compared with 12 (63 percent) of 19 patients receiving two grafts and only two (16 percent) of 13 patients with a single graft. Sheldon et al.[10] reported similar results. Consequently, the frequency of a second coronary bypass operation for recurrence of angina pectoris also is much greater in patients having one or two grafts inserted in the first aortocoronary bypass procedure compared with those having three or more grafts inserted in the first operation.[12–17] Assad-Morell et al.[11] found "positive" ischemic exercise responses with the exercise (stress) treadmill test in only 2 (9 percent) of 23 patients with three or more grafts, in 23 (70 percent) of 30 patients with two grafts and in 23 (96 percent) of 24 patients with only one graft.

Finally, progression of the atherosclerotic process in nonbypassed coronary arteries appears to be the major cause of recurrence of myocardial ischemia late after aortocoronary bypass operation. Seides et al.[18] restudied 22 patients 53 to 84 months after aortocoronary bypass grafting who had had at least one graft patent 3 to 9 months after the bypass operation. At the late study, 31 of 33 grafts were patent, but angina pectoris had reappeared in 11 of 16 patients who had become asymptomatic early after operation. Progression of narrowing in ungrafted coronary arteries accounted for the clinical deterioration in 9 of these 11 patients.

References

1. **Isner JM, Wu M, Virmani R, Jones A, Roberts WC.** Comparison of degrees of coronary arterial luminal narrowing determined by visual inspection of histologic sections under magnification among independent observers and comparison to that obtained by videoplanimetry: an analysis of 559 five-mm segments of 61 coronary arteries from eleven patients. Lab Invest 1980;42:566–70.
2. **Arnett EN, Isner JM, Redwood DR, et al.** Coronary artery narrowing in coronary heart disease: comparison of cineangiographic and necropsy findings. Ann Intern Med 1979;91:350–6.
3. **Roberts WC, Buja LM.** The frequency and significance of coronary arterial thrombi and other observations in fatal acute myocardial infarction. A study of 107 necropsy patients. Am J Med 1972; 52:425–43.
4. **Roberts WC, Virmani R.** Quantification of coronary arterial narrowing in clinically-isolated unstable angina pectoris. An analysis of 22 necropsy patients. Am J Med 1979;67:792–8.
5. **Roberts WC, Jones AA.** Quantitation of coronary arterial narrowing at necropsy in acute transmural myocardial infarction: analysis and comparison of findings in 27 patients and 22 control. Circulation 1980;61:789–90.
6. **Roberts WC, Jones AA.** Quantitation of coronary arterial narrowing at necropsy in sudden coronary death: an analysis of 31 patients and comparison of findings to those in 25 control subjects. Am J Cardiol 1979;44:39–45.
7. **Virmani R, Roberts WC.** Quantification of coronary arterial narrowing and of left ventricular myocardial scarring in healed myocardial infarction with chronic, eventually fatal, congestive heart failure. Am J Med 1980;68:831–8.
8. **Virmani R, Roberts WC.** Non-fatal healed myocardial infarction and fatal non-cardiac disease: qualification and quantification of coronary arterial narrowing and of left ventricular scarring in 18 necropsy patients. Br Heart J, in press.
9. **Stiles QR, Lindesmith GG, Tucker BL, Hughes RK, Meyer BW.** Long-term follow-up of patients with coronary artery bypass grafts. Circulation 1976;54:Suppl III:III-33–4.
10. **Sheldon WC, Rincon G, Pichard AD, Razavi M, Cheanvechai C, Loop FD.** Surgical treatment of coronary artery disease: pure graft operations, with a study of 741 patients followed 3–7 years. Prog Cardiovasc Dis 1975;18:237–53.
11. **Assad-Morell JL, Frye RL, Connolly DC, et al.** Aorto-coronary artery saphenous vein bypass surgery. Clinical and angiographic results. Mayo Clin Proc 1975;50:379–86.
12. **Stiles QR.** Reoperation for myocardial revascularization. Cleve Clin Q 1978;45:136–8.
13. **Johnson WD, Hoffman JF Jr, Flemma RJ, Tector AJ.** Secondary surgical procedure for myocardial revascularization. J Thorac Cardiovasc Surg 1972;64:524–9.
14. **Thomas CS, Alford WC, Burrus GR, Frist RA, Stoney WS.** Results of reoperation for failed aortocoronary bypass grafts. Arch Surg 1976;111:1210–3.
15. **Irarrazaval MJ, Cosgrove DM, Loop FD, Ennix CL Jr, Groves LK, Taylor PC.** Reoperation for myocardial revascularization. J Thorac Cardiovasc Surg 1977;73:181–8.
16. **Winkle RA, Alderman EL, Shumway NE, Harrison DC.** Results of reoperation for unsuccessful coronary artery bypass surgery (abstr). Circulation 1975;51:Suppl I:I-62.
17. **Culliford AT, Girdwood MD, Isom OW, Krauss KR, Spencer FC.** Angina following myocardial revascularization. Does time of recurrence predict etiology and influence results of operation? J Thorac Cardiovasc Surg 1979;77:889–95.
18. **Seides SF, Borer JS, Kent KM, Rosing DR, McIntosh CL, Epstein SE.** Long-term anatomic fate of coronary-artery bypass grafts and functional status of patients five years after operation. N Engl J Med 1978;298:1213–7.

Amount of Luminal Narrowing in Bypassed and Nonbypassed Native Coronary Arteries in Necropsy Patients Dying Early or Late after Aortocoronary Bypass Operations

B. F. Waller, W. C. Roberts

Pathology Branch, National Heart, Lung and Blood Institute, National Institutes of Health, Bethesda, Maryland, USA

Summary

From study at necropsy of 102 patients dying either early (≤60 d) or late [2.5–108 months (mean 35)] after aortocoronary bypass operations, the following observations seemed most important. (1) Both the bypassed and nonbypassed native coronary arteries had similar degrees of severe luminal narrowing by atherosclerotic plaques. In 213 (94%) of the 226 bypassed arteries and in 73 (91%) of 80 nonbypassed arteries, the degree of narrowing was >75%. (2) The percent of bypassed native coronary arteries severely narrowed distal to anastomotic sites was similar in the early- and late-death patients. In 82 (44%) of 187 arteries in the 65 early-death patients and in 49 (51%) of 97 arteries in the 37 late-death patients, the native arteries distal to the anastomotic sites were narrowed >75% in cross-sectional area by atherosclerotic plaques.

Introduction

Relatively little anatomic information is available on the status of the bypassed and nonbypassed native epicardial coronary arteries in necropsy patients dying after aortocoronary bypass operations. This report summarizes our observations on these arteries, the information being obtained from study of 102 necropsy patients dying either early (65 patients) or late (37 patients) after aortocoronary bypass operation.

Patients and Methods

From July, 1971 to August, 1980, we examined the hearts from 102 patients from 29 different institutions who died after an aortocoronary bypass operation: 65 (64%) died within 60 d of operation (mean 5)(*early*), and 37 (36%) from 2.5 to 108 months (mean 35)(*late*) after operation. Each patient had angina pectoris and a single aortocoronary bypass operation. None had associated left ventricular aneurysmectomy, closure of ventricular septal defect, or cardiac valve replacement, anuloplasty, or commissurotomy, and none had a primary disease of the ascending aorta such as dissection or aortitis.

The 102 patients ranged in age from 26 to 78 years (mean 55) and 75 (74%) were men. Of the 65 early-death patients, 30 (46%) died in the operating room (unable to be separated from the bypass pump); 25 (39%) died after varying intervals of the low cardiac output syndrome (2 h to 14 d); and 10 (15%) died 14–43 d later from infection (5 patients), acute myocardial infarction (3 patients), or suddenly (out of hospital) (2 patients). Of the late-death patients, 11 (30%) died 2.5–12 months postoperatively and the remaining 26 (70%) died 13–108 months after operation. Twenty-six patients died from coronary heart disease [sudden (15), chronic congestive heart failure (8), acute myocardial infarction (3)] and 11 patients died from noncoronary causes [cancer (6), infection (2), trauma (2), stroke (1)].

The early-death patients had 187 aortocoronary conduits (182 saphenous vein, 5 internal mammary arteries) to 147 major coronary arterial systems (left anterior descending, left circumflex, right), an average of 2.8 conduits/patient. The late-death patients had 79 major coronary arterial systems bypassed (97 saphenous veins), an average of 2.6/patient. Of the 80 major coronary systems not bypassed, 48 (60%) were in the 65 early-death patients and 32 (40%) in the late-death patients.

The coronary arteries (bypassed and nonbypassed) and the bypass conduits were removed from the hearts and cut transversely to the longitudinal axes into 5-mm-long segments. The degrees of luminal narrowing of the bypass conduits, anastomotic sites, and native coronary arteries proximal and distal to the anastomostic sites were based upon histologic examination of Movat-stained sections. The percent of cross-sectional area narrowing by thrombus, atherosclerotic plaques, or both was determined as follows: 0–25, 26–50, 51–75, 76–95, or 96–100.

Results

Both the bypassed and nonbypassed native coronary arteries had similar degrees of severe luminal narrowing by atherosclerotic plaques. In 213

(94%) of the 226 bypassed arteries and in 73 (91%) of 80 nonbypassed arteries, the degree of luminal narrowing was 76–100% in cross-sectional area. Findings from the analysis of the 5-mm coronary segments narrowed to various degrees of cross-sectional area by plaques in the bypassed and nonbypassed arteries in the early- and late-death patients are summarized in Tables I and II. No significant difference was present in the percent of 5-mm segments narrowed >75% in cross-sectional area in bypassed and nonbypassed arteries. In 2,799 (49%) of the 5,681 segments from the bypassed arteries and in 760 (48%) of the 1,595 segments from the nonbypassed arteries, the degree of luminal narrowing was 76–100% in cross-sectional area. Furthermore, the amount of narrowing in the bypassed and nonbypassed arteries in the patients dying early and late was similar. In 1,905 (50%) of the 3,795 segments from the bypassed arteries in the early-death patients and in 894 (48%) of the 1,886 segments from the bypassed arteries in the late-death patients, the cross-sectional area luminal narrowing was severe (>75%). In 413 (46%) of 893 coronary segments from nonbypassed arteries in the early-death patients and in 347 (49%) of 702 segments from the late-death patients, the cross-sectional area narrowing was 76–100%.

TABLE I Findings in patients dying early after an aortocoronary bypass operation[a]

	Percent cross-sectional area luminal narrowing					
Coronary artery	0–25 no. (%)	26–50 no. (%)	51–75 no. (%)	76–95 no. (%)	96–100 no. (%)	Totals no. (%)
LAD						
B	165 (9.5)	207 (12)	481 (28)	837 (48)	43 (2.5)	1733 (100)
NB	11 (13)	12 (14)	21 (24)	42 (48)	1 (1)	87 (100)
LC						
B	94 (12)	117 (15)	164 (21)	400 (51)	6 (1)	781 (100)
NB	56 (15)	63 (17)	86 (23)	166 (44)	2 (1)	373 (100)
R						
B	147 (11)	185 (14)	330 (26)	584 (46)	35 (3)	1281 (100)
NB	52 (12)	78 (18)	104 (24)	195 (45)	4 (1)	433 (100)
Totals						
B	406 (11)	509 (13)	975 (26)	1821 (48)	84 (2)	3795 (100)
NB	119 (13)	153 (17)	211 (24)	406 (45)	7 (1)	893 (100)

Abbreviations: LAD, left anterior descending coronary artery; LC, left circumflex coronary artery; R, right coronary artery; B, bypassed; NB, nonbypassed

[a] The number and percent of 5-mm segments of 147 bypassed and 48 nonbypassed major coronary arteries and the grade of cross-sectional area luminal narrowing by atherosclerotic plaque in 65 necropsy patients dying early (60 d, mean 5) after an aortocoronary bypass operation are given.

The percent of bypassed native coronary arteries severely (>75%) narrowed distal to anastomotic sites was similar in the early- and late-death patients. In 82 (44%) of 187 arteries in the 65 early-death patients and in 49 (51%) of 97 arteries in the 37 late-death patients, the native arteries distal to the anastomotic sites were narrowed 76–100% in cross-sectional area by atherosclerotic plaques. Of 996 5-mm coronary segments of the native arteries distal to the anastomotic sites in the early-death patients, 333 (34%) were severely narrowed, and of 479 segments in the late-death patients, 183 (39%) were narrowed >75% in cross-sectional area.

The amount of narrowing of the native coronary artery by atherosclerotic plaques at the anastomotic site of the bypass conduit also was similar in the early- and late-death patients. Of 121 anastomotic sites examined in the early-death patients, 27 (22%) were narrowed 76–100% in cross-sectional area by plaques, and of 63 anastomotic sites from the late-death patients, 11 (17%) were similarly narrowed.

Discussion

It is not surprising that our necropsy patients with angina pectoris and aortocoronary bypass operations had severe and diffuse coronary luminal

TABLE II Findings in patients dying late after an aortocoronary bypass operation[a]

Coronary artery	Percent cross-sectional area luminal narrowing 0–25 no. (%)	26–50 no. (%)	51–75 no. (%)	76–95 no. (%)	96–100 no. (%)	Totals no. (%)
LAD						
B	71 (7)	140 (15)	293 (31)	447 (46)	12 (1)	963 (100)
NB	7 (16)	8 (18)	11 (25)	18 (41)	0 (0)	44 (100)
LC						
B	52 (12)	85 (18)	107 (24)	194 (44)	7 (2)	445 (100)
NB	41 (16)	33 (13)	67 (26)	113 (44)	3 (1)	257 (100)
R						
B	57 (12)	57 (12)	130 (27)	223 (47)	11 (2)	478 (100)
NB	21 (5)	7 (19)	91 (23)	206 (51)	7 (2)	401 (100)
Totals						
B	180 (9)	282 (15)	530 (28)	864 (46)	30 (2)	1886 (100)
NB	69 (10)	117 (17)	169 (24)	337 (48)	10 (1)	702 (100)

Abbreviations: LAD, left anterior descending coronary artery; LC, left circumflex coronary artery; R, right coronary artery; B, bypassed; NB, nonbypassed

[a] The number and percent of 5-mm segments of 79 bypassed and 32 nonbypassed major coronary arteries and the grade of cross-sectional area luminal narrowing by atherosclerotic plaque in 37 necropsy patients dying late (2.5–108 months, mean 35) after an aortocoronary bypass operation are given.

narrowing by atherosclerotic plaques. Previous necropsy studies in our laboratory of nonoperated patients with fatal coronary heart disease [unstable angina pectoris (Roberts and Virmani, 1979), acute myocardial infarction (Roberts and Jones, 1980), and healed myocardial infarction with cardiac (Virmani and Roberts, 1980) or noncardiac death (Virmani and Roberts, 1981)] disclosed similarly severe and diffuse coronary narrowing of these arteries by atherosclerotic plaques. In our early- and late-death bypass patients, nearly half of the lengths of bypassed and nonbypassed coronary arteries were narrowed severely (>75%), and over 70% of the lengths were narrowed >50% in cross-sectional area by plaques. Thus, the odds are great that all three major coronary arteries will be considerably narrowed in necropsy patients with angina pectoris dying early or late after aortocoronary bypass operations.

Several clinical studies have demonstrated that the early postoperative mortality is lower, the frequency of postoperative acute myocardial infarction is lower, the frequency of disappearance of angina pectoris is higher, and improvement in exercise tolerance is higher in patients having three or more aortocoronary grafts as opposed to two grafts, and lower in patients having two grafts compared to those having only one graft inserted. Stiles *et al.* (1976) found the combined immediate and 6-month mortality in 445 patients receiving three grafts to be 4%; in the 416 patients receiving two grafts, 9%; and in the 85 patients receiving a single graft, 21%. Sheldon *et al.* (1975) observed clinical evidence of acute myocardial infarction early postoperatively in only 6 (3%) of 187 patients having multiple grafts and in 49 (17%) of 286 patients having single grafts. Of 58 patients followed 13–36 months by Assad-Morell *et al.* (1975), 21 (80%) of 26 receiving three or more grafts were free of angina pectoris; 12 (63%) of 19 patients receiving two grafts were pain-free, and only 2 (16%) of 13 patients with a single graft were pain-free. Sheldon *et al.* (1975) reported similar results. Consequently, the frequency of a second bypass operation for recurrence of angina pectoris also is much higher in the patients having one or two bypass conduits inserted at the first aortocoronary bypass procedure compared to those having three or more grafts inserted at the first operation (Culliford *et al.*, 1979; Irarrazaval *et al.*, 1977; Johnson *et al.*, 1972; Stiles, 1978; Thomas *et al.*, 1976; Winkle *et al.*, 1975). By exercise (stress) treadmill test performance, Assad-Morell *et al.* (1975) found "positive" ischemic exercise responses in only 2 (9%) of 23 patients with three or more bypass conduits, in 23 (70%) of 30 patients with two grafts, and in 23 (96%) of 24 patients with only one graft inserted. And finally, progression of the atherosclerotic process in nonbypassed coronary arteries appears to be the major cause of recurrence of myocardial ischemia late after an aortocoronary bypass operation. Seides *et al.* (1978) studied 22 patients 53–84 months after undergoing aortocoronary bypass who had had at least one graft patent 3–9 months after the bypass operation. At the late study, 31 of 33 bypass conduits were patent but angina pectoris had, nevertheless, reappeared in 11 of 16 patients who had become asymptomatic early after operation. Progression of narrowing in nonbypassed coronary arteries accounted for the clinical deterioration in 9 of these 11 patients.

In addition to similarly severe coronary arterial narrowing proximal to the anastomotic sites of the bypass conduits, the amounts of severe narrowing by atherosclerotic plaques *distal to* the anastomotic site also were similar. In 82 (44%) of 187 arteries [333 (34%) 5-mm segments] distal to the anastomotic sites in the early-death patients, the cross-sectional area luminal narrowing was >75%; in 49 (51%) of 97 arteries [183 (38.5%) 5-mm segments] distal to the anastomotic sites from the late-death patients, the lumina were similarly narrowed.

The amount of severe narrowing by atherosclerotic plaques *at* the anastomotic sites of the conduits also was similar in patients who died early and late after bypass operation. Of 121 anastomotic sites examined in 51 of 65 early-death patients, 27 (22%) were narrowed >75% in cross-sectional area; of 63 sites examined in 26 of 37 late-death patients, 11 (17%) were similarly narrowed. In each patient in whom the lumen at the site of anastomosis was severely narrowed, the native coronary artery distal to the anastomosis also was severely narrowed by plaque.

The fate of the bypass conduits appears to be dependent upon the status of the native coronary arteries *at* and *distal to* the anastomotic sites of the conduits. In 37 (39%) of 97 conduits in the 37 late-death patients, the lumina were narrowed 76–100% in cross-sectional area by thrombus, atherosclerotic plaques, or both; in all 37, the native coronary arteries distal to the severely narrowed conduits also were narrowed >75% by plaques. Of the remaining 40 conduits in the 37 late-death patients, the native coronary arteries were severely narrowed distal to the anastomotic sites in 12; the lumina of the associated conduits were narrowed 51–75% in 6 of them and 50% or less in the other 6.

Although it is easy to determine degrees of cross-sectional area narrowing in conduits of patients dying late (>60 d) after aortocoronary bypass operation, this determination may be extremely difficult if not impossible in many or most of the patients dying early after bypass operation. The reason for this difficulty lies in the fact that most patients dying early do so in the operating room at the time of the bypass or within a few days thereafter. Consequently, in the patients dying within 1 week of operation, it is rare to find organizing or organized thrombus within the lumen of a conduit. We believe what actually happens is that blood enters the conduit but is blocked from exiting the conduit because of severe narrowing of the native coronary artery at the site of or distal to the coronary–conduit anastomosis. Thus, the blood which initially fills the lumen of the conduit is never replaced and, therefore, the products necessary to form a true thrombus are not available. The clot in the conduits, therefore, consists nearly entirely of erythrocytes and has the appearance of a "postmortem clot." Among our 65 patients dying early, 51 died within 7 d of the bypass operation, and at necropsy none of the 151 conduits of these 51 patients contained organizing thrombi. In contrast, of the 36 conduits in the 14 patients dying from 8 to 60 d after bypass operations, 5 had lumina narrowed by organizing thrombi. It is likely but not probable that flow through many of the conduits in the patients dying early was minimal or absent because of the severe narrowing of the lumina of the native coronary arteries *at* or *distal to* the anastomotic sites of the conduits.

References

Assad-Morell JL, Frye RL, Connolly DC, Davis GD, Pluth JR, Wallace RB, Barhorst DA, *et al.*: Aorto-coronary artery saphenous vein bypass surgery. Clinical and angiographic results. *Mayo Clinic Proc* 50, 379 (1975)

Culliford AT, Girdwood MD, Isom OW, Krauss KR, Spencer FC: Angina following myocardial revascularization. Does time of recurrence predict etiology and influence results of operation? *J Thorac Cardiovasc Surg* 77, 889 (1979)

Irarrazaval MJ, Cosgrove DM, Loop FD, Ennix CL Jr, Groves LK, Taylor PC: Reoperation for myocardial revascularization. *J Thorac Cardiovasc Surg* 73, 181 (1977)

Johnson WD, Hoffman JF Jr, Flemma RJ, Tector AJ: Secondary surgical procedure for myocardial revascularization. *J Thorac Cardiovasc Surg* 64, 524 (1972)

Roberts WC, Jones AA: Quantitation of coronary arterial narrowing at necropsy in *sudden coronary death:* An analysis of 31 patients and comparison of findings to those in 25 control subjects. *Am J Cardiol* 44, 39 (1979)

Roberts WC, Jones AA: Quantitation of coronary arterial narrowing at necropsy in acute transmural myocardial infarction. Analysis and comparison of findings in 27 patients and 22 controls. *Circulation* 61, 786 (1980)

Roberts WC, Virmani R: Quantification of coronary arterial narrowing in clinically-isolated unstable angina pectoris. An analysis of 22 necropsy patients. *Am J Med* 67, 792 (1979)

Seides SF, Borer JS, Kent KM, Rosing DR, McIntosh CL, Epstein SE: Long-term anatomic fate of coronary-artery bypass grafts and functional status of patients five years after operation. *N Engl J Med* 298, 1213 (1978)

Sheldon WC, Rincon G, Pichard AD, Razavi M, Cheanvechai C, Loop FD: Surgical treatment of coronary artery disease: Pure graft operations, with a study of 741 patients followed 3-7 years. *Prog Cardiovasc Dis* 18, 237 (1975)

Stiles QR: Reoperation for myocardial revascularization. *Cleve Clin Q* 45(1), 136 (1978)

Stiles QR, Lindesmith GG, Tucker BL, Hughes RK, Meyer BW: Long-term follow-up of patients with coronary artery bypass grafts. *Circulation* 54 (suppl III), III-33 (1976)

Thomas CS, Alford WC, Burrus GR, Frist RA, Stoney WS: Results of reoperation for failed aortocoronary bypass grafts. *Arch Surg* 111, 1210 (1976)

Virmani R, Roberts WC: Quantification of coronary arterial narrowing and of left ventricular myocardial scarring in healed myocardial infarction with chronic, eventually fatal, congestive heart failure. *Am J Med* 68, 831 (1980)

Virmani R, Roberts WC: Non-fatal healed transmural myocardial infarction: Qualification and quantification of coronary arterial narrowing and of left ventricular scarring in 18 necropsy patients with fatal non-cardiac disease. *Br Heart J* 45, 434 (1981)

Winkle RA, Alderman EL, Shumway NE, Harrison DC: Results of reoperation for unsuccessful coronary artery bypass surgery. *Circulation* 51 (suppl I), I-62 (1975)

False Aneurysm of Ascending Aorta After Aortocoronary Bypass Grafting

JEFFREY E. SAFFITZ, MD
CHARLES E. GANOTE, MD
C. ERIC PETERSON, MD
WILLIAM C. ROBERTS, MD

Aortic tears with or without dissection may occur after aortocoronary artery bypass grafting (CABG).[1] We report 4 patients who had large false aneurysms of the ascending aorta after CABG (Table I, Fig. 1 to 4).

The sequence of events leading to formation of the aortic false aneurysm in Patients 1 to 3 appears to be: (1) initiation of a limited aortic dissection beginning at an aortocoronary bypass anastomosis; (2) rupture of the outer partition of the false channel; and (3) progressive enlargement of the false aneurysm, the wall of which was adventitial fibrous tissue with or without adjacent adherent parietal pericardium. In Patients 1 and 3, the aneurysm involved the right side of the ascending aorta and compressed the right atrium and superior vena cava (Fig. 1 and 3); in Patient 2, the aneurysm involved the left side of the aorta and compressed the left atrium and pulmonary trunk (Fig. 2). In none of these 3 patients was an aneurysm of the ascending aorta suspected clinically. Patient 1 developed substernal chest pain 3 days before death (37 days after CABG) and a pericardial friction rub was recorded. This man died with features of the low cardiac output syndrome. Patients 2 and 3 died from progressive worsening of chronic congestive heart failure and in each, ≥1 aortocoronary conduit was totally occluded. In Patient 3, Dressler's syndrome developed early after CABG. During the next 40 months she received prednisone almost daily.

Patient 4 had pseudoxanthoma elasticum. After CABG, she developed mediastinitis and died from consequences of a generalized infection. At necropsy, the metallic rings that had been placed to mark the aortic anastomosis of each of the 2 conduits had eroded through the wall of aorta to be visible from its interior. The proximal portions of the conduits were surrounded by thrombus and both conduits were occluded (Fig. 4). The rupture of the wall of aorta in this patient appears to have been the result of both mediastinitis and the underlying weakened aorta from pseudoxanthoma elasticum.

From the Pathology Branch, National Heart, Lung, and Blood Institute, National Institutes of Health, Bethesda, Maryland; the Department of Pathology, Northwestern Memorial Hospital, Chicago, Illinois; and the Department of Pathology, Florida Hospital, Orlando, Florida. Manuscript received and accepted April 21, 1983.

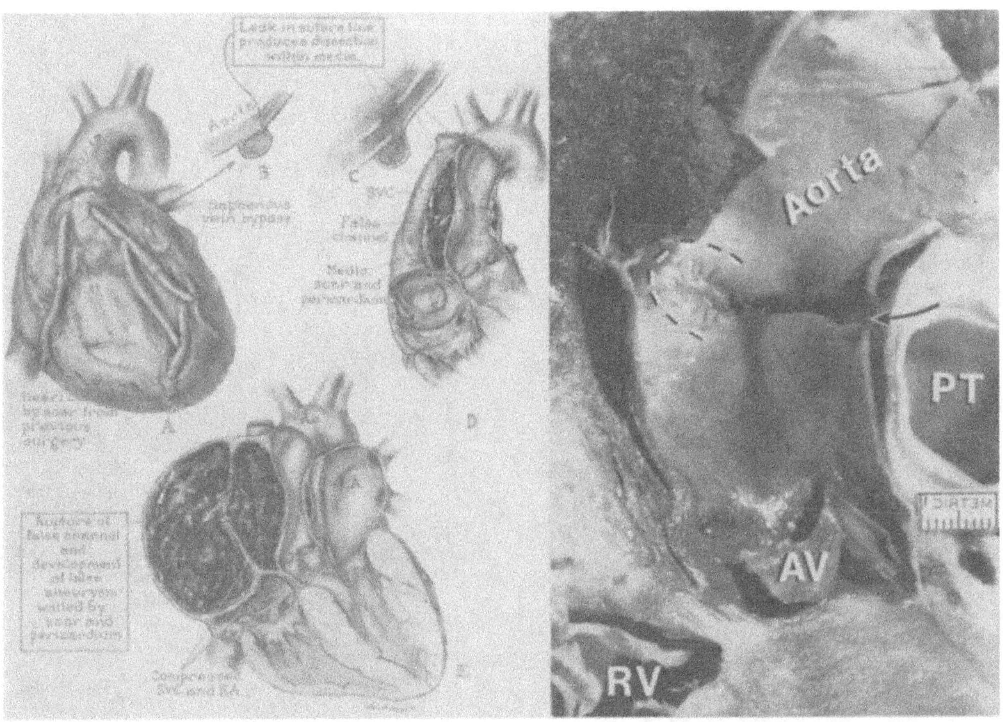

FIGURE 1. Patient 1. **Left,** the sequence of events leading to false aneurysm of the ascending aorta (Ao) after coronary artery bypass grafting (CABG). Repeat CABG was performed 9 years after the first CABG with saphenous vein grafts to the right and first diagonal coronary arteries and a jump-graft to the left anterior descending artery (**A**). False aneurysm was not present at the time of repeat operation. An aortic dissection originating at an aortic anatomosis (**B and C**) extended nearly to the origin of the innominate artery (**D**). The outer partition of the false channel ruptured, giving rise to a large false aneurysm contained by fibrous tissue (**E**). The aneurysm compressed the lumen of the superior vena cava (SVC) and the cavity of the right atrium (RA). **Right,** The heart at necropsy showing the aortic tear (**arrow**) originating at a saphenous vein anastomosis (**dashed semicircle**). AV = aortic valve; LA = left atrium; PT = pulmonary trunk; RV = right ventricle.

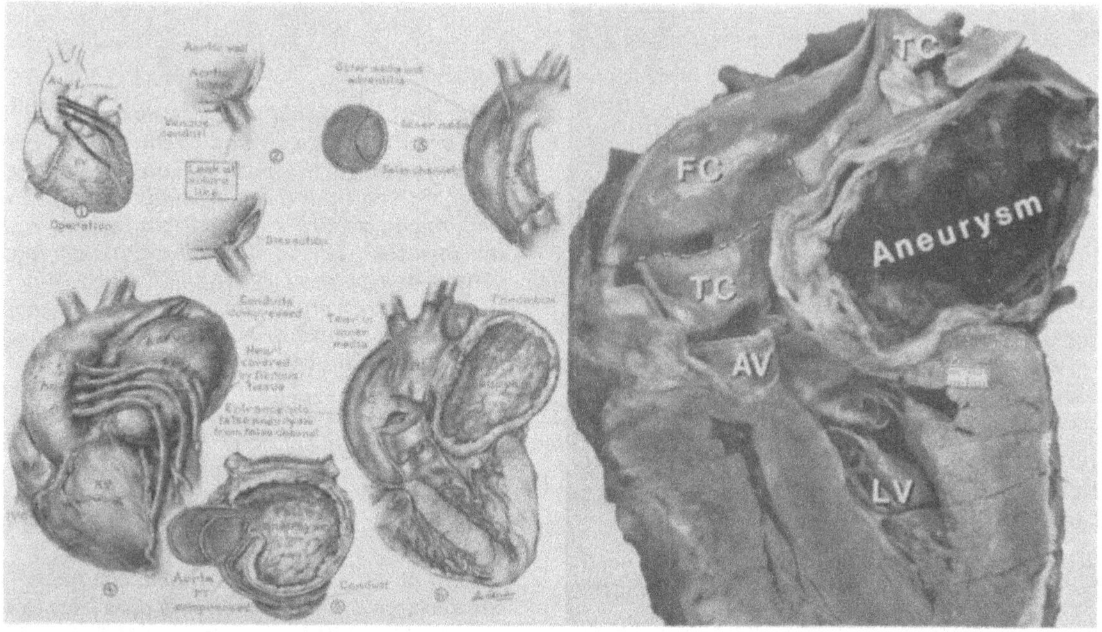

FIGURE 2. Patient 2. **Left,** the sequence of events leading to false aneurysm of the ascending aorta (Ao) after coronary artery bypass grafting. Saphenous vein conduits connect the ascending aorta to the left anterior descending, first diagonal, left obtuse marginal, and left circumflex coronary arteries (**1**). At operation, the aorta was described as dilated and more posterior than usual. Placement of the aortic anastomoses was technically difficult and required more than the usual amount of aortic manipulation. A limited dissection originated at an aortic anastomosis (**2**) and extended to the origin of the innominate artery (**3**). Rupture of the posterior wall of the false channel (FC) caused formation of a large false aneurysm, contained by fibrous tissue, which caused stretching of the saphenous vein conduits (**4**) and compression of the left atrium (LA) and pulmonary trunk (PT) (**5**). The walls of the aneurysm were focally calcified and lined by thrombus (**6**). **Right,** The heart at necropsy showing the large aortic tear (**dashed line**) and resulting true (TC) and false channels (FC). Rupture of the outer partition of the false channel led to formation of the large false aneurysm located in the left atrioventricular groove. AV = aortic valve; IVC = inferior vena cava; LV = left ventricle; RA = right atrium; RV = right ventricle.

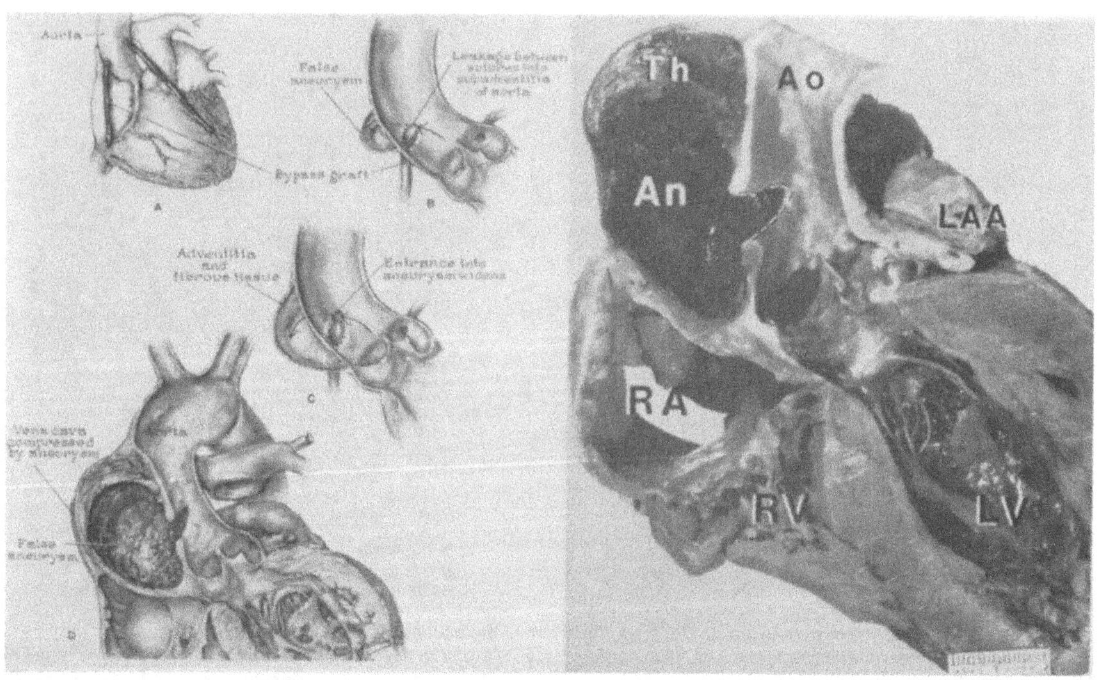

FIGURE 3. Patient 3: **Left,** the presumed sequence of events leading to false aneurysm of ascending aorta after coronary artery bypass grafting (CABG). Saphenous vein conduits connected the ascending aorta (Ao) to the right and left anterior descending coronary arteries (**A**). Postoperative Dressler's syndrome was treated with large doses of corticosteroids. The patient was taking 10 mg of prednisone daily 36 months after CABG. A healed tear adjacent to the site of the aortic anastomosis of the conduit (**B**) enlarged and ruptured through the aortic wall (**C**), giving rise to a false aneurysm which compressed the superior vena cava and right atrium (RA) (**D**). **Right,** the heart at necropsy. The aortic tear originated at a saphenous vein anastomosis (not shown) and forms the mouth of the large aneurysm (An), which contains thrombus (Th). LAA = left atrial appendage; LV = left ventricle; RV = right ventricle.

TABLE I Pertinent Clinical and Morphologic Findings in 4 Necropsy Patients with Ascending Aortic Aneurysms Developing After Aortocoronary Bypass Grafting (CABG)

Case	Age (yr)	No. of Aortic Anastomoses (no. occluded)	SH PO	C-S Rx	M	CTD	Interval (mo) Between CABG and Death	HW (g)	Healed MI
1	57	2 (1)	0	0	0	0	1.3	690	+
2	76	4 (2)	—	0	0	0	23	670	+
3	66	2 (1)	+	+	0	0	40	380	0
4	32	2 (2)	0	0	+	+	3.5	300	0

C-S Rx = corticosteroid therapy; CTD = connective tissue disease; HW = heart weight; M = acute mediastinitis; MI = myocardial infarction; SH PO = systemic hypertension postoperatively; + = present; 0 = absent; — = unknown.

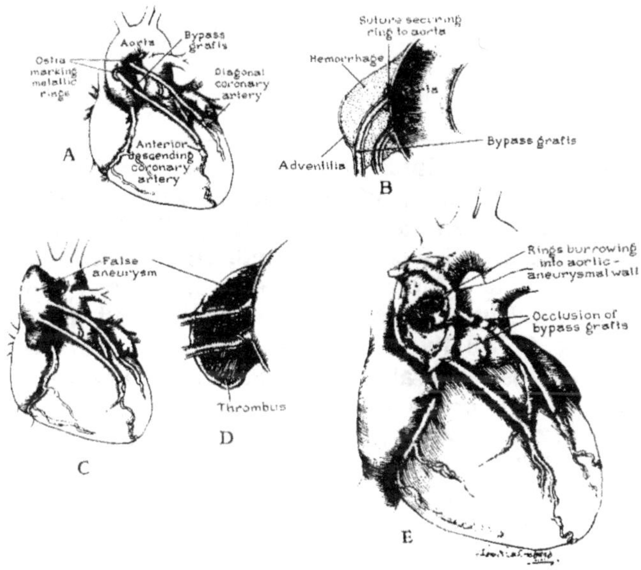

FIGURE 4. Patient 4. The sequence of events leading to false aneurysm after coronary artery bypass grafting in a 32-year-old woman with pseudoxanthoma elasticum. Saphenous vein conduits, marked at the aortic anastomoses by metallic rings, connected the aorta to the left anterior descending and first diagonal coronary arteries (**A**). The postoperative course was complicated by mediastinal infection. Leakage of blood at the aortic anastomoses caused an adventitial hematoma (**B**), eventually leading to formation of a false aneurysm filled with thrombus (**C, D**). At necropsy, the metallic rings had burrowed through the aortic wall and the conduits were occluded (**E**).

The principle illustrated by each of the 4 patients described herein is that an incision into the wall of ascending aorta for any purpose potentially sets the stage for the aorta to form a medial dissection and/or a false aneurysm at or near the site of initial entrance into the aorta. The incision into the aorta may be an aortotomy for aortic valve replacement, a cannulation site for cardiopulmonary bypass, or an incision for insertion of a conduit between aorta and coronary artery. These incisions, if not perfectly closed, can allow leakage of blood into the adjacent well. The resulting dissecting hematoma may progressively enlarge and produce a false aneurysm as illustrated by the aforementioned 4 patients. The appearance on the chest roentgenogram of a dilated aorta after any open heart operation that includes an incision into the aorta or the insertion of an instrument into the aorta suggests that a dissection or false aneurysm has occurred and has the potential to rupture.

Reference

1. **Roberts WC.** Aortic dissection: anatomy, consequences, and causes. Am Heart J 1981;101:195–214.

Arrhythmogenic Right Ventricular Dysplasia Associated with Atrioventricular Conduction Disturbance

LEE B. BEERMAN, MD
JAMES R. ZUBERBUHLER, MD
WILLIAM H. NECHES, MD
DONALD R. FISCHER, MD
FREDERICK J. FRICKER, MD
ROBERT A. MATHEWS, MD
SANG C. PARK, MD
CORA C. LENOX, MD

From the Department of Pediatrics, Children's Hospital of Pittsburgh, University of Pittsburgh School of Medicine, Pittsburgh, Pennsylvania.

Manuscript received February 24, 1983; revised manuscript received May 10, 1983, accepted May 16, 1983.

Right ventricular (RV) dysplasia is an unusual entity that consists of partial or complete replacement of the RV musculature by fibrous or adipose tissue.[1] When there are focal areas of RV dysplasia and hypo- or dyskinesia associated with recurrent ventricular dysrhythmias that originate from the right ventricle, the syndrome has been called arrhythmogenic RV dysplasia (ARVD).[1,2] A few children with ventricular ectopic activity and ARVD have been reported; however, most cases have occurred in adults.[1–3] Atrioventricular (AV) conduction disturbances have only rarely been mentioned.[1] This report describes a boy with syncope, complex ventricular ectopic activity and infra-His conduction system disease associated with ARVD.

The 16-year-old white boy with the Hallerman-Streiff syndrome had no cardiac symptoms until syncope occurred while boarding a bus. Frequent ventricular ectopic activity

Remnant Saphenous Veins After Aortocoronary Bypass Grafting: Analysis of 3,394 Centimeters of Unused Vein from 402 Patients

BRUCE F. WALLER, MD, and WILLIAM C. ROBERTS, MD

To assess the status of a saphenous vein (SV) excised for coronary artery bypass grafting (CABG), 3,394 cm of remnant SV from 402 patients who underwent CABG were examined. The SV remnants were 0.5 to 52 cm long (mean 8.4). They were sectioned into 5-mm-long segments, and the resulting 6,788 five-millimeter segments were examined histologically: 5,896 (87%) were narrowed 0 to 25% in cross-sectional area by fibrous tissue; 853 (12%) were narrowed 26 to 50%; 23 (0.6%), 51 to 75%, and 16 (0.4%) segments were narrowed 76 to 100%. Of the 16 segments severely narrowed, 7 (44%) were nearly totally occluded by fibrous tissue. In 17 patients who died within 24 hours of CABG, similar degrees of luminal narrowing were observed in remnant segments and in utilized segments of SV. Thus, significant preexisting luminal narrowing of SV used for CABG is infrequent. The intimal fibrous thickening is variable within the same vein when each 5-mm-long segment is analyzed; it is variable from 1 vein to another in the same patient, and it varies among patients.

(Am J Cardiol 1985;55:65–71)

Many studies describing early and late morphologic changes occurring in the saphenous vein (SV) used for coronary artery bypass grafting (CABG) have been published.[1–17] Little attention has been focused, however, on the status of the excised SV not used for CABG.[18–20] This study describes morphologic findings in remnant portions of excised SV from 402 patients who underwent CABG.

Methods

Veins studied: Remnants of operatively excised SVs were examined from 402 patients who underwent CABG at the National Heart, Lung, and Blood Institute between January 1972 and December 1981. At the time of CABG, the SV to be used for bypass grafting was isolated between the ankle and knee or thigh or both areas from 1 or both legs. After attached veins were ligated, the SV was removed and washed with heparinized saline solution. All unused segments of SV were submitted for gross and histologic examination. The submitted remnant SV was not simply discarded portions of abnormal SV, but represented all unused segments of SV. The length of the unused segment was measured (in centimeters) and the entire SV remnant was sectioned into 5-mm-long segments (Fig. 1 and 2). The segments were dehydrated, embedded in paraffin, sectioned and stained by the Movat pentachrome method. The percent of cross-sectional area (XSA) luminal narrowing of each SV segment was graded histologically, after magnification to about 40 times, into 4 categories: 0 to 25, 26 to 50, 51 to 75 and 76 to 100 (Fig. 1, 3 and 4). The internal elastic membrane was considered the normal outer rim of the lumen. A total of 3,394 cm of remnant SV were examined (Table I).

Patients: The 402 patients were 34 to 75 years old (mean 56): 16 (4%) were 34 to 40; 77 (19%) were 41 to 50; 184 (46%) were 51 to 60; 115 (29%) were 61 to 70; and 10 (2%) were 71 to 80 (Table I). Of the 402 patients, 337 (84%) were men, from whom 2,789 (82%) cm of remnant SV were examined. No patient had previous CABG, a known history of phlebitis or other diseases of the leg veins, and none had preoperative venograms.

Comparison of unused segments of saphenous vein with segments used as aortocoronary bypass grafts: Of the 402 patients who underwent CABG, 17 (4%) died within 24 hours of operation, and a necropsy was performed (Table II). Of these 17 patients, 13 (76%) could not be separated from the bypass pump, 1 died 6 hours and 3 died 24 hours after operation. These 17 patients had 327 cm of aortocoronary SV bypass conduit available for comparison with 169 cm of their respective SV remnants (Table II). The 17 necropsy patients were of similar age (34 to 68 years, mean 54) and sex (12 men, 71%) to the remaining 385 living patients. The percent of 5-mm segments of SV narrowed to various degrees was similar in 654 SV segments from bypass grafts compared with 338 SV segments from submitted remnants: 0 to 25%: graft = 94%,

From the Pathology Branch, National Heart, Lung, and Blood Institute, National Institutes of Health, Bethesda, Maryland. Manuscript received and accepted September 5, 1984.

Address for reprints: Bruce F. Waller, MD, Department of Pathology, University Hospital, N340, Indiana University School of Medicine, Indianapolis, Indiana 46223.

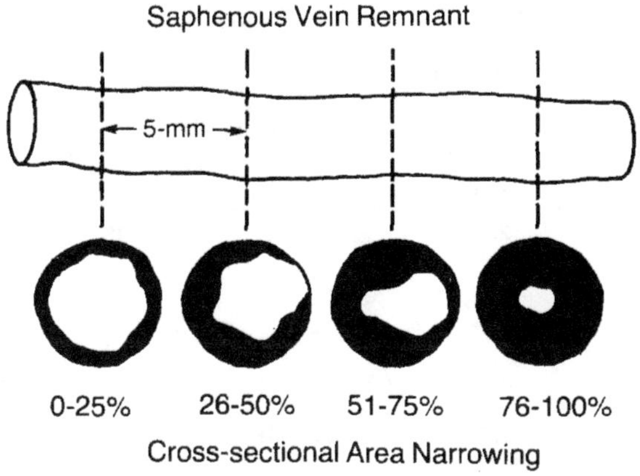

FIGURE 1. The method of sectioning of saphenous vein remnants at 5-mm intervals and the 4 grades of luminal cross-sectional area narrowing.

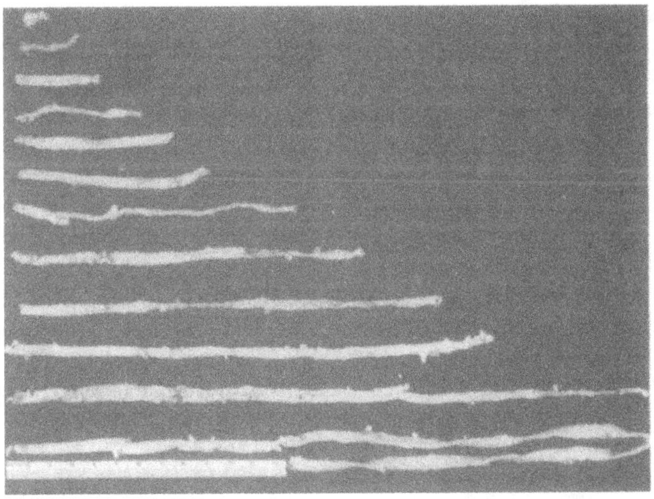

FIGURE 2. Twelve saphenous vein remnants showing the wide range in specimen lengths. The remnants in these 12 patients were 1 to 52 cm long.

remnant = 92%; 26 to 50%: graft = 6%, remnant = 8%; 51 to 100%: graft and remnant = 0 (Table II).

Histology of normal saphenous vein: The wall of the human SV contains a thin intima, separated from media by a rudimentary, fragmented internal elastic membrane. The media consists of 2 layers of smooth muscle cells: an internal longitudinal layer mixed with bundles of collagen and an external circular layer. The adventitia is composed of bundles of collagen, scattered foci of smooth muscle cells and vasa vasorum. At the insertion of venous valves, the medial longitudinal layer usually is thickened.

Results

Remnant length: The SV remnants were from 0.5 to 52 cm long (mean 8.4) (Table I, Fig. 2). The average length of unused portions of SV was similar in men (8.3 cm) and women (9.3 cm), and in younger (50 years or younger [8.8 cm]) and older (older than 50 years [8.4 cm]) patients.

Degrees of cross-sectional area luminal narrowing: SV luminal narrowing consisted of various degrees of intimal fibrous thickening composed of acellular connective tissue. The amount of luminal XSA narrowing in 6,788 five-millimeter SV segments graded histologically was: 0 to 25% XSA = 5,896 (87%) segments; 26 to 50% = 853 (12%); 51 to 75% = 23 (0.6%); and 76 to 100% = 16 (0.4%) segments (Table I, Fig. 3 to 6). Of 5,896 segments narrowed 0 to 25% in XSA by fibrous tissue, only 649 (11%) segments were narrowed to 0 to 5% (i.e., virtually normal). Of 16 segments (from 10 patients) narrowed 76 to 100% in XSA, 7 (44%) segments (from 7 patients) were narrowed 95 to 100% (i.e., virtually occluded) (Fig. 4D, 5 and 7).

Relation of amounts of saphenous vein intimal thickening to sex: The relation between various amounts of XSA narrowing and sex is summarized in Table I and Figure 8. Of 5,578 SV segments from 337 men, 13 (0.5%) segments were narrowed 76 to 100% in

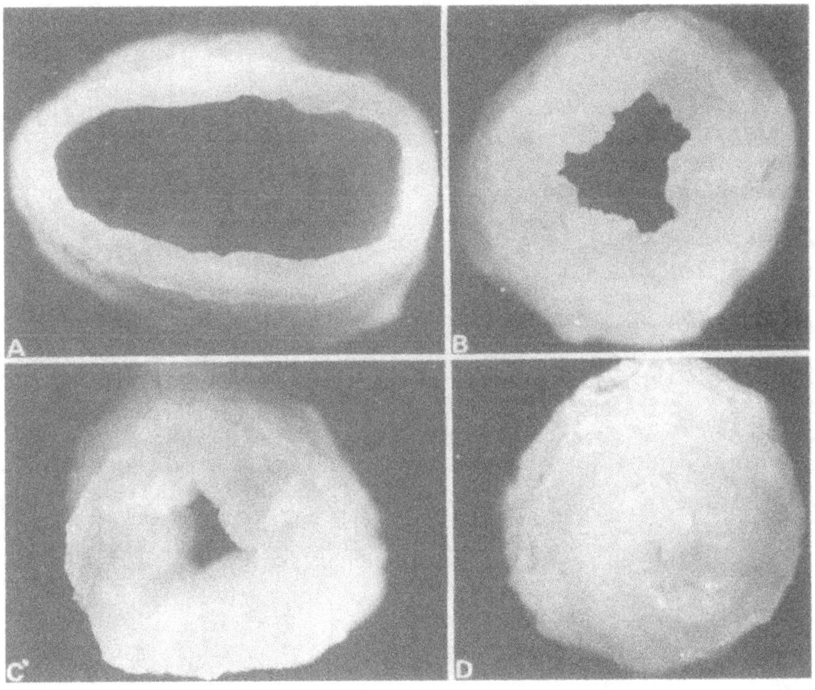

FIGURE 3. Photomacrographs of 4 saphenous vein remnants showing the 4 grades of cross-sectional area narrowing: **A,** (S80-2) 0 to 25%; **B,** (S78-103) 26 to 50%; **C,** (S77-17) 51 to 75%; **D,** (S80-92) 76 to 100%.

TABLE I Certain Clinical Findings in 402 Patients Undergoing Aortocoronary Bypass Grafting and Morphologic Observations in 3,394 CM of Remnant Saphenous Vein

Age (yr) (range, mean)	No. of Pts	Sex M:F	L of SV Remnant (cm)	Total L (cm)	Total 5-mm Seg	No. (%) Narrowed to Various Amounts in XSA by Intimal Fibrosis 0–25	26–50	51–75	76–100
34–40 (38)	16	15:1	4–24 (9.4)	150	300	231 (77)	65 (22)	3 (0.6)	1 (0.4)
41–50 (47)	77	69:8	0.5–35 (8.1)	620.5	1,241	1,087(87)	146(12)	1 (0.2)	7 (0.8)
51–60 (56)	184	150:34	0.5–52 (8.2)	1,500	3,000	2,640 (88)	346 (11)	10 (0.6)	4 (0.4)
61–70 (65)	115	96:19	1–34 (9.1)	1,046	2,092	1,818 (87)	264 (12)	6 (0.5)	4 (0.5)
71–80 (72)	10	7:3	3–10 (7.8)	77.5	155	120 (77)	32 (21)	3 (2)	0
Subtotal									
Men: 34–73 (55)		337 M (84%)	0.5–52 (8.3)	2,789	5,578	4,889 (87)	658 (12)	18 (0.5)	13 (0.5)
Women: 40–75 (58)		65 F (16%)	1–34 (9.3)	605	1,210	1,007 (83)	195 (16)	5 (0.6)	3 (0.4)
Total 34–75 (56)	402	337:65	0.5–52 (8.4)	3,394	6,788	5,896 (87)	853 (12)	23 (0.6)	16 (0.4)

L = length; Seg = segments; SV = saphenous vein; XSA = cross-sectional area.

XSA, 18 (0.5%) were narrowed 51 to 75%, and 5,547 (99%) segments were narrowed 0 to 50%. Similarly, of 1,210 SV segments from 65 women, 3 (0.4%) segments were narrowed 76 to 100% in XSA, 5 (0.6%) were narrowed 51 to 75%, and 1,202 (99%) were narrowed 0 to 50% (Fig. 8). Significant differences in amounts of XSA narrowing between men and women occurred only in the 0 to 50% category. Compared with men, women had a significantly greater percent of SV narrowed 26 to 50% in XSA (16 vs 12%), but a significantly lower percent of SV segments narrowed 0 to 25% in XSA ($p < 0.05$) (Fig. 8).

Relation of amounts of saphenous vein narrowing to age: The relation between patient age and various

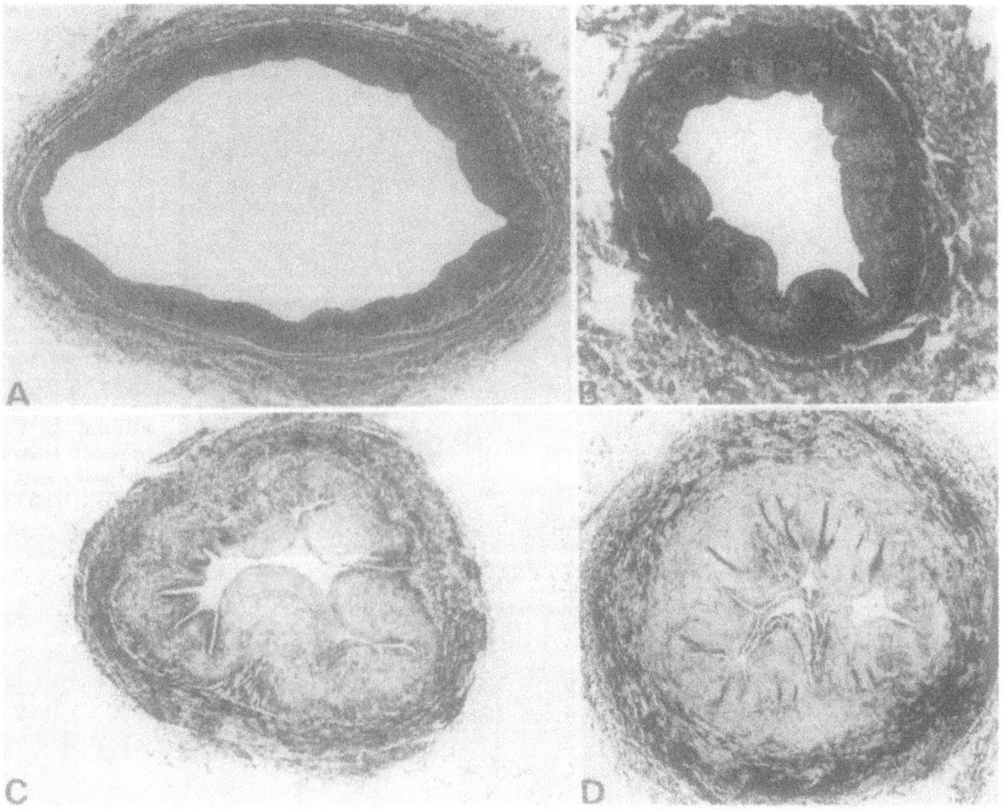

FIGURE 4. Photomicrographs of histologic sections of the 4 saphenous vein remnants illustrated in Figure 3. Movat stain.

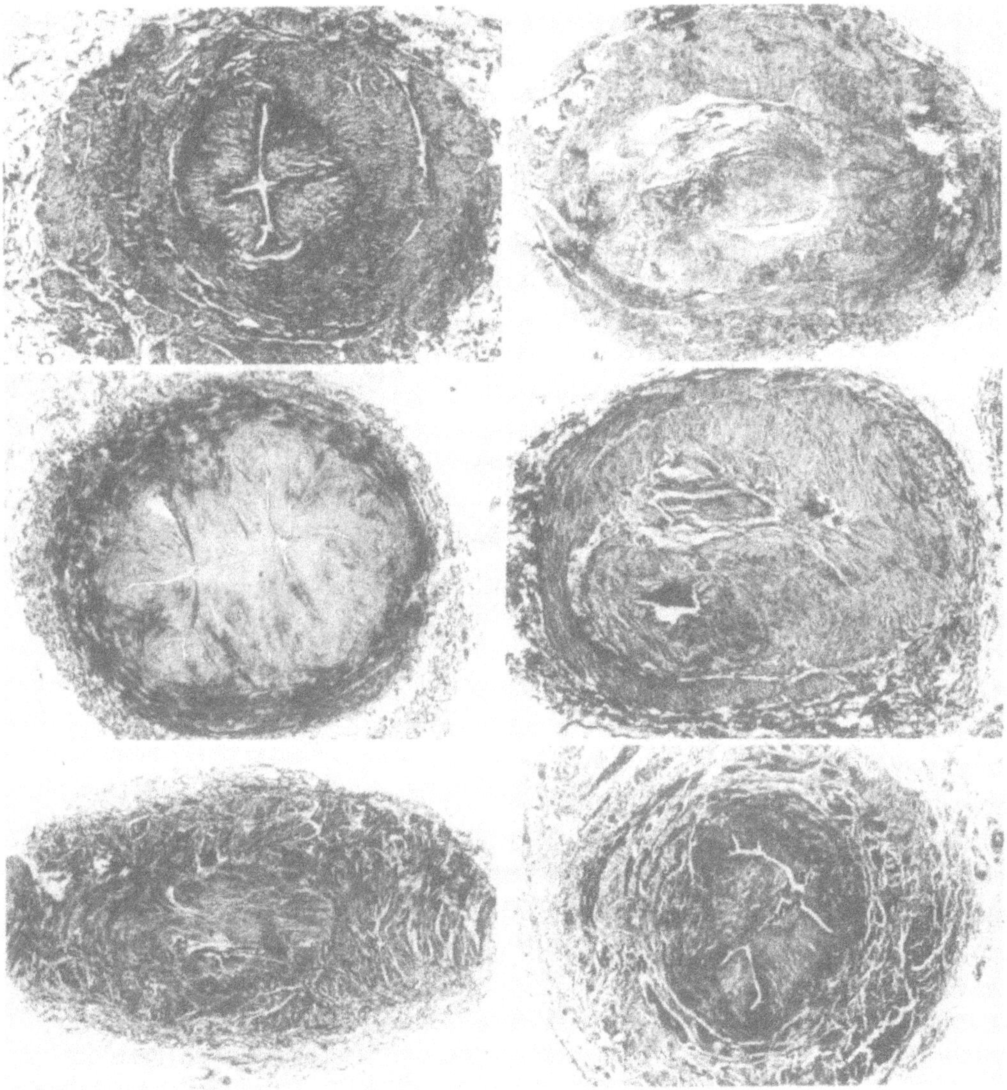

FIGURE 5. Photomicrographs of sites of maximal narrowing in saphenous vein remnants from 6 patients undergoing bypass operation (S79-162, S79-165, S81-63, S81-71, S81-175 and S81-202). All 6 remnants have severe luminal cross-sectional area narrowing by intimal fibrosis. Movat stain.

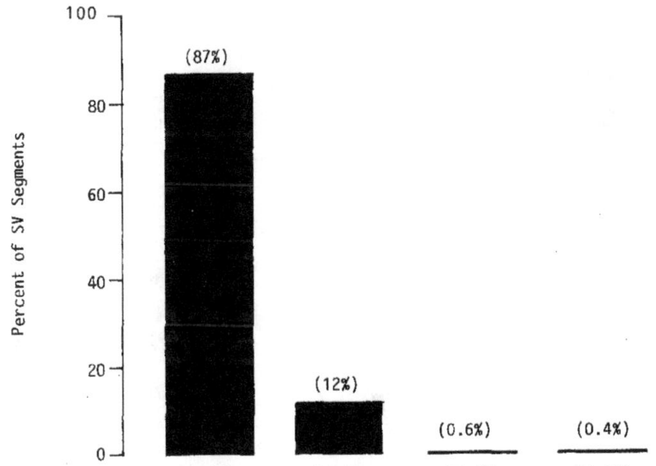

FIGURE 6. Percent of 6,788 five-millimeter-long segments of saphenous vein (SV) remnant from 402 patients undergoing aortocoronary bypass operation, narrowed to various degrees in cross-sectional area by intimal fibrosis.

amounts of luminal XSA narrowing is summarized in Table I and in Figure 9. Of 1,541 SV segments from 93 patients aged 50 years and younger, 8 (0.5%) segments were narrowed 76 to 100% in XSA by intimal fibrous tissue, compared with 8 (0.1%) of 5,247 segments from 309 patients aged older than 50 years. Analysis of luminal narrowing by age decade (Table I, Fig. 9) disclosed a similar frequency of severe (>75% XSA) narrowing between the fourth and seventh decades. No patient in the eighth decade of life had severe (>75% XSA) SV remnant luminal narrowing.

Relation of amount of saphenous vein luminal narrowing to sex and age: Analysis of SV remnants disclosed a similar frequency of severe luminal narrowing in men (7 of 1,392 [0.5%]) and women (1 of 149 [0.7%]) aged 50 years and younger and a similar frequency in men (6 of 4,186 [0.1%]) and women (2 of 1,061 [0.2%]) aged 50 years and older (Fig. 10).

Varicosity of saphenous vein remnants: Of 402 patients, 20 (5%) had focally or diffusely dilated SV remnants. The wall of the SV at sites of dilation were

TABLE II Comparison of Number of Segments and Percent Cross-Sectional Area Narrowing by Intimal Fibrosis in Saphenous Vein Aortocoronary Bypass Grafts and Their Respective Unused Saphenous Vein Remnants in 17 Necropsy Patients Dying Within 1 Day of Bypass Operation

No.	Age (yr) & Sex	Interval (days) Op → D	Length (cm) of SV		Total 5-mm SV Seg		No. (%) of Seg and XSA Narrowing by Intimal Fibrosis							
							0–25		26–50		51–75		76–100	
			G	R	G	R	G	R	G	R	G	R	G	R
1	34M	OR	22	6	44	12	40 (91)	10 (83)	4 (9)	2 (17)	0	0	0	0
2	40M	0.5	7.5	8	13	16	11 (85)	14 (88)	2 (15)	2 (12)	0	0	0	0
3	40F	OR	30	9	60	18	50 (83)	13 (72)	10 (17)	5 (18)	0	0	0	0
4	42M	OR	12	9	24	18	24 (100)	18 (100)	0	0	0	0	0	0
5	47F	1	9	14	18	28	18 (100)	27 (96)	0	1 (4)	0	0	0	0
6	49M	OR	21	11	42	22	38 (90)	19 (86)	4 (10)	3 (14)	0	0	0	0
7	56F	OR	12	17	24	34	20 (83)	27 (79)	4 (17)	7 (21)	0	0	0	0
8	56M	1	22	7	44	14	40 (91)	14 (100)	4 (9)	0	0	0	0	0
9	57M	OR	21	10	42	20	35 (83)	15 (75)	7 (17)	5 (25)	0	0	0	0
10	57M	OR	29	5	58	10	58 (100)	10 (100)	0	0	0	0	0	0
11	59M	OR	20.5	16	41	32	41 (100)	32 (100)	0	0	0	0	0	0
12	60M	OR	29.5	12	59	24	59 (100)	24 (100)	0	0	0	0	0	0
13	60M	OR	26	7	52	14	52 (100)	14 (100)	0	0	0	0	0	0
14	61F	OR	20.5	9	41	18	39 (95)	18 (100)	2 (5)	0	0	0	0	0
15	62M	1	16	11	32	22	32 (100)	21 (95)	0	1 (5)	0	0	0	0
16	64M	OR	13	10	26	20	24 (92)	19 (92)	2 (8)	1 (5)	0	0	0	0
17	68F	OR	17	8	34	16	34 (100)	15 (94)	0	1 (6)	0	0	0	0
Total range (Avg) 34–68 (54)	12M 5F	0–1 (0.2)	327 (19)	169 (10)	654	338	615 (94%)	310 (92%)	39 (6%)	28 (8%)	0	0	0	0

Avg = average; D = death; G = aortocoronary bypass graft; Op = operation; OR = operating room; R = remnant of excised SV; 0 = none; other abbreviations as in Table I.

thinner than normal in 16 patients and thicker than normal in 4 patients.

Discussion

Fibrous thickening of lumens of SV grafts studied early after CABG generally has been regarded as an acquired change rather than as a preexisting preoperative occurrence.[2–5,7] In the present study, analysis of unused portions of operatively excised SV disclosed varying degrees of intimal fibrous thickening in over 90% of SV segments before their use for CABG. Of 402 patients studied, the luminal narrowing was severe (>75% XSA) in 10 patients (16 segments [0.4%]) with near-total occlusion of segments from 7 patients.

Although intimal fibrous thickening is a common finding in the SV used as an aortocoronary conduit for more than 1 month,[2–5,7] considerable variation in amounts of intimal thickening is observed in grafts in

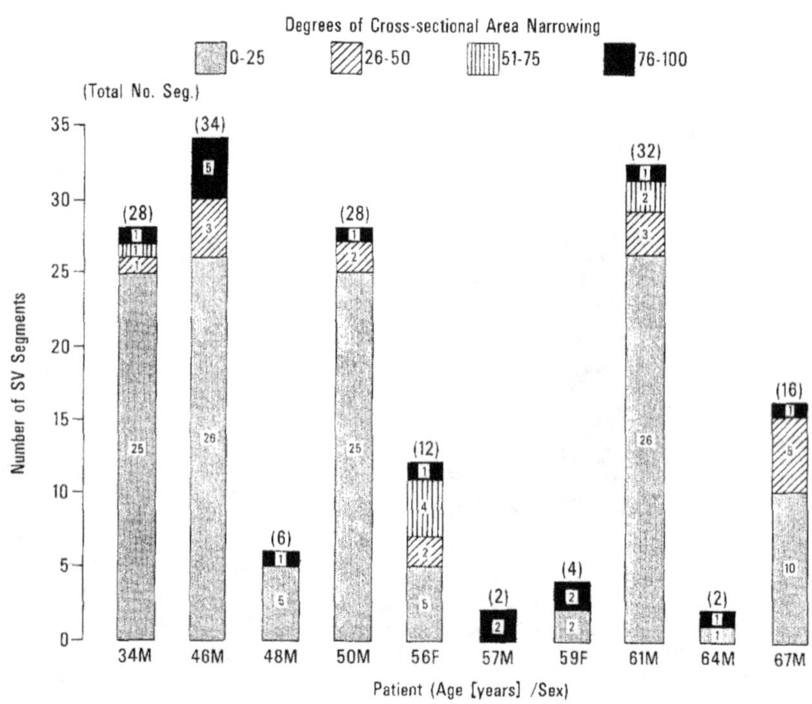

FIGURE 7. The variability in luminal cross-sectional area narrowing within the same saphenous vein (SV) remnant from the 10 patients having at least 1 five-millimeter SV segment (Seg.) narrowed 76 to 100% in cross-sectional area by intimal thickening.

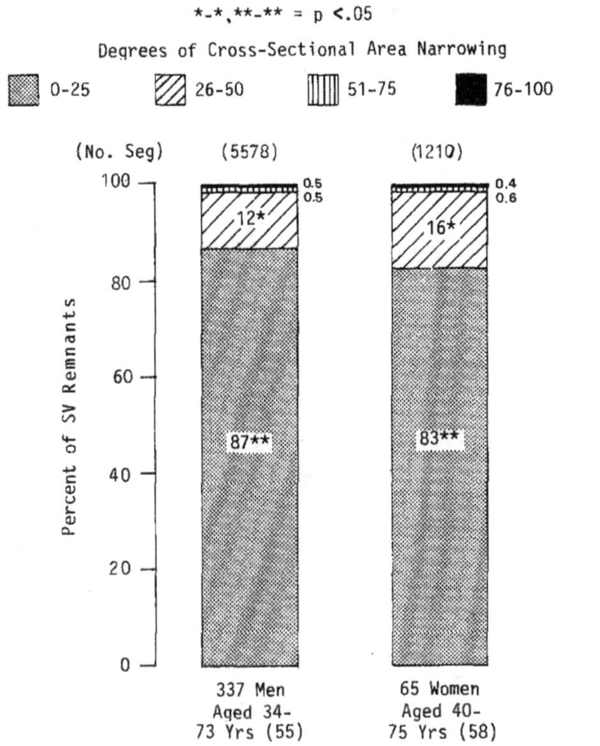

FIGURE 8. Relation between sex and degrees of cross-sectional area luminal narrowing by intimal fibrosis in 6,788 five-millimeter segments (Seg) of saphenous vein (SV) remnant from 337 men and 65 women who underwent aortocoronary bypass grafting.

place for a similar length of time. The variability in degree and extent of the luminal narrowing among different patients has been attributed to such factors as differing systemic arterial pressures,[4] vein damage during SV excision or manipulation before implantation,[21,22] and vein damage from agents used in preparation of the SV for implantation.[23] The high frequency of fibrous thickening in unused SV in the present study, and a similar distribution of these changes in remnant SV segments and their corresponding aortocoronary bypass graft segments suggests that preexisting intimal fibrous thickening may account for some of the variability. Preexisting severe narrowing of the SV used as a conduit of course may impede graft flow.

Two previous studies[18,20] have commented on morphologic changes observed in excised SV intended for use as aortocoronary bypass grafts. Cheanvechai et al[18] examined "representative pieces" of SV not used for grafting procedures from 1,179 patients undergoing CABG. Of 1,179 SV segments, 861 (73%) were "normal" and 318 (27%) were "abnormal." Of the 318 abnormal veins, 280 (88%) were "mildly phlebosclerotic" and 38 (12%) were "moderately sclerotic." Of the 1,170 patients, 391 underwent postoperative conduit angiography 1.5 to 24 months after operation (295 patients with normal SV remnants, 86 patients with abnormal SV remnants); no significant differences were observed in graft patency rates, graft stenoses, or luminal irregularities between the 2 groups. They concluded that the phlebosclerotic vein could be used as a bypass conduit without adverse results. Their study, however, did not define "mild" or "moderate" amounts of phlebosclerosis, and it did not correlate changes in unused (nonimplanted) segments of SV with those in used (implanted) segments.

Thiene et al[20] examined SV from 150 consecutive patients who underwent CABG. Intimal fibrous thickening was observed in 93%, but it was rarely severe enough to narrow the lumen more than 50% (unit not stated). These investigators graded amounts of intimal sclerosis as 1 to 4 with grade 4 representing luminal narrowing greater than 50%. Of 150 veins, 105 (70%) had intimal fibrous thickening but no SV segment had more than 50% luminal narrowing.

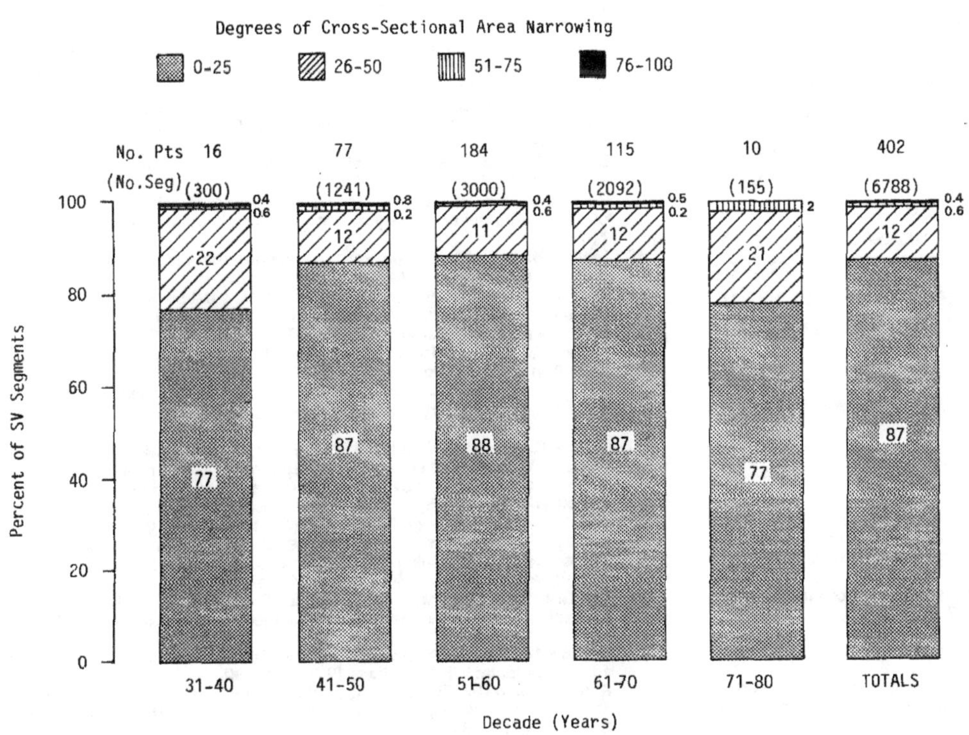

FIGURE 9. Relation between age and degrees of cross-sectional area luminal narrowing by intimal fibrosis in 6,788 five-millimeter segments (Seg) of saphenous vein (SV) remnant from 402 patients aged 31 to 75 years (mean 56) who underwent aortocoronary bypass grafting.

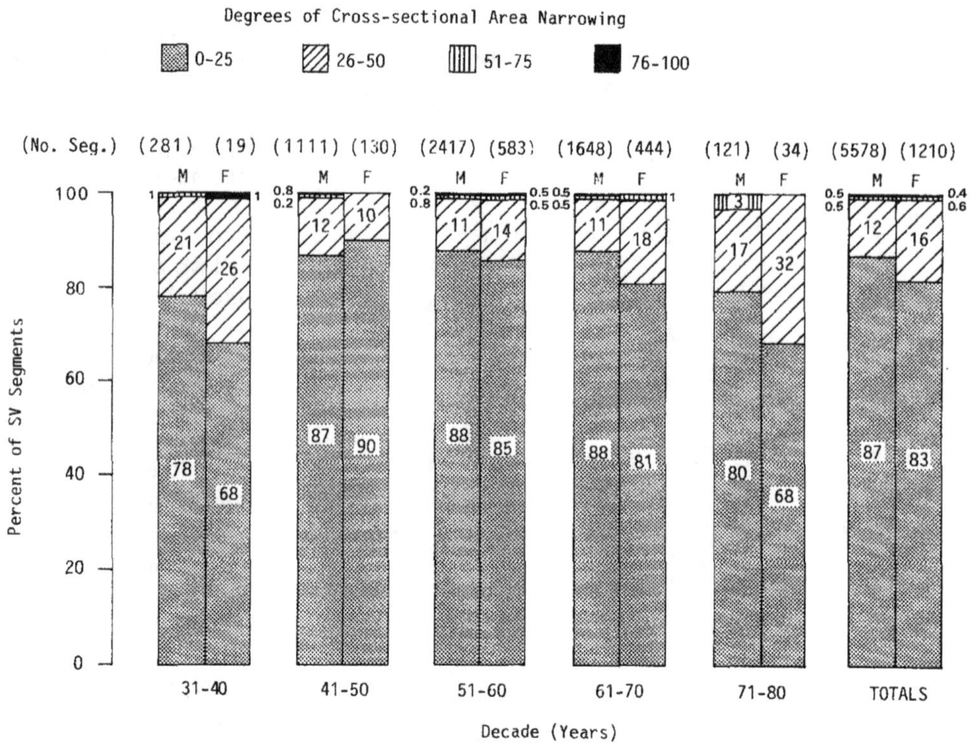

FIGURE 10. Relation between sex, age and degrees of cross-sectional area luminal narrowing by intimal fibrosis in 6,788 five-millimeter segments (Seg.) of saphenous vein (SV) remnants from 402 patients who underwent aortocoronary bypass grafting.

Saphenous vein intimal fibrous thickening has been stated to increase with advancing age and to occur more frequently in women.[24] In our study and in the study by Thiene et al,[20] age did not correlate with the amount of intimal fibrous thickening. Furthermore, in the present study, severe (>75% XSA) intimal fibrous thickening was similar in both men and women.

About 5% of SV remnants examined in our study had varicoses. Although focal aneurysmal dilation of an implanted aortocoronary SV bypass graft has been reported,[25] its rarity suggests that focal graft aneurysm formation probably represents focal varicoses of the SV present at the time of graft insertion.

Of our 402 patients who underwent CABG, nearly 3,500 cm of SV (about 8.5 cm per patient) was not implanted. The length of unused SV ranged from 0.5 to 52 cm per patient; 45 patients (11%) had at least 15 cm of remnant vein. Repeat CABG is increasing and, correspondingly, the need for additional autogenous bypass graft material is increasing. Perhaps unused excised SV could be "stored" for future use in the same patient, or "denatured" and used as homologous bypass grafts in patients with depleted or diseased SV systems.

Acknowledgment: We thank Filippina Giacometti for her countless hours of tissue embedding, sectioning and staining.

References

1. **Marti MC, Bouchardy B, Cox JN.** Aorto-coronary bypass with autologous saphenous vein grafts: Histopathologic aspects. Virchows Arch [A] 1971;352:255–266.
2. **Vlodaver Z, Edwards JE.** Pathologic changes in aortic-coronary arterial saphenous vein grafts. Circulation 1971;44:719–728.
3. **Kern WH, Dermer GB, Lindesmith GG.** The intimal proliferation in aorto-coronary saphenous vein grafts: light and electron microscopic studies. Am Heart J 1972;84:771–777.
4. **Brody WR, Kosek JC, Angell WW.** Changes in vein grafts following aorto-coronary bypass induced by pressure and ischemia. J Thorac Cardiovasc Surg 1972;64:847–854.
5. **Vlodaver Z, Edwards JE.** Pathologic analysis in fatal cases following saphenous vein coronary arterial bypass. Chest 1973;64:555–563.
6. **Unni KK, Kottke BA, Titus JL, Frye RL, Wallace RB, Brown HL.** Pathologic changes in aortocoronary saphenous vein grafts. Am J Cardiol 1974;34: 526–531.
7. **Lawrie GM, Brawley RK.** Vein graft patency and intimal proliferation after aorto-coronary bypass: early and long-term angiopathologic correlations. Am J Cardiol 1976;38:856–862.
8. **Spray TL, Roberts WC.** Status of the grafts and the native coronary arteries proximal and distal to coronary anastomotic sites of aortocoronary bypass grafts. Circulation 1977;55:741–749.
9. **Spray TL, Roberts WC.** Changes in saphenous veins used as aortocoronary bypass grafts. Am Heart J 1977;94:500–516.
10. **Griffith LSC, Bulkley BH, Hutchins GM, Brawley RK.** Occlusive changes at the coronary artery-bypass graft anastomosis. J Thorac Cardiovasc Surg 1977;73:668–679.
11. **Roscher AA, Kern WH.** Aortocoronary bypass surgery from the pathologist's point of view. A clinicopathologic study of 240 cases with 26 autopsies. Intern Surg 1977;62:282–293.
12. **Lie JT, Lawrie GM, Morris GC.** Aortocoronary bypass saphenous vein graft atherosclerosis. Anatomic study of 99 vein grafts from normal and hyperlipoproteinemic patients up to 75 months postoperatively. Am J Cardiol 1977;40:906–914.
13. **Batayias GE, Barboriak JJ, Korns ME, Pintar K.** The spectrum of pathologic changes in aortocoronary saphenous vein grafts. Circulation 1977;56:Suppl II:II-18–II-22.
14. **Bulkley BH, Hutchins GM.** Pathology of coronary artery bypass graft surgery. Arch Pathol Lab Med 1978;102:273–280.
15. **Bulkley BH, Hutchins GM.** Acute post-operative graft phlebitis: a rare cause of saphenous vein-coronary artery bypass failure. Am Heart J 1978;95: 757–760.
16. **Smith SH, Geer JC.** Morphology of saphenous vein-coronary artery bypass grafts. Arch Pathol Lab Med 1983;107:13–18.
17. **Dye TE, Izquierdo P.** Abnormal venous valves: a cause of early obstruction of saphenous vein bypass grafts. Tex Heart Inst J 1983;10:365–369.
18. **Cheanvechai C, Effler DB, Hooper JR, Eschenbruch EM, Sheldon WC, Sones FM Jr, Levin HS, Hawk WA.** The structural study of the saphenous vein. Ann Thorac Surg 1975;20:636–645.
19. **Mills NL, Ochsner JL.** Valvulotomy of valves in the saphenous vein graft before coronary artery bypass. J Thorac Cardiovasc Surg 1976;71:878–879.
20. **Thiene G, Miazzi P, Valsecchi M, Valente M, Bortolotti U, Casarotto D, Gallucci V.** Histologic survey of the saphenous vein before its use as autologous aortocoronary bypass graft. Thorax 1980;35:519–522.
21. **Abbott WM, Wieland S, Austen WG.** Structural changes during preparation of autogenous venous grafts. Surgery 1974;76:1031–1040.
22. **Gundry SR, Jones M, Ishihara T, Ferrans VJ.** Intraoperative trauma to human saphenous veins: scanning electron microscopic comparison of preparation techniques. Ann Thorac Sur 1980;30:40–47.
23. **MacGregor DC, Agarwal VK, Silver MD.** Changes produced in the wall of the saphenous vein of dogs by distending media and pressures. Surg Forum 1972;23:135–137.
24. **Robbins SL, Cotran RS.** Blood vessels. In: Pathologic Basis of Disease. 2nd ed. Philadelphia: WB Saunders, 1979:628–630.
25. **Riahi M, Vasu CM, Tomatis LA, Schlosser RJ, Zimmerman G.** Aneurysm of saphenous vein bypass graft to coronary artery. J Thorac Cardiovasc Surg 1975;70:358–359.

Illogical Use of Saphenous Veins for Aortocoronary Bypass Grafting

WANDA M. LESTER, MD
WILLIAM C. ROBERTS, MD

The saphenous vein (SV) is usually a wonderful structure for use as a conduit for bypassing 1 or more severe narrowings in a coronary artery. If, however, the lumen of the SV is small, because of superimposed phlebosclerosis or simply initial small size, the SV may not serve as an adequate conduit. The January 1 issue of the AJC contains a report describing the frequency of phlebosclerosis and the degrees of luminal narrowing produced by it in SV remnants not used for coronary bypass grafts.[1] The present report was prompted by observing 2 SVs at necropsy, a small-sized one containing considerable phlebosclerosis anastomosed directly to the aorta, and a good-sized one with a good lumen anastomosed not to the aorta, but to the small phlebosclerotic SV. This type of use of the SV does not appear reasonable.

From the Pathology Branch, National Heart, Lung, and Blood Institute, National Institutes of Health, Bethesda, Maryland. Dr. Lester was on a fellowship from the Canadian Heart Foundation. Manuscript received and accepted October 29, 1984.

W.G., a 74-year-old man who had nonfatal cardiac arrest at age 62 and onset of angina pectoris at age 68 years underwent angiography because of worsening angina. The amount of coronary arterial narrowing as percent of diameter reduction was as follows: right = 100; left anterior descending = 95; left circumflex = 60, and left main = 0. Left ventricular angiography disclosed no abnormalities. Aortocoronary bypass grafting was performed (at another hospital) with insertion of 1 SV graft (12 cm long) between the aorta and left anterior descending coronary artery (graft no. 1) with sequential grafting to a diagonal coronary artery. A second SV (graft no. 2) was 18 cm long and coursed around the left side

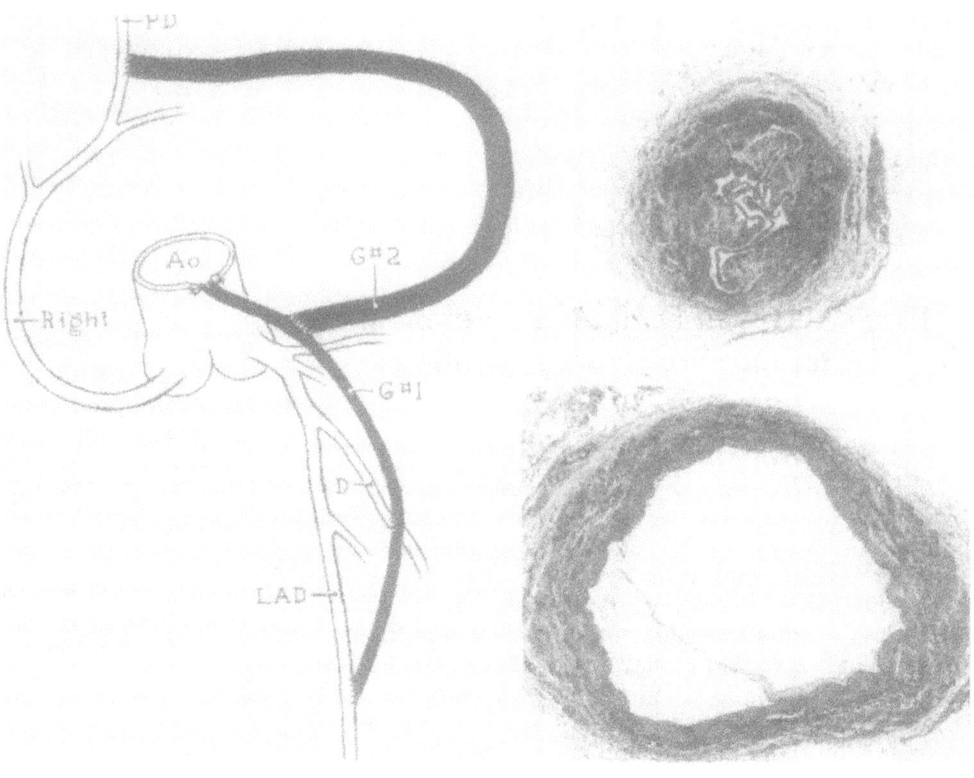

FIGURE 1. Left, drawing of portion of aorta and coronary arteries with saphenous vein grafts. Graft no. 1 (G#1) is much smaller than graft no. 2 (G#2). **Upper right,** photomicrograph of a section of graft no. 1 proximal to anastomosis to graft no. 2. The graft is small, its wall is thick, and its lumen is small. A valve is present within the lumen at this site. **Lower right,** photomicrograph of a section of graft no. 2 just distal to anastomosis to graft no. 1. The lumen is wide open. Ao = aorta; D = diagonal branch; LAD = left anterior descending artery; PD = posterior descending. (Movat stain × 23 [**upper and lower right**], reduced 39%.)

of the heart and connected a posterior descending coronary artery to graft no. 1 as shown in Figure 1. During the entire 8-hour postoperative period the patient was hypotensive and had complete heart block.

At necropsy, the lumens of the native coronary arteries distal to the SV anastomotic sites were insignificantly narrowed and the 3 coronary anastomotic sites were wide open. The lumen of graft no. 1 was very small as a result of both phlebosclerosis and the initial small size of the vein (Fig. 1). The lumen of graft no. 2 was large (Fig. 1). Study of 22 histologic sections (1 from each 5-mm segment) of graft no. 1 disclosed phlebosclerosis and a very narrowed lumen. Study of 31 histologic sections of graft no. 2 disclosed virtually no phlebosclerosis and a wide open lumen. Foci of coagulation and contraction-band necrosis were present in the walls of both cardiac ventricles.

In 1984, it appears unwise to graft 1 SV to another when each is used as a bypass conduit. Ample arguments against use of Y grafting of SVs were made as early as 1974.[2,3] In the present patient, the small graft was the only conduit connected to the aorta and the large graft was anastomosed directly to the small one. It would appear more reasonable in the present patient to have anastomosed graft no. 2 directly to the aorta. Had the graft been placed around the right side of the heart rather than the left, the graft could easily have reached the ascending aorta to be anastomosed directly to it. Because the small graft with an inadequate lumen was the only graft connected to the aorta, neither graft was perfused adequately.

References

1. **Waller BF, Roberts WC.** Remnant saphenous veins after aortocoronary bypass grafting: analysis of 3,394 centimeters of unused vein from 402 patients. Am J Cardiol 1985;55:65–71.
2. **Sewell WH.** Improved coronary vein graft patency rates with side-to-side anastomoses. Ann Thorac Surg 1974;17:538–544.
3. **Sewell WH.** Should we do Y- and sequential grafts for coronary bypass? Ann Thorac Surg 1979;27:397–398.

Additional Evidence for Relative Resistance to Atherosclerosis of the Internal Mammary Artery Compared to Saphenous Vein When Used to Increase Myocardial Blood Supply

DEBORAH J. BARBOUR, MD
WILLIAM C. ROBERTS, MD

Since the advent of coronary artery bypass grafting in 1967, ventricular intramyocardial implantation of an internal mammary artery (IMA) directly into left ventricular (LV) myocardium (Vineberg procedure)[1] has been supplanted. We recently studied the heart of a patient who had undergone concomitant aortocoronary bypass grafting with a saphenous vein (SV) and implantation of an IMA into LV myocardium nearly 16 years earlier. This case provided an opportunity to examine 2 types of vessels used for myocardial revascularization.

J.S., a 63-year-old man in whom angina pectoris developed at age 46 years (1967), had coronary arteriography at age 48 years and it disclosed severe narrowing of the left main, left circumflex and right coronary arteries. In July 1969 an SV was anastomosed to the aorta and left anterior descending coronary artery and the left IMA was implanted into LV myocardium. He had no further chest pain until age 62 years (1 year before death), when angina reappeared. He died in December 1984 of pneumonia. At necropsy, the heart weighed 345 g and there was no LV necrosis or fibrosis. The IMA, which had been inserted into LV wall, SV graft and the epicardial coronary arteries were divided into 5-mm segments and 1 histologic section was prepared from each segment. The left main, left anterior descending, left circumflex and dominant right coronary arteries were all narrowed >75% in cross-sectional area at some point by atherosclerotic plaque. Although widely patent, the SV walls were focally calcified and contained considerable atherosclerotic plaque (Fig. 1). The extramyocardial portions of the IMA was normal and its intramyocardial portion was mildly thickened by intimal fibrous tissue (Fig. 1).

From the Pathology Branch, National Heart, Lung, and Blood Institute, National Institutes of Health, Bethesda, Maryland 20205. Manuscript received January 22, 1985, accepted February 25, 1985.

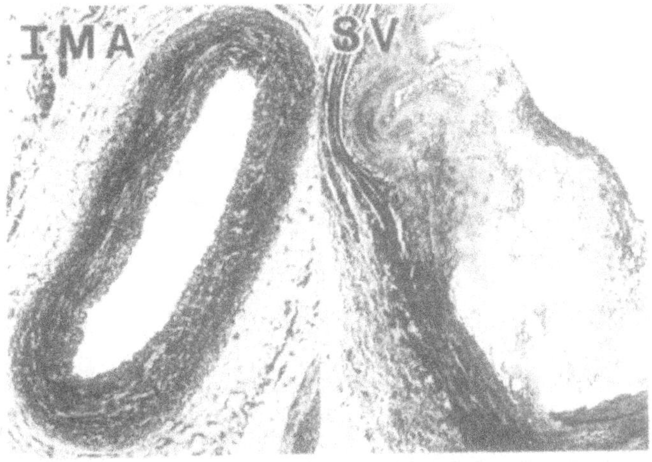

FIGURE 1. Cross-section of internal mammary artery (IMA) (extramyocardial portion) and portion of wall of saphenous vein (SV) in the patient described. The IMA is normal and the SV contains atherosclerotic plaque. Movat stains; original magnification × 54, reduced 46%.

Vineberg described necropsy findings in 3 patients who had had an IMA implanted into LV myocardium 6 to 14 years before death. In all 3 patients the IMA was normal in its extramyocardial segment and it had only mild intimal thickening in its intramyocardial portion. In all 3, postmortem angiography with injection of contrast material into the IMA resulted in retrograde filling of the proximally totally occluded native coronary arteries.[2]

Long-term patency of an IMA as an aorta-to-coronary-arterial graft is superior to that of SV grafts. A recent study cited an 84% 10-year patency for IMA grafts and 53% for SV grafts.[3] The lack of atherosclerotic plaque in the IMA and the presence of plaque in the concurrently placed SV graft in our patient gives further support to the apparent resistance of the IMA to atherosclerotic plaquing.[3]

References

1. **Vineberg A.** Revascularization of the entire heart through myocardial anteriolar networks. J Cardiovasc Surg 1970;11:suppl 3:168–194.
2. **Vineberg A.** Evidence that revascularization by ventricular-internal mammary artery implants increases longevity. Twenty-four year, nine month follow-up. J Thorac Cardiovasc Surg 1975;70:381–397.
3. **Grondin CM, Campeau L, Lesperance J, Enjalbert M, Bourassa MG.** Comparison of late changes in internal mammary artery and saphenous vein grafts in two consecutive series of patients 10 years after operation. Circulation 1984;70:suppl I:I-208–I-212.

Spasm of Saphenous Veins Used as Conduits for Aortocoronary Bypass Grafting

JESSICA M. MANN, MD
CHARLES L. McINTOSH, MD
WILLIAM C. ROBERTS, MD

Spasm of native epicardial coronary arteries early postoperatively after aortocoronary bypass grafting has been described.[1-3] Spasm of saphenous veins used as aortocoronary conduits has not been reported. This report describes such a case.

From the Pathology and Surgery Branches, National Heart, Lung, and Blood Institute, National Institutes of Health, Bethesda, Maryland 20892. Manuscript received and accepted November 4, 1986.

J.K., a 64-year-old white man who had smoked about 20 cigarettes daily for 30 years, had a stroke followed by carotid endarterectomy at age 60, and the onset of "burning" substernal chest pain unrelated to exertion but relieved quickly by nitrates at age 63 (9 months before death). One month before death, an exercise stress test result was positive (2 mm of ST-segment depression). The pressures (in mm Hg) were the following: pulmonary arterial wedge mean, 10; pulmonary artery, 30/13; left ventricle, 160/12; and systemic artery, 160/72. The cardiac index was 2.9 liters/min/m^2. Left ventricular angiography disclosed a normal-sized and normally contracting left ventricle without mitral regurgitation. The amount of diameter

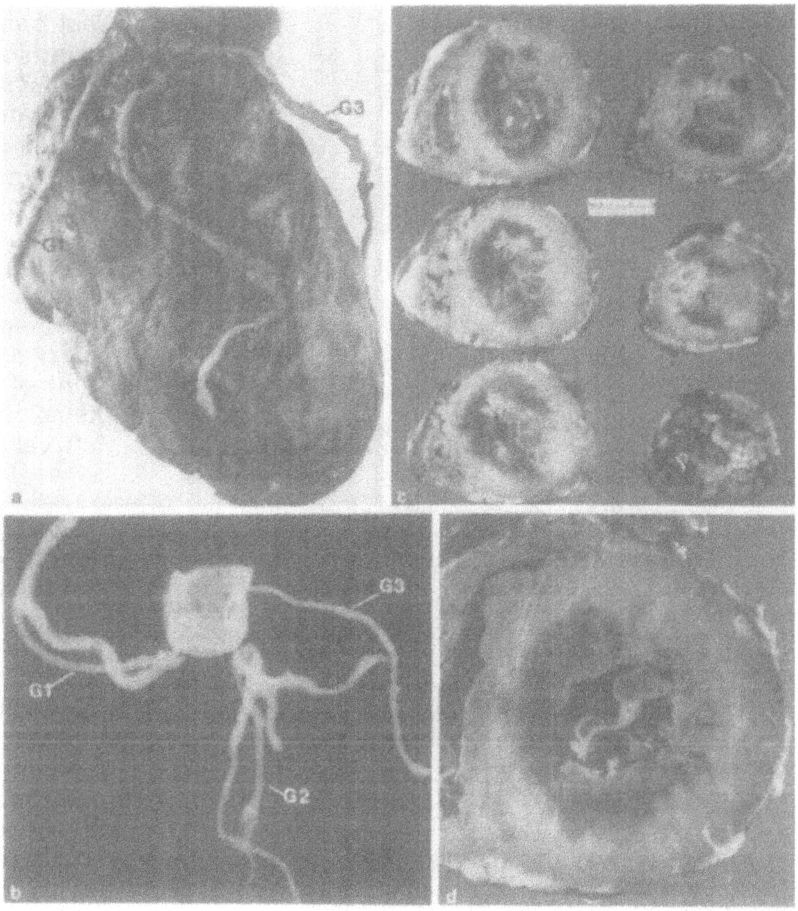

FIGURE 1. *a*, view of anterior portion of heart showing the saphenous vein grafts. G1, graft to the right coronary artery. G2, graft to the diagonal and left anterior descending. G3, graft to the left obtuse marginal. *b*, radiograph of ascending aorta, native coronary arteries and saphenous vein grafts. *c*, view of transverse cuts of the cardiac ventricles showing transmural left ventricular circumferential necrosis from apex to base. *d*, close-up view of the basal portion of left ventricle showing the circumferential hemorrhagic necrosis. A portion of mitral leaflet is visible in the normal-sized left ventricular cavity.

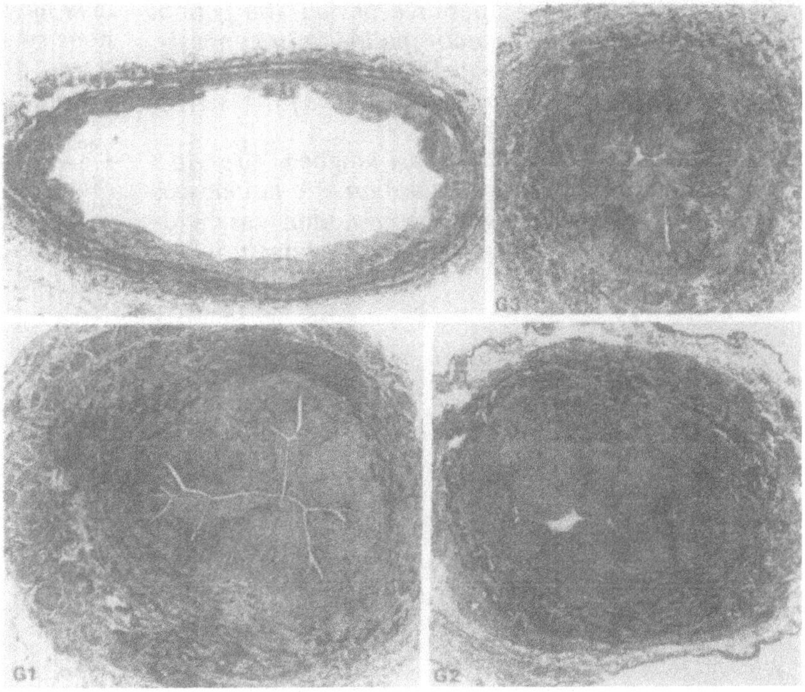

FIGURE 2. Photomicrographs of saphenous veins. *Top left*, section of saphenous vein remnant, which was excised but unused from this patient. G1, graft to the right coronary artery. G2, graft to the left anterior descending. G3, graft to the left obtuse marginal. The unused saphenous vein is wide open. Each of the 3 saphenous veins used as conduits, in contrast, is virtually occluded. (Movat stain, each × 40, reduced 38%.)

narrowing (in percent) of the major epicardial coronary arteries was as follows: left main, 50; left anterior descending, 50; first diagonal 50; left circumflex, 50; first left obtuse marginal, 75; and right, 80. Twenty-three hours before death, aortocoronary bypass grafting with saphenous veins was performed. There were 3 aortic anastomotic sites, 3 conduits, and 4 coronary arterial anastomotic sites: right (GI), left obtuse marginal (G3), and sequential to diagonal and then to left anterior descending (G2) (Fig. 1). Great difficulty was

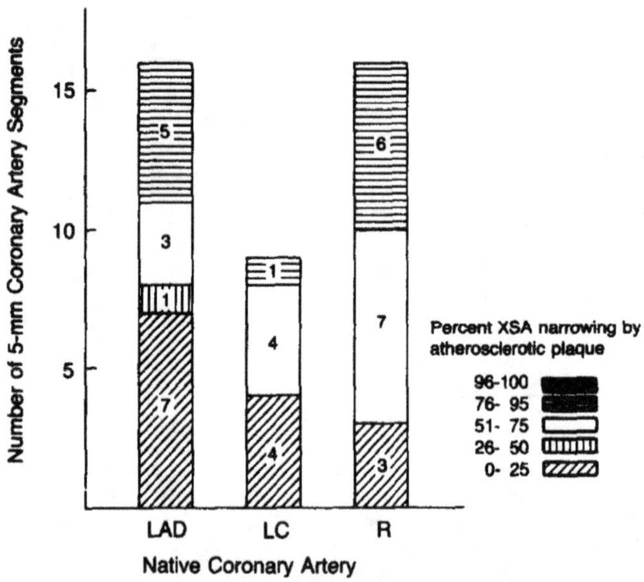

FIGURE 3. Bar graph showing the amount of narrowing in the cross-sectional area (XSA) by atherosclerotic plaque in the native left anterior descending (LAD), left circumflex (LC) and right (R) coronary arteries. Of the 41 five-mm segments of these 3 arteries, none was narrowed 96 to 100%; 12 arteries (29%) were narrowed 76 to 95%; 14 (34%), 51 to 75%; 1 (2%), 26 to 50%; and 14 (34%), 25% or less.

encountered weaning the patient from cardiopulmonary bypass. The operation and weaning period occupied 9 hours. Because of hypotension, an intraaortic balloon was inserted in the operating room. During the entire 14-hour postoperative period, the patient received vasopressors (noradrenaline) intravenously. About 4 hours before death a left ventricular assist device was inserted. Death resulted from progressively diminishing cardiac output.

At necropsy (A86-68), the heart weighed 540 g. All 3 conduits were firm and no sensation of a lumen was detected by palpation (Fig. 1). Each conduit was divided into 5-mm-long segments, cut transversely to the longitudinal axis, and the lumina were obliterated at many sites in all 3 conduits (Fig. 2). A 12-cm-long remnant of saphenous vein from this patient was not used as an aortocoronary conduit and it served as a control for the saphenous veins used as conduits (Fig. 2). In comparison to the saphenous vein used as conduit, the lumen of the remnant saphenous vein was wide open (Fig. 2). The native coronary arteries were divided into 5-mm-long segments and a section stained by Movat's method was prepared from each 5-mm segment. The amount of narrowing in the native epicardial coronary arteries is shown in Figure 3. Transverse sections of the cardiac ventricles disclosed extensive hemorrhagic necrosis of the ventricular septum and left ventricular free wall. Both ventricular cavities were of normal size.

The surprise finding at necropsy in this patient was the obliteration of the lumina of each of the 3 saphenous veins used as aortocoronary conduits. At the time of operation, the surgeon (CLM) considered the saphenous veins to be normal and no difficulty was encountered in making either the aortic or coronary arterial anastomoses. Support for the accuracy of this observation was the presence of normal luminal size in the remnant saphenous vein in this patient (not used for aortocoronary conduits). The luminal obliteration of the saphenous vein conduits was not the result of phlebosclerosis, which was absent. Thus, spasm appears to be the explanation of the luminal obliteration of the saphenous vein conduits in this patient. The constant intravenous infusion of vasopressors postoperatively may have contributed to or caused the saphenous venous spasm.

1. Buxton AE, Goldberg S, Harken A, Hirshfeld J, Kastor JA. *Coronary artery spasm immediately after myocardial revascularization. Recognition and management. N Engl J Med 1981;304:1249–1252.*

2. Buxton AE, Hirshfeld JW, Untereker WJ, Goldberg S, Harken AH, Stephenson LW, Edie RN. *Perioperative coronary arterial spasm: long-term follow-up. Am J Cardiol 1982;50:444–451.*

3. Nussmeier NA, Slogoff S. *Verapamil treatment of intraoperative coronary artery spasm. Anesthesiology 1985;62:539–541.*

Comparison of Morphologic Changes and Luminal Sizes of Saphenous Vein and Internal Mammary Artery After Simultaneous Implantation for Coronary Arterial Bypass Grafting

JAY M. KALAN, MD
WILLIAM C. ROBERTS, MD

It has now been demonstrated repeatedly by angiography that the long-term patency rate of internal mammary artery (IMA) when used as a coronary arterial bypass conduit is far better than that of the saphenous vein (SV) when used as an aortocoronary conduit.[1–10] It also has been demonstrated from morphologic studies that the wall of SV when used as an aortocoronary conduit changes enormously compared to its appearance at implantation.[11] These changes include conversion of the medial wall containing large numbers of smooth muscle cells to a wall composed predominantly of fibrous tissue; deposition on the intima of fibrous tissue devoid of elastic fibrils, and occasionally deposition of lipid material. Although much data exist from these reported angiographic and morphologic studies, little attention has been focused on morphologic changes and comparative sizes of both IMA and SV when used in the same patient as coronary bypass conduits. This report compares these 2 types of conduits when both were used for coronary artery bypass in each of 4 patients.

From the Pathology Branch, National Heart, Lung, and Blood Institute, National Institutes of Health, Bethesda, Maryland 20892. Manuscript received and accepted 18 March 1987.

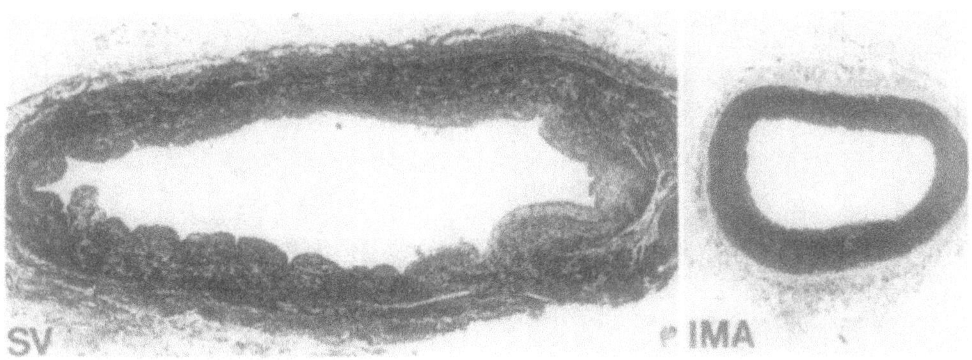

FIGURE 1. Patient 1 (Table I). Photomicrographs of saphenous vein (SV) from aorta to first obtuse marginal coronary artery and of *in situ* internal mammary artery (IMA) to left anterior descending coronary artery in a 64-year-old man (#A80-52) who died in the operating room after coronary artery bypass grafting. The lumen of the SV is about 2.6 times larger than that of the IMA. (Movat stains; original magnification, each × 20.)

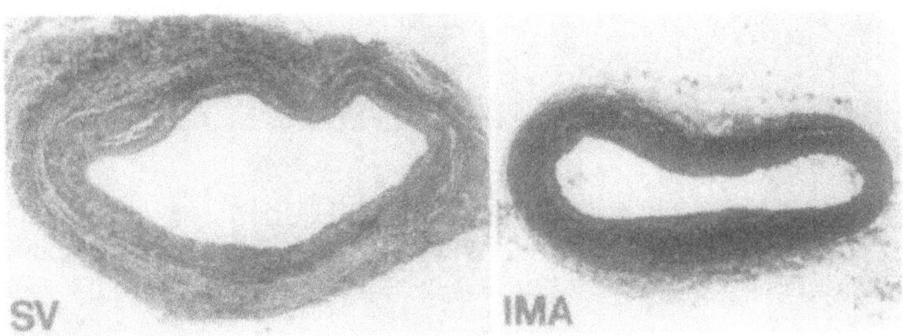

FIGURE 2. Patient 2 (Table I). Photomicrographs of saphenous vein (SV) from aorta to right coronary artery and *in situ* internal mammary artery (IMA) to first diagonal coronary artery in a 73-year-old woman (NNMC #A78-104) who died 4 months after coronary artery bypass grafting. The wall of the SV is mildly thickened. The mean size of the SV is about 1.6 times larger than that of the IMA. (Movat stains; original magnification, each × 20.)

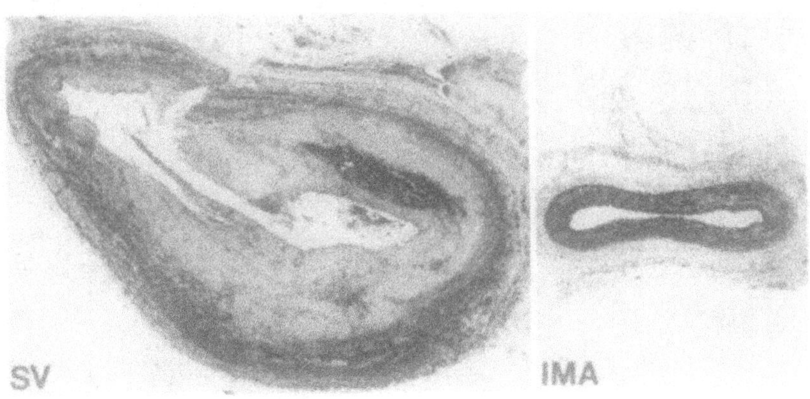

FIGURE 3. Patient 3 (Table I). Photomicrographs of saphenous vein (SV) from aorta to first obtuse marginal coronary artery and in situ internal mammary artery (IMA) to left anterior descending coronary artery in a 62-year-old man (WHC #A85-184) who died 8 years after coronary artery bypass grafting. The intima of the SV is thickened by fibrous tissue which contains an area of fibrin (dark colored). The mean size of the SV is about 4.9 times larger than that of the IMA. (Movat stains; original magnification, each × 20.)

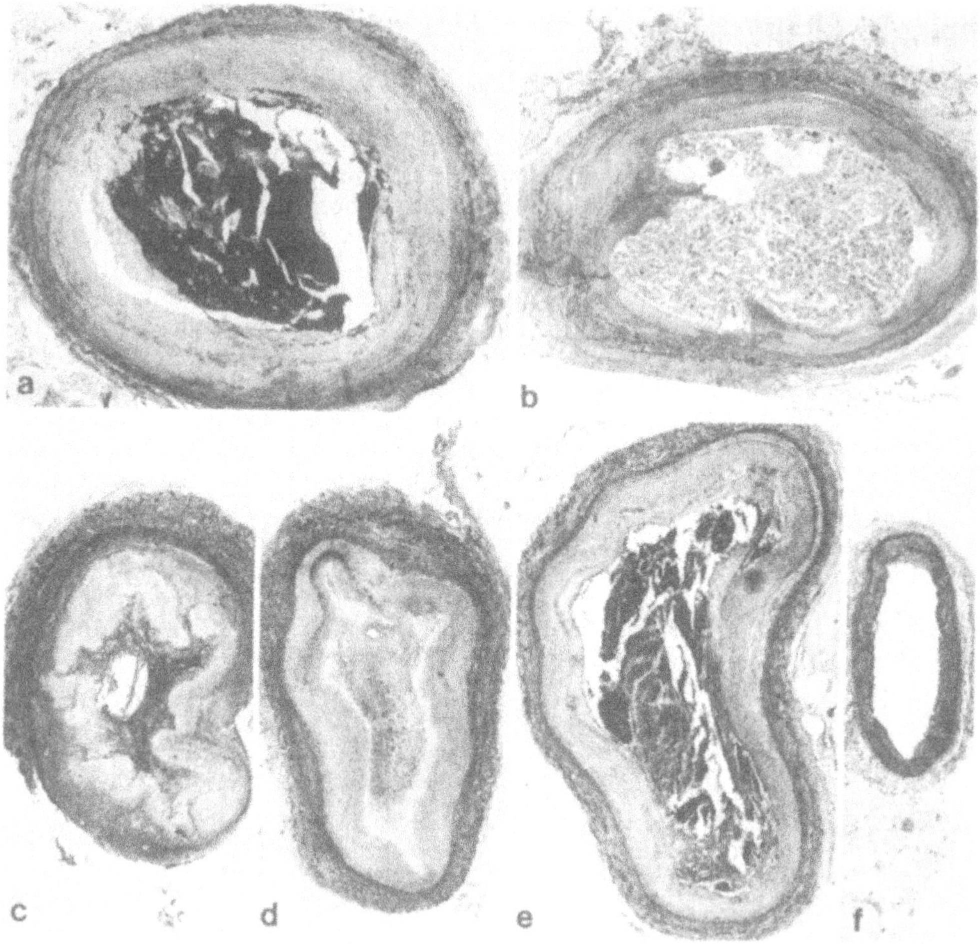

FIGURE 4. Patient 4 (Table I). Photomicrograghs of saphenous vein (SV) at 5 different sites (a to e) from aorta to right coronary artery and in situ internal mammary artery (f) to left anterior descending coronary artery in a 63-year-old man (GT #84A–137) who died 12 years after coronary artery bypass grafting. The SV lumen is almost totally occluded by thrombus (*a* and *c*) or pultaceous debris (*b*) or by fibrous tissue (*c* and *d*). The IMA (*f*) is nearly normal. The mean size of the SV is about 8.9 times larger than that of the IMA. (Movat stains; original magnification, each ×20.)

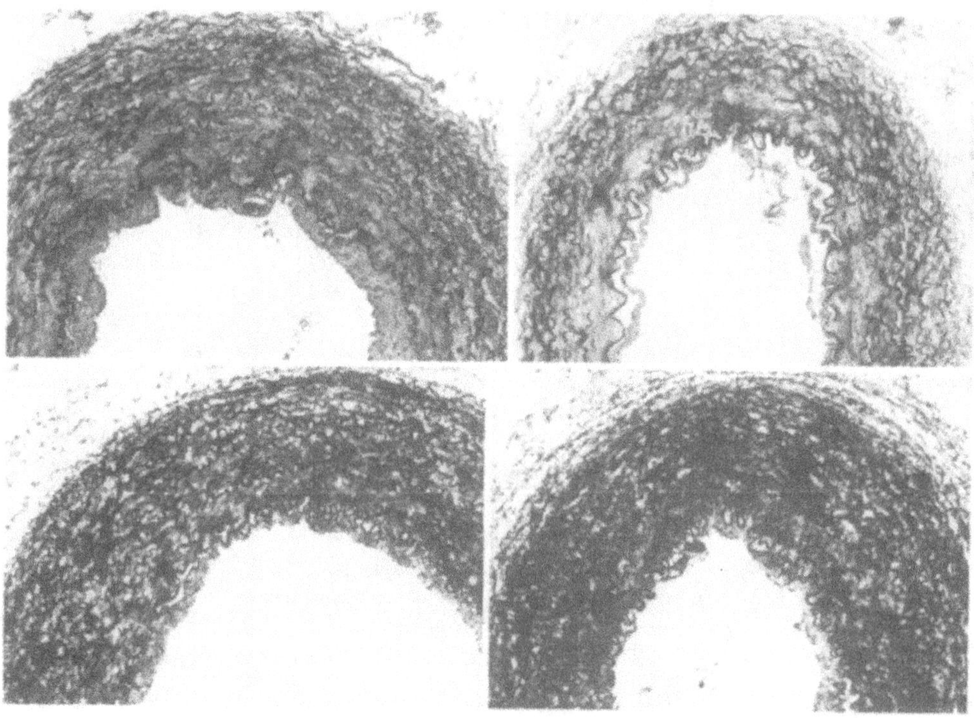

FIGURE 5. Patient 1 (*top*) and patient 2 (*bottom*) (Table I). Photomicrographs of portions of wall of the internal mammary artery of patient 1 (*top*), who died in the operating room after coronary artery bypass grafting, and of patient 2 (*bottom*), who died 4 months after operation. *Top*, abundant dark staining elastic fibers distributed uniformly. No medial or intimal thickening is present. *Bottom*, focal loss of elastic fibers and mild intimal thickening. (Movat stains; original magnification, each ×130.)

TABLE I Clinical and Morphologic Observations in Four Patients Who Died After Simultaneous Implantation of Both Saphenous Vein (SV) and Internal Mammary Artery (IMA) for Coronary Artery Bypass Grafting

Case	Age (yr)	Interval CABG to Death	Sex	DM	SH	No. of Anastomoses		CA Grafted		Maximal % CSA Narrowing		Thrombus		Maximal % CSA Narrowing of Native CA at or Within 2 cm Distal to Coronary Anastomotic Site		Ratio of Size of SV to IMA
						Aorta	CA	IMA	SV	IMA	SV	IMA	SV	Native CA with IMA	Native CA with SV	
1	64	0 days	M	+	0	2	3	LAD	OM	0	0	0	0	76–95	76–95	2.6
									R		0		0		76-95	
2	73	4 mo	F	0	+	2	3	D	OM	0	0	0	0	0	96–100	1.6
									R		26–50		0		76–95	
3	62	8 yr	M	0	+	1	2	LAD	OM	0	51–75	0	0	26–50	76–95	4.9
4	63	12 yr	M	0	0	1	2	LAD	R	0	96–100	0	+	51–75	96–100	8.9

CA = coronary artery; CABG = coronary artery bypass grafting; CSA = cross-sectional area; D = diagonal branch; DM = diabetes mellitus; LAD = left anterior descending; OM = obtuse marginal; R = right; SH = systemic hypertension.

Pertinent clinical and morphologic findings in the 4 patients are summarized in Table I. The conduits in patient 1 were inserted but the patient never left the operating room (Fig. 1); in patient 2 the conduits were in place for 4 months (Fig. 2); and in patients 3 and 4 the conduits were in place for 8 and 12 years, respectively (Fig. 3 and 4). All coronary artery anastomoses were end to side. All 4 patients had in situ left IMA grafts. No patient had narrowing of the IMA used as a coronary conduit. The configuration of the elastic fibers showed either no change or minor changes, specifically, mild focal loss of elastic fibers (Fig. 5 and 6). In contrast, all SV conduits in place for 4 months, 8 years, or 12 years had marked changes in their walls compared with the appearance of the SV at the time of implantation.

The sizes of the IMA in each of the 4 patients were smaller than the sizes of the SV when used as conduits. In all 4 patients both SV and IMA were divided into 5-mm-long segments, each segment was processed in alcohol and xylene and imbedded in paraffin. At least 1 histologic section was cut from each segment and stained by the Movat method. In all, 84 sections of SV and 48 sections of IMA were examined. In each of the 132 sections (84 + 48) the sizes of the SV or IMA were determined by magnifying all sections equally and projecting the magnified image onto paper. The circumference of the SV was determined by tracing the junction between media and adventitia, and the circumference of the IMA was determined by tracing the external elastic membrane. The area enclosed by the traced line was determined by computer planimetry. In patient 1 the mean size of the 21 sections of SV was 2.6 times larger than the mean size of the 7 sections of IMA; in patient 2 the mean size of the 36 sections of SV was 1.6 times larger than that of the 15 sections of IMA; in patient 3 the mean size of the 12 sections of SV was 4.9 times larger than that of the 6 sections of IMA; and in patient 4 the mean size of the 15 sections of SV was 8.9 times larger than that of the 20 sections of IMA.

The findings in these 4 patients indicate that the in situ IMA, when used as a coronary conduit changes little with time, and that the IMA is smaller than the SV when used as an aortocoronary conduit. The luminal size of the IMA when used as a coronary conduit does not appear to change with time. The wall of the SV becomes thicker with time and this thickening can narrow the lumen. Thus, despite its smaller size, the IMA when used as an *in situ* coronary conduit appears to remain normal or near normal histologically; intimal deposition did not occur, in contrast to striking changes in the SV used as an aortocoronary conduit in the same patient.

1. Kay EB, Naraghipour H, Beg RA, DeManey M, Tambe A, Zimmerman HA. *Internal mammary artery bypass graft—long term patency rate and follow-up. Ann Thorac Surg 1974;18:269–279.*

2. Geha AS, Baue AE. *Early and late results of coronary revascularization with saphenous vein and internal mammary artery grafts. Am J Surg 1979;137:456–463.*

3. Tyras DH, Barner HB, Kaiser GC, Codd JE, Pennington DG, Willman VL. *Bypass grafts to the left anterior descending coronary artery. Saphenous vein versus internal mammary artery. J Thorac Cardiovasc Surg 1980;80:327–333.*

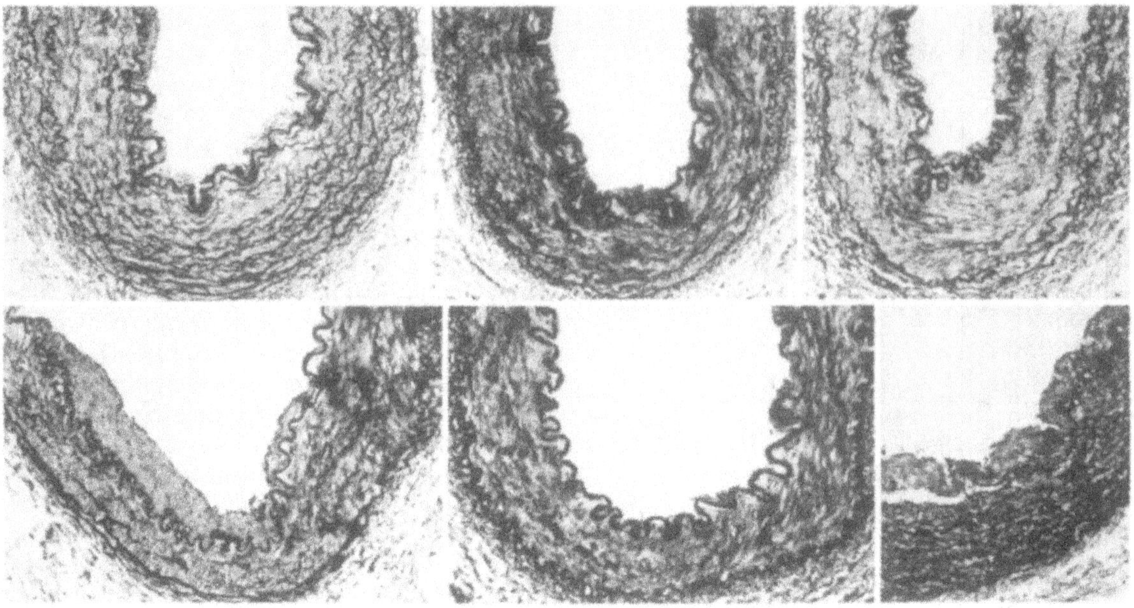

FIGURE 6. Patient 3 (*top*) and patient 4 (*bottom*). Photomicrographs of portions of wall of the IMA of patient 3 (*top*), who died 8 years after coronary artery bypass grafting, and of patient 4 (*bottom*), who died 12 years after operation. Variable amounts of elastic fiber loss are evident. The intima is focally thickened. (Movat stains; original magnification, each × 130.)

4. Bjork VO, Ivert T, Landou C. *Angiographic changes in internal mammary artery and saphenous vein grafts, two weeks, one year, and five years after coronary bypass surgery. Scand J Thorac Cardiovasc Surg 1981;15:23–30.*
5. Tector AJ, Schmahl TM, Janson B, Kallies JR, Johnson G. *Internal mammary artery graft. Its longevity after coronary bypass. JAMA 1981;246:2181–2183.*
6. Singh RN, Sosa JA, Green GE. *Long-term fate of the internal mammary artery and saphenous vein grafts. J Thorac Cardiovasc Surg 1983;86:359–363.*
7. Grondin CM, Campeau L, Lesperance J, Enjalbert M, Bourassa MG. *Comparison of late changes in internal mammary artery and saphenous vein grafts in two consecutive series of patients 10 years after operation. Circulation 1984;70:suppl I:I-208–I-212.*
8. Okies JE, Page US, Bigelow JC, Krause AH, Salomon NW. *The left internal mammary artery: the graft of choice. Circulation 1984;70:suppl I:I-213–I-221.*
9. Barner HB, Standeven JW, Reese J. *Twelve-year experience with internal mammary artery for coronary artery bypass. J Thorac Cardiovasc Surg 1985;90:668–675.*
10. Loop FD, Lytle BW, Cosgrove DM, Stewart RW, Goormastic M, Williams GW, Golding LAR, Gill CC, Taylor PC, Sheldon WC, Proudfit WL. *Influence of the internal-mammary-artery graft on 10-year survival and other cardiac events. N Engl J Med 1986;314:1–6.*
11. Spray TL, Roberts WC. *Changes in saphenous veins used as aortocoronary bypass grafts. Am Heart J 1977;94:500–516.*

Significance of Cardiac Weight in Patients Having Coronary Artery Bypass Grafting for Angina Pectoris

Jay M. Kalan, MD, and William C. Roberts, MD

Cardiac weight at necropsy in 211 patients who had coronary artery bypass grafting (CABG) for angina pectoris, and its relation to early (<60 days) and late (>60 days) death after CABG was sought. The 121 patients dying early had a lower mean heart weight than did the 90 patients dying late (444 ± 94 vs 498 ± 107 g; p <0.001). The mean heart weight of the 85 men dying early was less than that of the 75 men dying late (472 vs 506 g; p <0.05), and the mean heart weight of the 36 women dying early was less than that of the 15 women dying late (377 vs 459 g; p <0.005). Most patients with hearts of normal weight were in the early death group: of the 17 women with hearts of normal weight (≤350 g), 16 (94%) died early (p <0.01), and of the 34 men with hearts of normal weight (≤400 g), 21 (62%) died early (difference not significant). Conversely, most patients in the late death group had hearts of increased weight: of the 15 women dying late, 14 (93%) had hearts of increased weight, and of the 75 men dying late, 62 (83%) had hearts of increased weight. The mean cardiac weight of the 125 patients with left ventricular scars was larger than that of the 86 patients without scars (492 vs 432 g; p <0.01), and these differences were observed within each sex and in both early (463 vs 425 g) and late (520 vs 448 g) death groups. This study suggests that patients with normal or near normal sized hearts have a higher early mortality after CABG than do persons with hearts of increased weight.

(Am J Cardiol 1988;62:36–40)

Several groups of investigators have shown that the mortality rate early after coronary artery bypass grafting (CABG) is higher in women than in men.[1–11] It also is known that the mean heart weight of adult women is less than that of adult men.[12,13] Furthermore, the external diameter of the 4 major epicardial coronary arteries is proportional to cardiac mass.[14,15] Because coronary artery size may be a factor in early mortality after CABG and because cardiac mass is the major determinant of external coronary arterial dimensions, we examined cardiac weight at necropsy after CABG in 211 patients with angina pectoris to determine if a relation existed between cardiac weight and time of death postoperatively.

METHODS

Selection of patients: Cases selected for study included only patients who had CABG because of angina pectoris. Patients having CABG within 2 months of acute myocardial infarction were excluded from this study even when angina was the major reason for the CABG. During the past 17 years (November 1970 to March 1988), 449 patients having CABG have been studied at necropsy in the Pathology Branch, National Heart, Lung, and Blood Institute. Of these 449 patients, 238 (53%) were eliminated from the present study for the following reasons: (1) heart weights were unavailable (54 cases), (2) a cardiovascular operation in addition to CABG was performed simultaneously (118 cases) (cardiac valve replacement or anuloplasty [88 cases], left ventricular aneurysmectomy [25 cases] and carotid endarterectomy [5 cases]), (3) CABG was performed within 2 months of acute myocardial infarction (32 cases), (4) a CABG operation was performed on more than 1 occasion (21 cases), (5) a noncoronary type of cardiac disease also was present (11 cases) (hypertrophic cardiomyopathy [7 cases], aortic valve stenosis [3 cases] and cardiac amyloidosis [1 case]), (6) angina pectoris was never present (1 case) or (7) homozygous familial hyperlipoproteinemia was present (1 case). The presence of a previous myocardial infarct that healed did not prevent inclusion in the present study. After elimination of these 238 patients, 211 remained. The number of patients included in the study per year is shown in Figure 1.

Patient characteristics: The 211 patients ranged in age at death from 32 to 89 years (mean 60); 51 (24%) were women (mean age 58) and 160 (76%) were men (mean age 60). Of the 211 patients, 121 patients (57%) died <60 days after CABG (mean 7.4) (*early deaths*),

From the Pathology Branch, National Heart, Lung, and Blood Institute, National Institutes of Health, Bethesda, Maryland. Manuscript received March 21, 1988, and accepted April 4, 1988.

Address for reprints: William C. Roberts, MD, Building 10, Room 2N258, National Heart, Lung, and Blood Institute, National Institutes of Health, Bethesda, Maryland 20892.

and 90 patients (43%) died >60 days after CABG (range 63 days to 15 years [mean 45 months]) (*late deaths*). Ten patients (6 men and 4 women) had evidence of congestive heart failure before CABG. The mean number of coronary arterial anastomotic sites was similar in the early and late groups (2.8 vs 2.7), and in men and women (2.7 vs 2.7).

Heart weights: The hearts of all 211 patients were examined and weighed in our laboratory. The hearts were fixed in 10% formalin and weighed 3 to 30 days later. The cardiac weights were those recorded *after removal of all noncardiac tissues*, except for the aortocoronary grafts and portion of ascending aorta containing the anastomotic sites of the conduits. The hearts were weighed on a Mettler P1210 scale, which is accurate to 0.1 g.

Statistical analysis: Statistical testing between groups was done by chi-square analysis and the Student *t* test.

RESULTS

The mean weight of the heart in the 51 women was 401 g (Figure 2), and in the 160 men it was 488 g (p <0.01) (Figure 3) (Table I). The mean weight of the heart in the 121 patients dying early was 444 g, and in the 90 patients dying late it was 498 g (p <0.001). The mean weight of the heart of the 36 women dying early was 377 g, and of the 15 women dying late it was 459 g (p <0.005). The weight of the heart of the 85 men dying early was 472 g, and of the 75 men dying late it was 506 g (p <0.05).

Of the 51 patients with hearts of normal weight, 37 (73%) died early and 14 (27%) died late; of the 160 patients with hearts of increased weight, 84 (53%) died early and 76 (47%) died late (p <0.02). Of the 17 women with hearts of normal weight, 16 (94%) died early and 1 (6%) died late (p <0.01). Of the 34 men with hearts of normal weight, 21 (62%) died early and 13 (38%) died late.

Relation of cardiac weight to healed myocardial infarcts: Of the 211 patients, 125 (59%) had focal, grossly visible, left ventricular scars (Table I). These scars involved, at 1 or more sites, all of the inner one-half and a portion of the outer one-half of the wall (transmural) in 123 patients and only a portion of the inner one half of the wall (subendocardial) in 2 patients. The mean cardiac weight was larger in the 125 patients with left ventricular scars (492 g) than in the 86 patients without scars (432 g) (p <.001). This held true both in men (510 vs 454 g) and in women (425 vs 375 g) (p <0.05).

Relation of cardiac weight to mode of death: An attempt was made to characterize a single mode of death for each patient.

EARLY DEATHS: Of the 121 patients dying within 60 days of CABG, 34 patients (28%) could not be separated from cardiopulmonary bypass and they never left the operating room (Table II). The precise cause of death in these 34 patients is unclear. (At necropsy, none had evidence of left ventricular myocardial necrosis.) Of the 87 patients (72%) who left the operating room, the early postoperative period was characterized by evidence of the low cardiac output syndrome in 72 patients (83%).[16] Of them, excessive postoperative bleeding occurred in 13 (18%), and acute myocardial infarction involving the left ventricular wall was present at necropsy in 28 patients (39%), 17 of whom had the diagnosis of acute myocardial infarction established clinically during the early postoperative period. In the remaining 31 patients (43%), the cause of the inadequate cardiac output was unclear but none had evidence of myocardial necrosis. The remaining 15 patients did not have evidence of the low cardiac output syndrome early postoperatively:

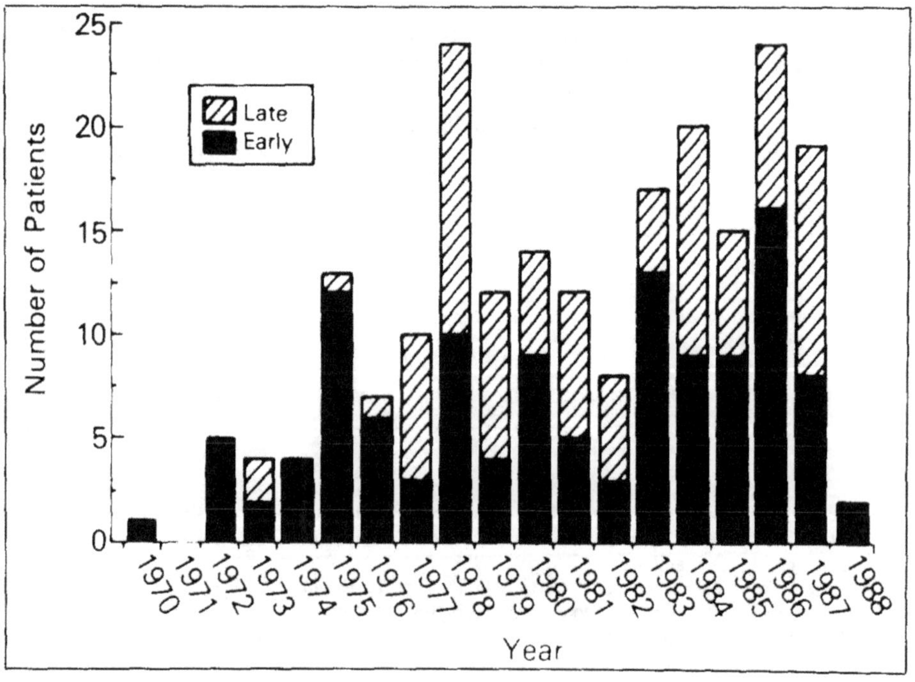

FIGURE 1. Number of patients studied at necropsy dying early (≤60 days) or late (>60 days) after coronary artery bypass grafting during each of 17 years.

TABLE I Relation of Heart Weight in Men and Women to Survival Period and to the Presence or Absence of Grossly Visible Left Ventricular Scars After Coronary Artery Bypass Grafting

		Heart Weight		Heart Weight (g)		Left Ventricular Scar			
						Present		Absent	
	No. (%)	Range	(Mean ± SD)	No. (%)	No. (%)	No. (%)	HW	No. (%)	HW
Women				<350	>350				
	51 (100)	270–640	(401 ± 85)	17 (33)	34 (67)	27 (53)	425	24 (47)	375
Early	36 (71)	270–605	(377 ± 68)	16 (94)	20 (59)	17 (63)	399	19 (79)	358
Late	15 (29)	310–640	(459 ± 96)	1 (6)	14 (41)	10 (37)	469	5 (21)	440
Men				<400	>400				
	160 (100)	305–865	(488 ± 99)	34 (21)	126 (79)	98 (61)	510	62 (39)	454
Early	85 (53)	320–690	(472 ± 89)	21 (62)	64 (51)	45 (46)	487	40 (65)	456
Late	75 (47)	305–865	(506 ± 107)	13 (38)	62 (49)	53 (54)	529	22 (35)	449
Total	211 (100)	270–865	(467 ± 103)	51 (24)	160 (76)	125 (59)	492	86 (41)	432
Early	121 (57)	270–690	(444 ± 94)	37 (73)	84 (53)	62 (50)	463	59 (69)	425
Late	90 (43)	305–865	(498 ± 107)	14 (27)	76 (47)	63 (50)	520	27 (31)	448

HW = heart weight; SD = standard deviation.

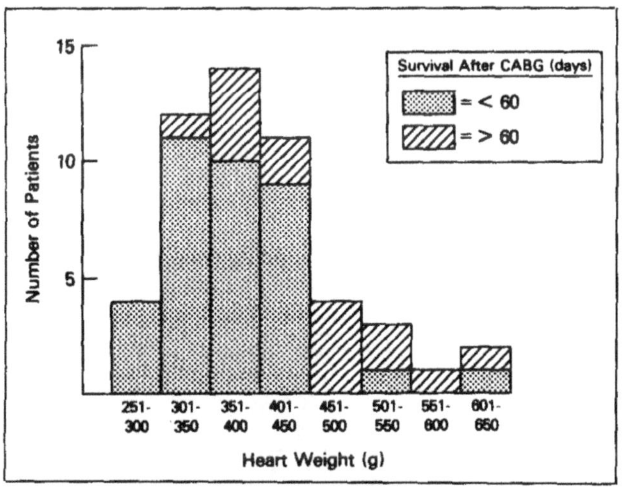

FIGURE 2. Heart weight in 51 women dying early (<2 months) (36 patients) or late (>2 months) (15 patients) after coronary artery bypass grafting (CABG).

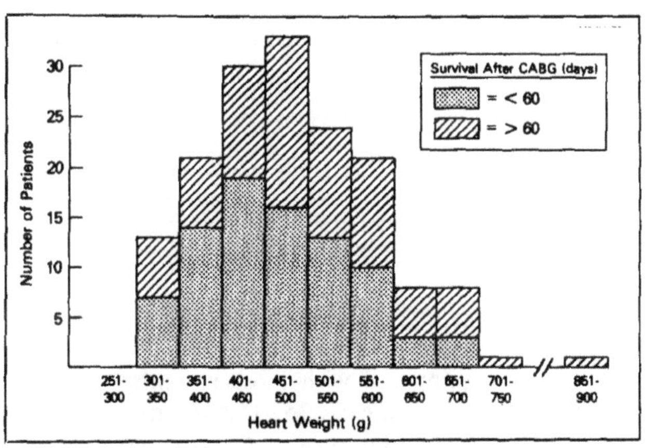

FIGURE 3. Heart weight in 160 men dying early (<2 months) (85 patients) or late (>2 months) (75 patients) after coronary artery bypass grafting (CABG).

4 died suddenly and unexpectedly; 4 had aortic dissection arising either at an aortic anastomotic site or at the aortic cannulation site; 3 had sepsis from wound infections; 2 had massive pulmonary embolism; 1 had rupture of a fusiform aneurysm of the abdominal aorta; and 1 had a stroke after CABG.

LATE DEATHS: Of the 90 patients dying >60 days after CABG, 21 (23%) died suddenly and unexpectedly, and at necropsy none had myocardial necrosis or dilated left ventricular cavities (Table II). Another patient had cardiac arrest during a period of unstable angina pectoris. Fourteen patients (17%) had chronic congestive heart failure: 13 of them had large left ventricular transmural scars and dilated left ventricular cavities (ischemic cardiomyopathy), and 1 patient had papillary muscle dysfunction. Death was attributed to acute myocardial infarction in 7 patients (8%), and to a vascular, but noncardiac, cause in 13 patients (14%): stroke in 6; massive pulmonary embolus in 3; complications early after resection of an abdominal aortic aneurysm in 2; aortic dissection in 1 and complications of carotid endarterectomy (performed 10 years after CABG) in 1. A nonvascular and noncardiac condition caused death in 34 patients (38%): cancer in 18 (14 different types of cancer in the 18 patients); trauma in 6 (murder [2 patients], suicide [1 patient], auto accident [1 patient], fall [1 patient] and electrocution [1 patient]); bleeding peptic ulcers in 2; sepsis in 2; and in 1 patient each, chronic obstructive lung disease, interstitial pulmonary fibrosis, hepatitis, pancreatitis, Parkinson's disease and complications following noncardiac surgery.

DISCUSSION

The major findings in the present study are summarized in Table III. Mean heart weights were smaller in the patients dying early (<60 days) after CABG for angina pectoris than in those dying later. A higher per-

TABLE II Modes of Death of 211 Patients Dying Early (≤60 days) (121 Patients) or Late (>60 days) (90 Patients) After Coronary Artery Bypass Grafting (CABG) for Angina Pectoris

Modes of Death	Pts No. (%)	Women	Men	Mean Age (yrs)	Mean Interval CABG to Death	Heart Weight (g) Range	(Mean)
Early Deaths (days)							
Intraoperative	34 (28)	9	25	54	0	275–690	(424)
Low cardiac output with:							
Acute myocardial infarct	28 (23)	10	18	60	13	330–635	(462)
Bleeding	13 (11)	4	9	60	7	300–685	(424)
Undetermined cause	31 (26)	11	20	61	7	270–680	(443)
Sudden	4 (3)	0	4	56	13	400–585	(506)
Aortic dissection	4 (3)	0	4	62	1	450–565	(506)
Wound infection	3 (2)	1	2	66	45	400–440	(418)
Pulmonary embolism	2 (2)	1	1	55	6	340–460	(400)
Stroke	1 (1)	0	1	53	3	510	
Abdominal aortic aneurysm rupture	1 (1)	0	1	60	32	510	
Total	121 (100)	36	85	59	7.5	270–685	(444)
Late Deaths (months)							
Sudden	21 (23)	3	18	57	44	370–695	(523)
Congestive heart failure	14 (16)	4	10	57	49	380–865	(582)
Acute myocardial infarct	7 (8)	3	4	54	35	310–525	(402)
Unstable angina pectoris	1 (1)	0	1	72	84	590	
Noncardiac							
Vascular	13 (14)	2	11	65	45	330–695	(493)
Nonvascular	34 (38)	3	31	62	47	305–710	(467)
Total	90 (100)	15	75	60	46	310–865	(498)

cent of patients dying early had normal sized hearts compared with those dying late (>60 days) after CABG. A lower percentage of patients dying early had left ventricular scars (healed myocardial infarcts) compared with those dying late.

The explanation for the smaller heart weights in the patients dying early is uncertain, but at least 3 possibilities need to be considered. The first is that hearts of the patients dying late contained more extraneous noncardiac tissues than did the hearts of the patients dying early. Of course more fibrous adhesions were present in the hearts of the patients dying late but every attempt was made to remove them before the heart was weighed. Therefore, this explanation is highly unlikely. The second possibility is that patients dying late had a longer interval between CABG and death and therefore a greater period of time to develop an increased myocardial mass. The mean ages, however, of the patients dying early and late were not significantly different (58 vs 60 years) and, more important, among the patients dying late there was no significant change in mean heart weight as the interval increased from time of CABG to death. Thus, this possibility also appears to be an unlikely explanation. The third possibility is that patients dying late had a longer period in which to develop evidence of myocardial ischemia, assuming that the evidence is sound that myocardial ischemia per se produces an increased myocardial mass. As shown in Table III, the patients dying late had a higher frequency of left ventricular scars (healed myocardial infarcts) compared to those patients dying early (70 vs 51%). The patients dying late with a left ventricular scar had a higher mean heart weight compared with those patients with a left ventricular scar dying early (520 vs 463 g) ($p < 0.005$). Thus, this explanation is a possibility. Nevertheless, comparison of early and late death groups of women without left ventricular scars still showed the late death group to have significantly higher mean heart weight

TABLE III Cardiac Weight in Necropsy Patients Having Coronary Artery Bypass Grafting (CABG) for Angina Pectoris Unassociated with Acute Myocardial Infarction

	Time of Death After CABG ≤60 Days (n = 121)	>60 Days (n = 90)	p Value
Mean heart weight (g)	444	498	<0.001
Men (n = 160)	472	506	<0.05
Women (n = 51)	377	459	<0.005
No. (%) with normal sized heart	37 (31)	14 (16)	<0.05
Men (≤400 g)	21/85 (25)	13/75 (17)	NS
Women (≤350 g)	16/36 (44)	1/15 (7)	<0.01
No. (%) with left ventricular scar	62/121 (51)	63/90 (70)	<0.01
Mean heart weight (g)	463	520	<0.005
Men (%)	45/85 (53)	53/75 (71)	<0.05
Mean heart weight (g)	487	529	<0.05
Women (%)	17/36 (47)	10/15 (67)	NS
Mean heart weight (g)	399	469	<0.06

NS = difference not significant.

than did the early death group (440 vs 358 g; $p \leq 0.01$). The presence of scar, therefore, does not fully explain the lower mean heart weight in women dying early after CABG.

REFERENCES

1. Bolooki H, Vargas A, Green R, Kaiser GA, Ghahramani A. *Results of direct coronary artery surgery in women. J Thorac Cardiovasc Surg 1975;69:271–277.*

2. Wukasch DC, Hall RJ, Cooley DA, Reul GJ, Oglietti JM, Kyger ER, Sandiford FM, Hallman GL. *Surgical versus medical treatment of coronary artery disease: long-term survival. Vasc Surg 1976;10:300–314.*

3. Tyras DH, Barner HB, Kaiser GC, Codd JE, Laks H, Willman VL. *Myocardial revascularization in women. Ann Thorac Surg 1978;25:449–453.*

4. Wukasch DC, Cooley DA, Hall RJ, Reul GJ, Sandiford FM, Zillgitt SL. *Surgical versus medical treatment of coronary artery disease. Nine year follow-up of 9,061 patients. Am J Surg 1979;137:201–207.*

5. Kennedy JW, Kaiser GC, Fisher LD, Maynard C, Fritz JK, Myers W, Mudd JG, Ryan TJ, Coggin J. *Multivariate discriminant analysis of the clinical and angiographic predictors of operative mortality from the collaborative study in coronary artery surgery (CASS). J Thorac Cardiovasc Surg 1980;80:876–887.*

6. Douglas JS Jr, King SB III, Jones EL, Craver JM, Bradford JM, Hatcher CR Jr. *Reduced efficacy of coronary bypass surgery in women. Circulation 1981; 64(suppl II):II-11–II-16.*

7. Fisher LD, Kennedy JW, Davis KB, Maynard C, Fritz JK, Kaiser G, Myers WO. *Association of sex, physical size, and operative mortality after coronary artery bypass in the Coronary Artery Surgery Study (CASS). J Thorac Cardiovasc Surg 1982;84:334–341.*

8. Killen DA, Reed WA, Arnold M, McCallister BD, Bell HH. *Coronary artery bypass in women: long-term survival. Ann Thorac Surg 1982;34:559–563.*

9. Loop FD, Golding LR, MacMillan JP, Cosgrove DM, Lytle BW, Sheldon WC. *Coronary artery surgery in women compared with men: analyses of risks and long-term results. JACC 1983;1:383–390.*

10. Gardner TJ, Horneffer PJ, Gott VL, Watkins L Jr, Baumgartner WA, Borkon AM, Reitz BA. *Coronary artery bypass grafting in women. Ann Surg 1985;201:780–784.*

11. Myers WO, Davis K, Foster ED, Maynard C, Kaiser GC. *Surgical survival in the coronary artery surgery study (CASS) registry. Ann Thorac Surg 1985;40:245–260.*

12. Zeek PM. *Heart weight. I. The weight of the normal human heart. Arch Pathol 1942;34:820–832.*

13. Reiner L, Mazzoleni A, Rodriguez FL, Freudenthal RR. *The weight of the human heart. I. Normal cases. AMA Arch Pathol 1959;68:58–73.*

14. Roberts CS, Roberts WC. *Cross-sectional area of the proximal portions of the three major epicardial coronary arteries in 98 necropsy patients with different coronary events: relationship to heart weight, age and sex. Circulation 1980; 62:953–959.*

15. O'Keefe JH Jr, Owen RM, Bove AA. *Influence of left ventricular mass on coronary artery cross-sectional area. Am J Cardiol 1987;59:1395–1397.*

16. Walston A, Hackel DB, Estes EH. *Acute coronary occlusion and the "power failure" syndrome. Am Heart J 1970;79:613–619.*

Morphologic Findings in Patients Undergoing Coronary Artery Bypass Grafting for Acute Myocardial Infarction

Jay M. Kalan, MD, and William C. Roberts, MD

Although available for patients undergoing coronary artery bypass grafting (CABG) for angina pectoris,[1-3] necropsy data are lacking on patients undergoing CABG shortly after an acute myocardial infarction (AMI). Herein, we describe certain clinical and necropsy findings in 15 patients who underwent CABG within 1 month of onset of an AMI.

The records of all patients having had CABG and studied subsequently at the Pathology Branch, National Heart, Lung, and Blood Institute, were reviewed. Fifteen patients had CABG without simultaneous left ventricular aneurysmectomy or cardiac valve replacement within 30 days of onset of AMI, and they form the basis of this study. All 15 patients had the AMI before admission to a hospital. Patients who were admitted to the hospital for angina pectoris and then developed an AMI during or shortly after cardiac catheterization were excluded from this analysis. The presence of AMI was confirmed at necropsy in all 15 patients. Pertinent findings in each patient are listed in Table I. Two patients (patients 2 and 6, Table I) received tissue plasminogen activator and 1 patient (patient 4) received streptokinase (2, 15 and 1 days, respectively) before CABG. Coronary angioplasty was performed on 1 patient (patient 5).

From the Pathology Branch, National Heart, Lung, and Blood Institute, National Institutes of Health, Bethesda, Maryland 20892. Manuscript received November 30, 1987; revised manuscript received and accepted March 24, 1988.

The major reason for CABG in 9 patients was persistent chest pain after AMI without recognized AMI extension. Four of these patients also had congestive heart failure. Extension of the AMI was the major reason for performing CABG in 2 of these 3 patients. Severe narrowing of the left main coronary artery was the reason for CABG in 2 patients (nos. 2 and 13). One patient (no. 9) had CABG because of severe 3-artery narrowing un-

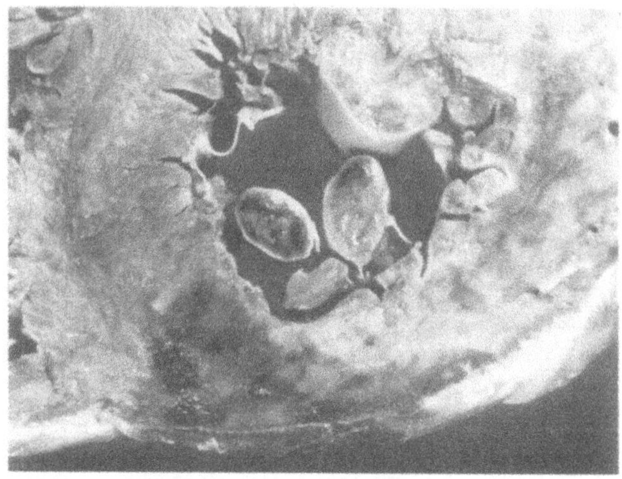

FIGURE 1. Patient 9 (Table I). Photograph of transverse slice of ventricular myocardium showing an area of hemorrhagic necrosis in the posterior wall. The necrosis involves the posteromedial papillary muscle and the lateral wall.

TABLE I Clinical and Morphologic Observations in 15 Necropsy Patients Having Coronary Artery Bypass Grafting During Acute Myocardial Infarction

Pt	Age (yrs), Sex	Reason for CABG	Interval (days): AMI to CABG	Interval (days): CABG to Death	Mode of Death	HW (g)	LV Scar (Location)	Preoperative AMI: Location	Preoperative AMI: Large	No. CA ↓ >75% in CSA by Plaque	CA T (Location)	No. of Anastomotic Sites: AA	No. of Anastomotic Sites: CA	No. of C (T in C)
1	65, F	CP	1	OR	OR	375	+ (L)	A	+	2	+ (LAD)	3	3	3
2	65, M	LM↓	15	OR	OR	450	0	P	+	4	0	3	5	3
3	68, M	LM↓	19	OR	OR	690	0	P	+	2	+ (R)	3	4	3
4	74, M	New AMI	5 + 1	0	Bleeding	560	+ (L)	A	0	3	0	2	3	2
5	61, M	PTCA Failure	7	0	↓CO	630	0	P	+	2	+ (R)	1	1	1
6	65, F	CP	2	1	↓CO	630	0	A	+	2	0	2	5	3
7	71, M	CP	14	1	↓CO	380	0	L	0	2	0	1	2	2
8	52, M	CP + CHF	28 + 14	3	↓CO	460	+ (P)	A	+	3	+ (LC)	2	3	2 (1)
9	69, M	3-VD	27	3	Bleeding	640	+ (L)	P	+	3	+ (R)	2	3	2
10	76, F	CP + CHF	8	8	↓CO	410	0	A	+	2	0	2	2	2 (2)
11	48, M	CP + CHF	12	9	Sudden	665	0	P	+	3	+ (FD)	2	3	3 (1)
12	75, M	New AMI	30 + 1	20	↓CO	410	0	P	+	3	+ (R)	3	4	3
13	59, M	CP	17	21	↓CO	570	0	A	+	3	+ (R)	3	4	3
14	61, F	CP	4	23	↓CO	410	+ (P)	A	0	3	0	3	3	3
15	75, F	CP + CHF	2	51	↓CO	480	0	A	+	2	0	2	2	2

A = anterior; AA = ascending aorta; AMI = acute myocardial infarct; C = conduits; CA = coronary artery; CABG = coronary artery bypass grafting; CHF = congestive heart failure; CO = cardiac output; CP = chest pain; CSA = cross-sectional area; FD = first diagonal; HW = heart weight; L = lateral; LAD = left anterior descending; LC = left circumflex; LM = left main; LV = left ventricle; OR = operating room; P = posterior; PTCA = percutaneous transluminal coronary angioplasty; R = right; T = thrombus; VD = vessel disease; + present; 0 = absent.

associated with persistent evidence of myocardial ischemia, and 1 patient had CABG immediately after unsuccessful coronary angioplasty.

The interval between CABG and death ranged from 0 (operating room death) to 51 days (mean 9, median 3). Three patients were unable to maintain a blood pressure after being removed from cardiopulmonary bypass and died in the operating room; 9 had cardiogenic shock (low cardiac output syndrome) presumably in part because of the earlier AMI; 2 patients had low cardiac output due to excessive bleeding; and 1 developed ventricular fibrillation during a previously uncomplicated postoperative course.

The heart weights ranged from 375 to 690 g (mean 517). Fourteen hearts (93%) were of increased weight

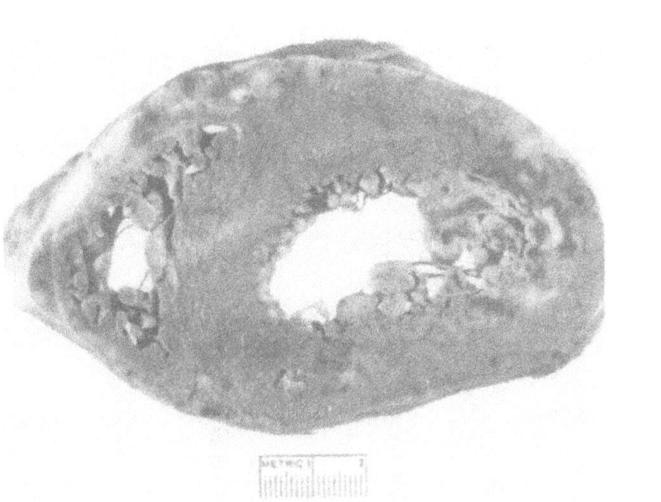

FIGURE 2. Patient 11 (Table I). Photograph of transverse slice of left and right ventricles showing an area of ischemic (nonhemorrhagic) necrosis in the posterior and lateral walls. The left ventricular cavity is mildly dilated, with moderate thinning of the lateral wall.

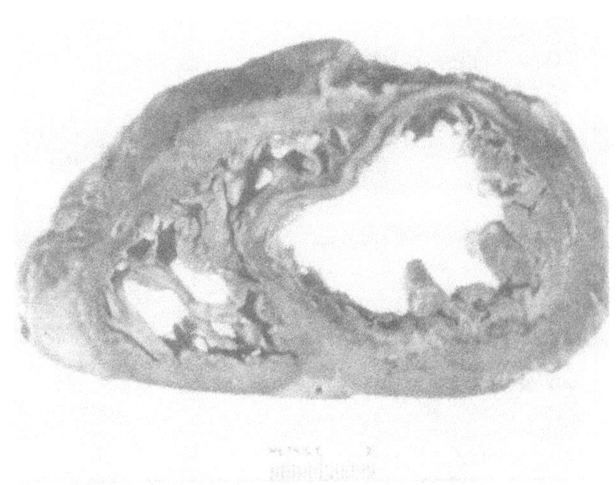

FIGURE 3. Patient 13 (Table I). Photograph of transverse slice of ventricular myocardium showing extensive transmural necrosis of the anterior wall. The necrosis extends through the septum and involves the subendocardial half of the posterior wall. The anterior wall is markedly thinned and the ventricular cavities are dilated.

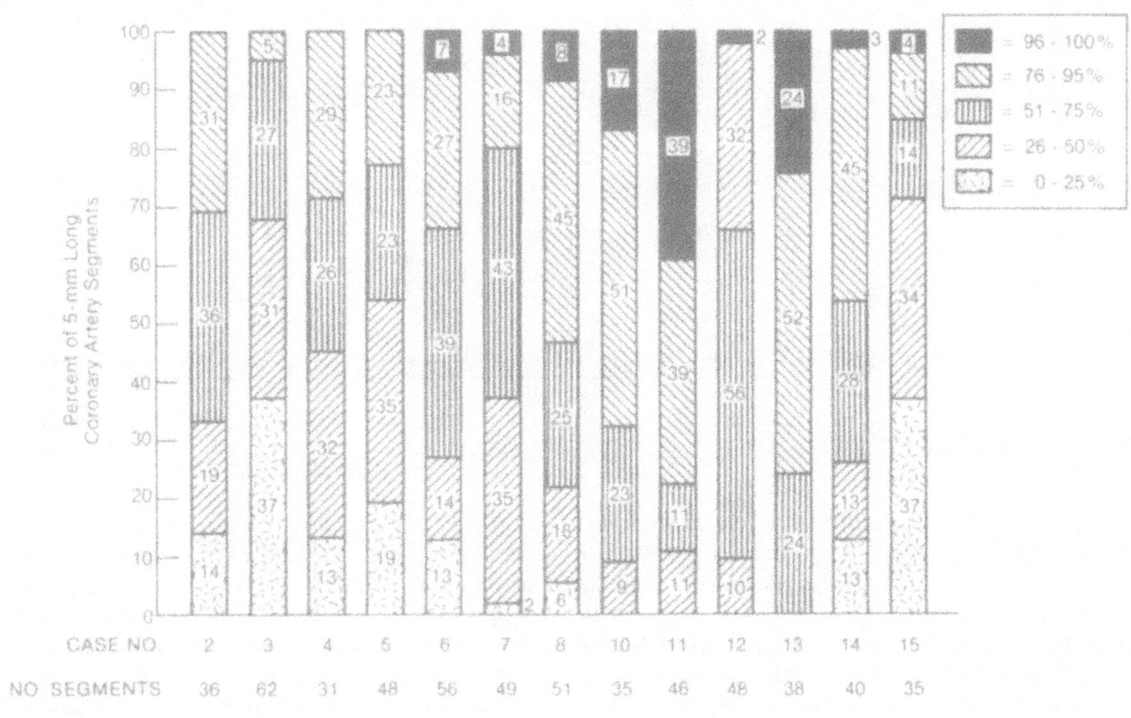

FIGURE 4. Amount of cross-sectional area narrowing by atherosclerotic plaque in 5-mm long segments of the 4 major (left main, left anterior descending, left circumflex and right) epicardial coronary arteries in each of 13 necropsy patients having coronary artery bypass grafting within 30 days of acute myocardial infarction. All 13 patients had narrowing >75%, and 9 patients had an artery narrowed >95% of cross-sectional area.

TABLE II Comparison of Clinical and Morphologic Findings in Patients Dying <60 Days after Coronary Artery Bypass Grafting for Angina Pectoris or Acute Myocardial Infarction

	AMI (n = 15)	AP (n = 121)	p Value
Mean age (years)	66	59	<0.05
Men	10 (67%)	85 (70%)	NS
Diabetes mellitus	6 (40%)	31 (26%)	NS
Systemic hypertension	9 (60%)	56 (46%)	NS
Interval (days) CABG to death (mean)	0–51 (9)	0–59 (7.4)	NS
Mode of death			
Operating room	3 (20%)	34 (28%)	NS
Inadequate cardiac output			
Without anatomic cause	0	31 (26%)	<0.05
Acute myocardial infarction	9 (60%)*	28 (23%)	<0.01
Bleeding	2 (13%)	13 (11%)	NS
Sudden	1 (7%)	4 (3%)	NS
Ascending aortic dissection	0	4 (3%)	NS
Other	0	7 (6%)	NS
Heart weight (g) (mean)	375–690 (517)	270–690 (444)	<0.05
Men	380–690 (545)	320–690 (472)	<0.05
Women	375–630 (461)	270–605 (377)	<0.05
Left ventricular scar	5 (33%)	62 (51%)	NS
Mean no. of 3 major CAs ↓ >75% CSA by plaque	2.6	2.6	NS
Left main ↓ >75% by plaque	2 (13%)	32 (26%)	NS
Mean no. of conduits	2.5	2.4	NS
Mean no. of aortic anastomotic sites	2.3	2.2	NS
Mean no. of CA anastomotic sites	3.1	2.9	NS

* All 15 patients, however, had transmural myocardial necrosis before CABG and at necropsy.
AP = angina pectoris; CA = coronary artery; CABG = coronary artery bypass grafting; CSA = cross-sectional area; NS = not significant.

TABLE III Composite of Data on Early Mortality in Patients Having Coronary Artery Bypass Grafting Within 30 days of Acute Myocardial Infarction

Study	Year	First Author	Pts (n)	Mean Age (yrs)	Men No. (%)	Interval (days) AMI to CABG	Mean No. of CA Anastomoses	Early Mortality No. (%)
1	1971	Favaloro	11	—	—	4–10 hrs	1.7	1
2	1971	Pifarre	8	54	5	0–17	—	1
3	1972	Sustaita	7	57	7	0–3	1.4	1
4	1974	Dawson	74	—	—	0–30	—	17 (23)
5	1978	Levine	33	—	—	0–10	—	3 (9)
6	1981	Jones	116	53	88 (76)	0–30	2.6	0 (0)
7	1982	Hines	7	—	—	0–21	2.0	1
8	1983	Roberts	20	57	—	2–28	2.8	0 (0)
9	1983	Nunley	80	58	65 (81)	0–14	2.2	4 (5)
10	1983	DeWood	701	56	551 (79)	0–24 hrs	—	31 (4)
11	1983	Phillips	181	—	—	1–36 hrs	3.8	8 (4)
12	1984	Baumgartner	34	59	26 (76)	6–29	—	3 (9)
13	1984	Hochberg	104	59	—	0–28	2.9	23 (22)
14	1986	Katz	145	61	111 (77)	0–28	2.9	5 (3)
Total			1,521	57	841/1,091 (77)	0–30	3.0	98 (6)

AMI = acute myocardial infarction; CA = coronary artery; CABG = coronary artery bypass grafting.

(>350 g in women, >400 g in men). The myocardial infarct that occurred before CABG involved predominantly the anterior wall in 8, the posterior wall in 6 and the lateral wall in 1 patient. The necrosis was extensive in 12 patients. It was hemorrhagic in 6, and ischemic in 9 patients (Figures 1 and 2). Healed myocardial infarcts (scars) were present in 5 patients. The left ventricular cavity was dilated in 5 patients (Figure 3).

The coronary arteries in 13 patients were removed from the heart, decalcified if necessary, cut transversely into 5-mm long segments, processed in alcohols and xylene, embedded in paraffin, cut into 6-μ thick sections, stained by the Movat pentachrome method and examined by 1 of us (JMK) at a magnification × 40. Luminal narrowing by atherosclerotic plaque was graded in 5 categories: 0 to 25%; 26 to 50%; 51 to 75%; 76 to 95% and 96 to 100% of the cross-sectional area enclosed by the internal elastic membrane.

The 13 patients in whom the 4 major epicardial coronary arteries were examined in detail had at least 2 major (left main, left anterior descending, left circumflex or right) arteries narrowed >75% in cross-sectional area by atherosclerotic plaque (mean 2.6 per patient). Eight patients (53%) had at least 3 arteries narrowed

>75%. The left main coronary artery was narrowed >75% in 2 patients (nos. 2 and 13). Additionally, 8 patients had an occluding thrombus in the "infarct-related" coronary artery. The amounts of cross-sectional area narrowing in the 575 five-mm long coronary segments in 13 patients are shown in Figure 1. The infarct-related coronary artery was narrowed >75% in cross-sectional area by plaque in all 13 patients. The non-infarct-related coronary artery (left anterior descending coronary artery for posterior wall AMI, dominant left circumflex or dominant right coronary artery for anterior wall AMI) was narrowed >75% in 12 of the 13 patients. The percentage of segments narrowed >75% in cross-sectional area for each artery was greater in the infarct-related artery than in the noninfarct-related artery in 9 of the 13 patients. Thrombus was present in a saphenous vein conduit in 3 (20%) of 15 patients or in 4 (11%) of 37 conduits.

Findings in these 15 patients who had AMI before entering the cardiac catheterization laboratory and operating room (for CABG) and who survived <60 days postoperatively were compared with those in 121 previously reported[3] necropsy patients who did not have an AMI (angina pectoris only) before CABG and who survived <60 days (Table II). Comparison between these 2 groups showed 1 important significant difference: the mean heart weight in the AMI group was significantly larger than that of the angina group (517 vs 444 g). Of the 15 patients, 14 (93%) in the AMI group had hearts of increased weight compared with 84 of 121 patients (69%) in the angina group ($p < 0.05$).

Table III summarizes previously published reports of results of CABG during AMI.[4-11] None of these 14 reports described cardiac morphologic findings in the fatal cases. The present study attempts to fill that void.

1. Spray TL, Roberts WC. *Changes in saphenous veins used as aorto-coronary bypass grafts. Am Heart J 1977;94:500–516.*

2. Roscher AA, Kern WH. *Aortocoronary bypass surgery from the pathologist's point of view. A clinicopathologic study of 240 cases with twenty-six autopsies. Int Surg 1977;62:282–293.*

3. Kalan JM, Roberts WC. *Significance of cardiac weight in patients having coronary artery bypass grafting for angina pectoris. Am J Cardiol 1988;62:36–40.*

4. Favaloro RG, Effler DB, Cheanvechai C, Quint RA, Sones FM, Jr. *Acute coronary insufficiency (impending myocardial infarction and myocardial infarction). Surgical treatment by the saphenous vein graft technique. Am J Cardiol 1971;28:598–607.*

5. Pifarre R, Spinazzola A, Nemickas R, Scanlon PJ, Tobin JR. *Emergency aortocoronary bypass for acute myocardial infarction. Arch Surg 1971;103:525–528.*

6. Sustaita H, Chatterjee K, Matloff JM, Marty AT, Swan HJC, Fields J. *Emergency bypass surgery in impending and complicated acute myocardial infarction. Arch Surg 1972;105:30–35.*

7. Dawson JT, Hall RJ, Hallman GL, Cooley DA. *Mortality in patients undergoing coronary artery bypass surgery after myocardial infarction. Am J Cardiol 1974;33:483–486.*

8. Levine FH, Gold HK, Leinbach RC, Daggett WM, Austen WG, Buckley MJ. *Management of acute myocardial ischemia with intraaortic balloon pumping and coronary bypass surgery. Circulation 1978;58(suppl I):I-69–I-72.*

9. Jones EL, Waites TF, Craver JM, Bradford JM, Douglas JS, King SB, Bone DK, Dorney ER, Clements SD, Thompkins T, Hatcher CR, Jr. *Coronary bypass for relief of persistent pain following acute myocardial infarction. Ann Thorac Surg 1981;32:33–43.*

10. Hines GL, Mohtashemi M. *Delayed operative intervention in cardiogenic shock after myocardial infarction. Ann Thorac Surg 1982;33:132–138.*

11. Roberts AJ, Sanders JH, Jr, Moran JH, Spies SM, Lesch ML, Michaelis LL. *The efficacy of medical stabilization prior to myocardial revascularization in early refractory postinfarction angina. Ann Surg 1983;197:91–98.*

12. Nunley DL, Grunkemeier GL, Teply JF, Abbruzzese PA, Davis JS, Khonsari S, Starr A. *Coronary bypass operation following acute complicated myocardial infarction. J Thorac Cardiovasc Surg 1983;85:485–491.*

13. DeWood MA, Spores J, Berg R, Jr, Kendall RW, Grunwald RP, Selinger SL, Hensley GR, Sutherland KI, Sheilds JP. *Acute myocardial infarction: a decade of experience with surgical reperfusion in 701 patients. Circulation 1983;68(suppl II):II-8–II-16.*

14. Phillips SJ, Kongtahworn C, Skinner JR, Zeff RH. *Emergency coronary artery reperfusion: a choice therapy for evolving myocardial infarction. Results in 339 patients. J Thorac Cardiovasc Surg 1983;86:679–688.*

15. Baumgartner WA, Borkon AM, Zibulewsky J, Watkins L, Jr, Gardner TJ, Bulkley BH, Achuff SC, Baughman KL, Traill TA, Gott VL, Reitz BA. *Operative intervention for postinfarction angina. Ann Thorac Surg 1984;38:265–267.*

16. Hochberg MS, Parsonnet V, Gielchinsky I, Hussain SM, Fisch DA, Norman JC. *Timing of coronary revascularization after acute myocardial infarction. Early and late results in patients revascularized within seven weeks. J Thorac Cardiovasc Surg 1984;88:914–921.*

17. Katz NM, Kubanick TE, Ahmed SW, Green CE, Pearle DL, Satler LF, Rackley CE, Wallace RB. *Determinants of cardiac failure after coronary bypass surgery within 30 days of acute myocardial infarction. Ann Thorac Surg 1986;42:658–663.*

Morphologic Changes in Coronary Artery Seen Late After Endarterectomy

Amy H. Kragel, MD, Charles M. McIntosh, MD, PhD, and William C. Roberts, MD

Coronary endarterectomy occasionally is performed in conjunction with coronary artery bypass grafting. While information is available regarding the morphologic changes occurring late in the carotid artery after endarterectomy,[1–7] there is no information on histologic changes in coronary arteries late following endarterectomy. Herein we describe morphologic findings in a man who died 4.5 years after coronary endarterectomy.

From the Pathology and Surgery Branches, National Heart, Lung, and Blood Institute, National Institutes of Health, Bethesda, Maryland 20892. Manuscript received November 18, 1988; revised manuscript received and accepted December 19, 1988.

W.N., a 77-year-old man, had his purely regurgitant mitral valve replaced and an endarterectomy of the right coronary artery followed by insertion of a saphenous vein conduit at age 73. Preoperatively, the left ventricular pressure was 144/14 mm Hg. Left ventricular angiography showed 4+/4+ mitral regurgitation. Coronary artery cineangiography before operation showed total occlusion of the right coronary artery distal to the second right ventricular branch. At operation, the mitral valve was typical of mitral valve prolapse. An endarterectomy was performed in the right coronary artery distal to the first right ventricular branch with removal of an 8-cm segment (Figure 1) of atheromatous plaque. A saphenous vein graft was inserted in the right coronary artery near the crux of the heart. He died

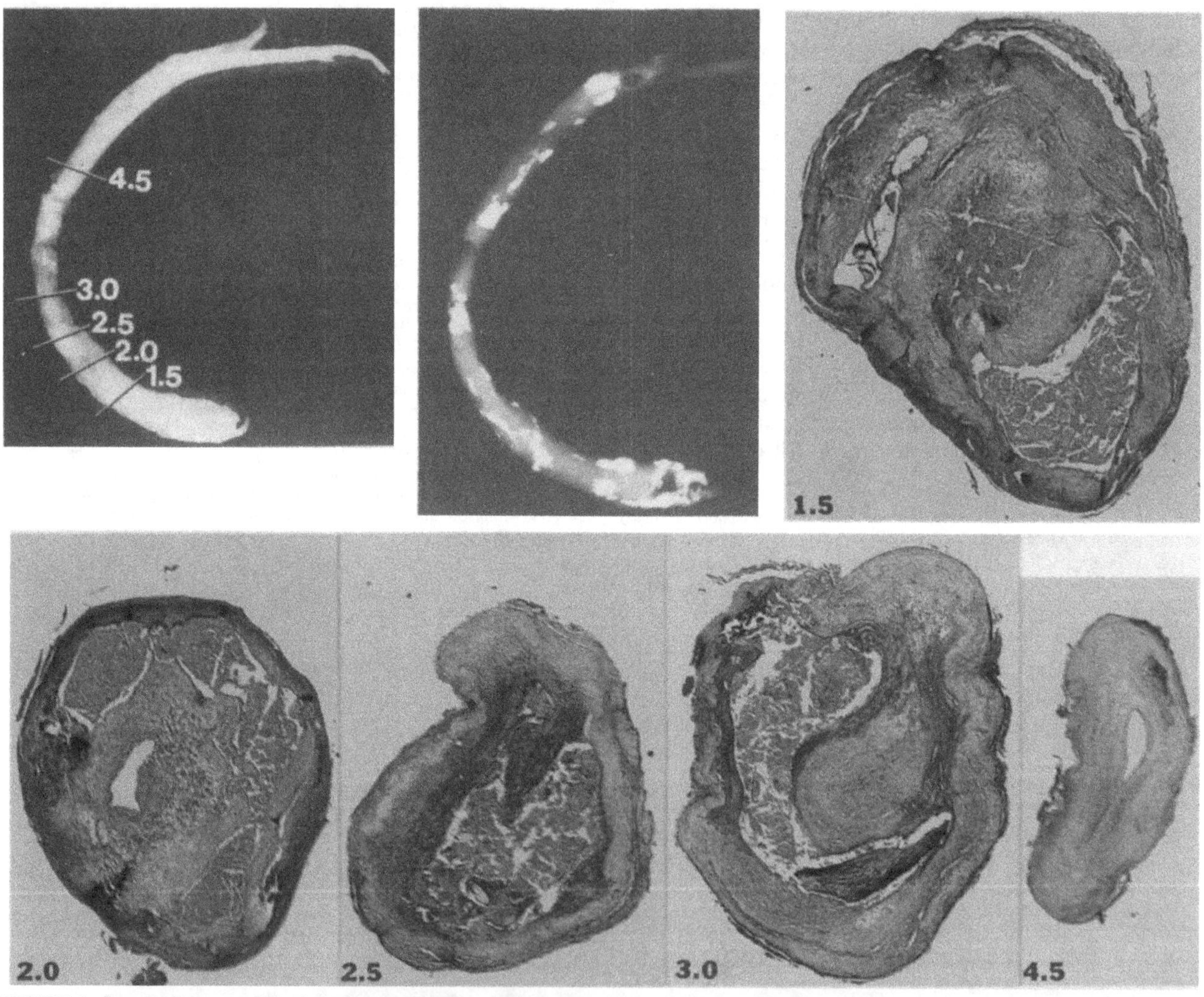

FIGURE 1. Gross photograph (original magnification × 2), radiograph (original magnification × 2) and Movat-stained sections (original magnification × 20) of the endarterectomy specimen. The approximate distance from the most proximal portion of the specimen (in cm) at which the histologic section was taken is noted on the gross photograph and in the corresponding panels. The specimen contains an atheromatous "core," which includes portions of internal elastic lamina and media (*arrow*). There is near total occlusion of the lumen by atherosclerotic plaque. The plaque contains large lipid "lakes" surrounded by fibrous tissue. In addition, foci of calcium, inflammatory infiltrates and small vascular channels are present.

suddenly at home 4.5 years after cardiac operation.

At necropsy, the heart weighed 970 g. A radiograph of the heart showed calcium in the mitral anulus and in the epicardial coronary arteries. There was no gross or histologic evidence of myocardial necrosis or fibrosis. The Hancock bioprosthesis in the mitral position appeared grossly free of any evidence of significant degeneration and no paravalvular communications were present.

The 4 major epicardial coronary arteries and the saphenous vein bypass graft were excised, decalcified, sectioned at 5-mm intervals and examined histologically. The left anterior descending, left circumflex and right coronary arteries were all narrowed >75% in cross-sectional area by atherosclerotic plaque. Movat-stained sections of the native right coronary artery showed the proximal 3 cm (where endarterectomy presumably had not *been performed) to be narrowed by calcified fibrous tissue containing scattered inflammatory infiltrates. The distal 8 cm (the presumed site of endarterectomy) was narrowed by a homogenous mixture of spindle cells and collagen. The internal elastic membrane could not be identified and the "media" were indistinguishable from intima (Figure 2). The saphenous vein graft was virtually occluded throughout its course by fibrous tissue containing small vascular channels (Figure 3).*

Studies of the morphologic changes in surgical endarterectomy specimens removed for restenosis of the carotid artery have shown that restenosis occurring within 2 years of

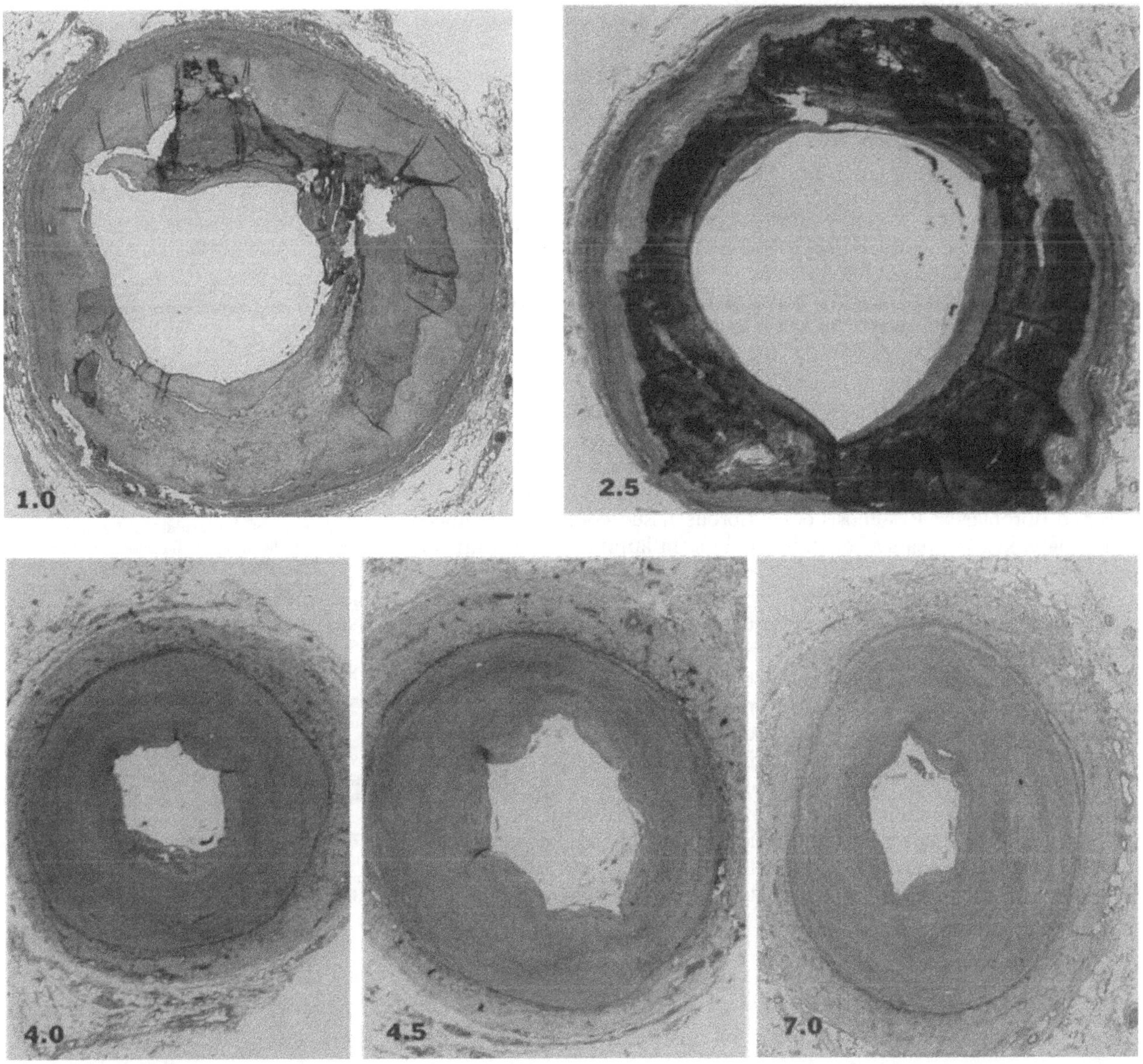

FIGURE 2. Movat-stained sections (each × 60) of the right coronary artery at necropsy. The distance (in cm) from the aortic ostium at which the section was taken is indicated on each section. Sections 1.0 and 2.5 were proximal to the endarterectomy site and they are composed of calcified fibrous tissue. Sections 4.0, 4.5 and 7.0 were taken from the site of endarterectomy and they are composed of a homogeneous mixture of spindle cells admixed with collagen. The internal elastic membrane cannot be identified in these distal sections.

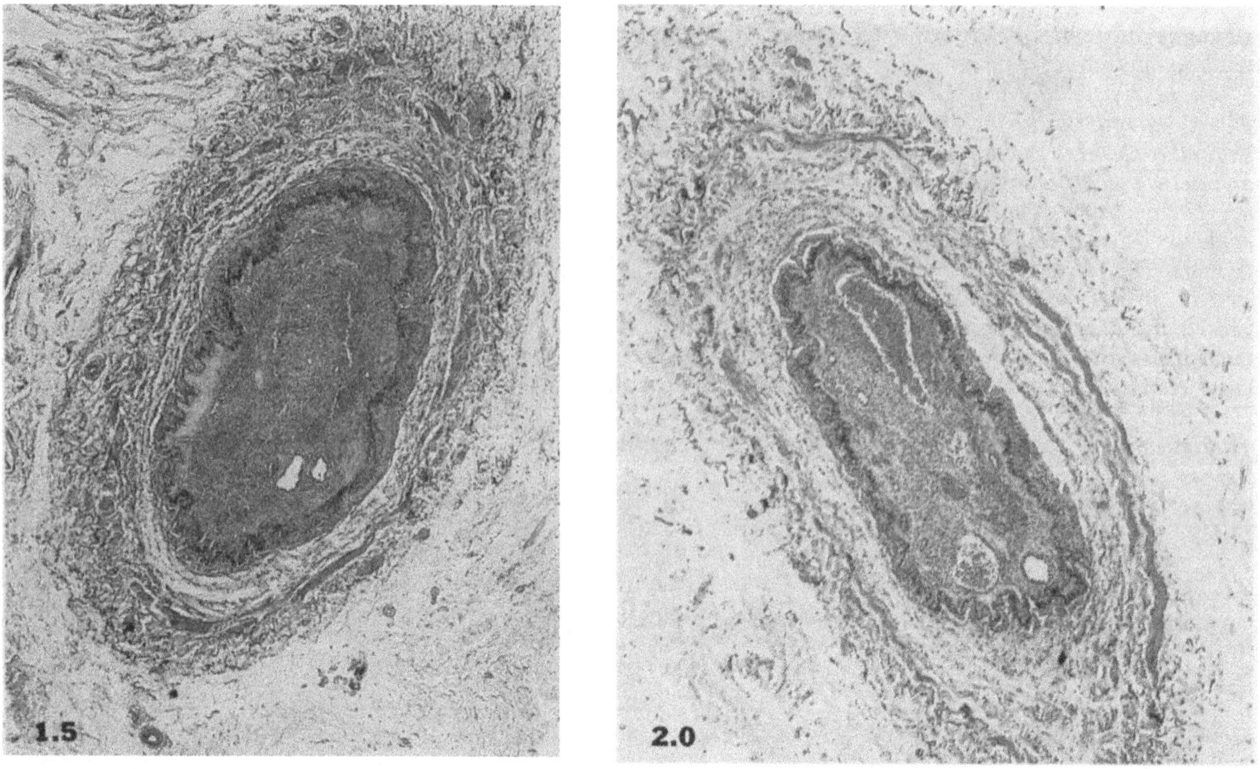

FIGURE 3. Movat-stained sections of the saphenous vein graft (× 60) taken at 1.5 cm and 2.0 cm from the proximal ostium showing near total obliteration of the lumen by fibrous tissue containing small vascular channels.

the initial surgical procedure is usually, but not always, due to a diffuse proliferation of spindle cells.[1,3,5] These cells, by electron microscopy, have features of both smooth muscle cells and fibroblasts.[2] Restenosis occurring late, i.e., >2 years after endarterectomy, is usually, but not always, due to "typical atherosclerotic plaque" containing various elements including fibrous tissue, hemosiderin and calcium.[1,3,5] Cases of early restenosis secondary to typical atherosclerotic plaque and late restenosis secondary to a proliferation of myofibroblasts have been described.[2,4,6,7]

In our patient, we studied plaque morphology of the native coronary artery at the site of endarterectomy and compared it to plaque morphology of the surgical endarterectomy specimen removed 4.5 years previously. The lumen of the endarterectomy specimen was narrowed by plaque composed of heavily calcified fibrous tissue containing pultaceous debris, inflammatory infiltrates and multiple small vascular channels. In contrast, the native coronary artery that had been the site of endarterectomy had no internal elastic membrane and its lumen was narrowed by nearly homogenous connective tissue containing spindle cells. While it is impossible to say when these changes occurred, they resemble those associated with early restenosis of the carotid artery. To our knowledge, this is the first description of coronary artery plaque morphology in a patient dying late after coronary endarterectomy.

1. Stoney RJ, String ST. Recurrent carotid stenosis. *Surgery 1976;80:705–710.*

2. French BN, Rewcastle NB. Recurrent carotid stenosis at the site of carotid endarterectomy. *Stroke 1977;8:597–605.*

3. Cossman D, Callow D, Stein A, Matsumoto G. Early restenosis after carotid endarterectomy. *Arch Surg 1978;113:275–278.*

4. Hertzer NR, Martinez BD, Beven EG. Recurrent stenosis after carotid endarterectomy. *Surg Gynecol Obstet 1979;149:360–364.*

5. Cantelmo NL, Cutler BS, Wheeler HB, Herrmann JB, Cardullo PA. Noninvasive detection of carotid stenosis following endarterectomy. *Arch Surg 1981;116:1005–1008.*

6. Das MB, Hertzer NR, Ratliff NB, O'Hara PJ, Bebin EG. Recurrent carotid stenosis: a five-year series of 65 reoperations. *Ann Surg 1985;202:28–35.*

7. Shumway SJ, Edwards WH, Jenkins JM, Mulherin JL Jr, Edwards WH Jr. Recurrent carotid stenosis: incidence and management. *Am Surg 1987; 53:61–65.*

Coronary Arterial Morphology 10 Years After "Endarterectomy"

A. H. KRAGEL, M.D., C. L. MCINTOSH, M.D., Ph.D., W. C. ROBERTS, M.D.

Pathology and Cardiac Surgery Branches, National Heart, Lung, and Blood Institute, National Institutes of Health, Bethesda, Maryland, USA

Summary: Little information is available regarding coronary artery morphology after endarterectomy. In this report, we describe coronary artery morphology seen at necropsy 10 years after coronary artery endarterectomy and compare it with the morphology of the original endarterectomy specimen. Surprisingly, in some areas, all of the internal elastic membrane and most of the media were observed in the "endarterectomy" specimen.

Key words: coronary artery disease, coronary artery bypass surgery

Introduction

Coronary artery endarterectomy is performed on occasion as an adjunct to coronary artery bypass surgery. While there is extensive information regarding the morphology of changes in saphenous vein grafts and native coronary arteries following coronary artery bypass grafting, only two previous reports have described morphologic findings in the coronary arteries which have been sites of endarterectomy.[1,2] In this report we compare the histologic changes in the native coronary artery seen at necropsy 10 years after "endarterectomy" with those seen in the surgical "endarterectomy" specimen.

Address for reprints:

A. H. Kragel, M.D.
Pathology Branch
National Heart, Lung, and Blood Institute
Building 10, Room 2N258
Bethesda, MD 20892, USA

Received: November 7, 1989
Accepted: November 20, 1989

Case Report

G.O., a 62-year-old man with systemic hypertension, diabetes mellitus, and hypercholesterolemia, first developed angina pectoris at age 48. After a 4-year period of stable exertional angina, the angina worsened to functional class 4/4. Angiography disclosed 50–75% diameter narrowing of the left main and left obtuse marginal, 75–99% narrowing of the left circumflex, total occlusion of the right, and less than 50% narrowing of the left anterior descending coronary arteries. The left ventricular pressure was 145/10 mmHg. Saphenous vein grafts were placed to the left anterior descending, left obtuse marginal, and distal right coronary arteries, with endarterectomy of the distal right and proximal posterior descending coronary arteries (Fig. 1). Cardiac catheterization per-

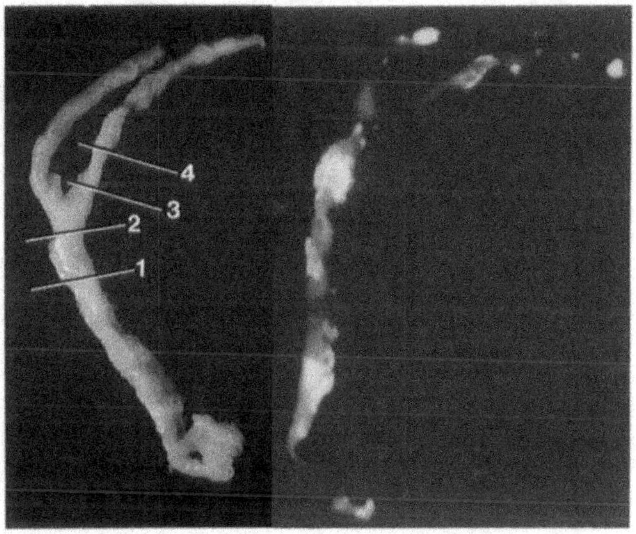

FIG. 1. Photograph (left) and radiograph (right) of the endarterectomy specimen removed 10 years before death from the distal right and proximal posterior descending coronary artery. The numbers approximate locations of the corresponding sections from the distal right (1 and 2), and proximal posterior descending (3 and 4), coronary arteries illustrated in Fig. 2.

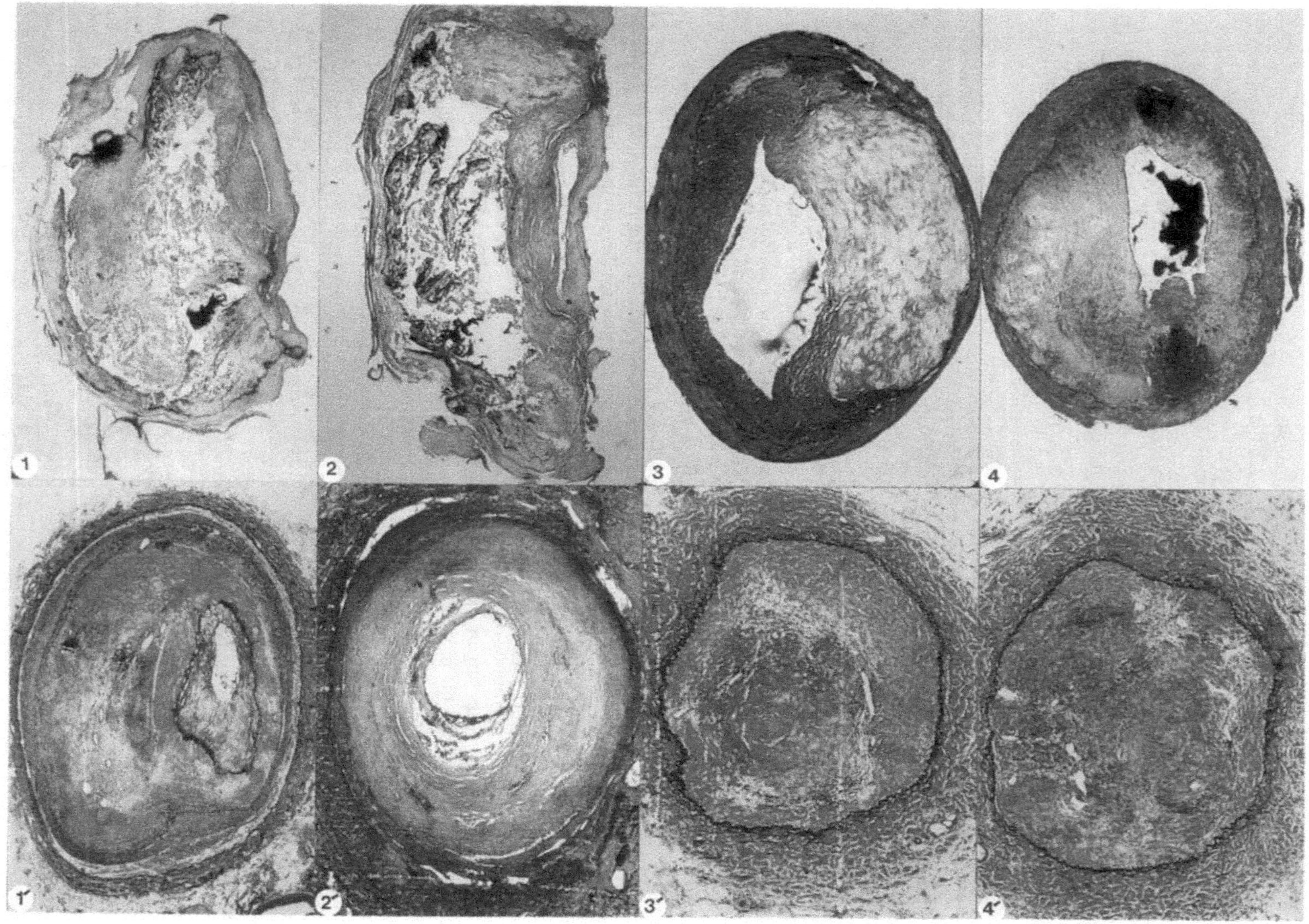

FIG. 2. Photomicrographs of cross-sections of the endarterectomy specimen (1–4) removed 10 years before death, and the corresponding sites in the distal right and proximal posterior descending coronary artery at necropsy (1′–4′). The lumen of the endarterectomy specimen is severely narrowed by focally calcified atherosclerotic plaque. The sections from the proximal posterior descending coronary artery portion (3 and 4) of the surgical specimen contain internal elastic membrane plus media. The lumen of the distal right coronary artery (1′, 2′) at necropsy also is severely narrowed by focally calcified plaque. Sections of proximal posterior descending coronary artery (3′ and 4′), show that internal elastic membrane and media are absent, but there is severe luminal narrowing by a nearly homogeneous proliferation of spindle cells admixed with collagen and containing small vascular channels and scattered inflammatory cells. Movat stains; ×5.2[1], ×3.9[2], ×9.75[3], ×9.75[4], ×4.88[1′], ×6.5[2′], ×9.75[3′], ×9.75[4′].

formed 6 months postoperatively showed all three saphenous vein grafts to be patent. At age 58, the angina returned and by age 60 he was reclassified as functional class 3/4. Repeat catheterization disclosed the saphenous vein grafts to the left anterior descending and the right coronary arteries to be completely occluded. He continued to be severely limited by angina and underwent repeat coronary artery bypass surgery. Saphenous vein grafts were placed to the distal posterior descending, the second diagonal, and the first obtuse marginal coronary arteries, and a left internal mammary graft was placed in the distal left anterior descending coronary artery. The saphenous vein grafts placed 10 years previously were resected. He developed severe pump failure and sepsis and died 26 days after this second operation.

The "endarterectomy" specimen (Fig. 1) removed 10 years before death measured 7 cm in length and consisted of distal right coronary artery and two posterior descending branches. The native right and posterior descending coronary arteries were dissected from the epicardial surface of the heart and, using the bifurcation of the right coronary artery as a landmark, corresponding areas of the surgical and necropsy specimens were identified. Both specimens were decalcified, sectioned transversely at 5 mm intervals, processed in xylene, cleared in alcohol, and stained using the Movat method.

Sections from the proximal endarterectomy specimen (Fig. 2), corresponding to the distal portion of the right coronary artery, showed severe luminal narrowing by calcified atherosclerotic plaque. Small portions of internal elastic membrane and media also were present in these segments. Distal portions of the "endarterectomy" specimen, corresponding to the posterior descending coronary artery, not only showed severe luminal narrowing by calcified atherosclerotic plaque, but also contained large portions of internal elastic membrane and media.

Movat-stained sections of the native distal right coronary artery, examined 10 years after endarterectomy, showed severe luminal narrowing by atherosclerotic plaque composed of admixtures of focally calcified cellular and acellular connective tissue containing small vascular channels and chronic inflammatory cells. The internal elastic membrane and media were focally disrupted. Sections of the proximal posterior descending coronary artery showed near total occlusion of the lumen by cellular fibrous tissue composed of a homogeneous admixture of spindle cells and collagen which contained small vascular channels and chronic inflammatory cells. Both the internal elastic membrane and media were absent (Fig. 2).

Comment

Comparison of features of the native coronary artery and the "endarterectomy" specimen removed 10 years previously showed differences in plaque morphology between segments devoid of internal elastic membrane and media (which had been removed along with plaque) and those segments containing internal elastic membrane and media. In areas where the internal elastic membrane was largely intact, the plaque was pleomorphic, and consisted of cellular and acellular fibrous tissue and calcium. In contrast, where the internal elastic membrane and media had been excised at the time of "endarterectomy," the plaque was much more homogeneous in appearance, and consisted of an admixture of spindle cells and collagen containing only a few inflammatory cells and a few small vascular channels. This homogeneous proliferation of spindle cells admixed with collagen in the absence of the internal elastic membrane is similar to what we reported in a previous case in which death occurred 4.5 years after endarterectomy of the right coronary artery.[2] Byard and associates earlier had described similar changes in 6 of 9 patients who died 6 to 9 years after coronary endarerectomy.[1] Similar changes also have been described in operative specimens in association with early restenosis of the carotid artery after endarterectomy.[3-6] The spindle cells in these plaques have been shown by electron microscopy to have features of both smooth muscle cells and fibroblasts.[7]

References

1. Byard RW, Keon WJ, Walley VM: Coronary endarterectomy: The long-term local effects. *Am J Cardiovasc Pathol* 2, 31 (1988)
2. Kragel AH, McIntosh CL, Roberts WC: Morphologic changes in coronary artery seen late after endarterectomy. *Am J Cardiol* 63, 757 (1989)
3. Stoney RJ, String ST: Recurrent carotid stenosis. *Surgery* 80, 705 (1976)
4. Cossman D, Callow AD, Stein A, Matsumoto G: Early restenosis after carotid endarterectomy. *Arch Surg* 113, 275 (1978)
5. Cantelmo NL, Cutler BS, Wheeler HB, Herrmann JB, Cardullo PA: Noninvasive detection of carotid stenosis following endarterectomy. *Arch Surg* 116, 1005 (1981)
6. Palmaz JC, Hunter G, Carson SN, French SW: Postoperative carotid restenosis due to neointimal fibromuscular hyperplasia. Clinical, angiographic and pathologic findings. *Radiology* 148, 699 (1983)
7. Hertzer NR, Martinez BD, Beven EG: Recurrent stenosis after carotid endarterectomy. *Surg Gynecol Obstet* 149, 360 (1979)

Morphologic findings in saphenous veins used as coronary arterial bypass conduits for longer than 1 year: Necropsy analysis of 53 patients, 123 saphenous veins, and 1865 five-millimeter segments of veins

Certain clinical and necropsy findings are described in 53 patients who died from 13 to 185 months (mean 58) after a single aortocoronary bypass operation. Of the 53 patients, 32 (60%) died of a cardiac cause and of their 72 saphenous vein aortocoronary conduits, 36 (49%) were narrowed at some point more than 75% in cross-sectional area by atherosclerotic plaque; the remaining 21 patients (40%) died of a noncardiac cause and of their 50 saphenous vein conduits, 10 (20%) were narrowed at some point more than 75% in cross-sectional area by plaque. Thus the noncardiac mode of death in a large percentage of the patients suggests that the bypass operation prolonged life to a degree sufficient for another condition to develop. The 123 saphenous vein conduits were divided into 5 mm segments, and a histologic section was prepared from each. Of the 1104 five-millimeter segments in the 32 patients dying as a consequence of myocardial ischemia, 291 (26%) were narrowed more than 75% in cross-sectional area by plaque; in contrast, of the 761 five-millimeter segments of veins in the 21 patients with a noncardiac mode of death, 86 (11%) were narrowed more than 75% by plaque. Of the total 1865 five-millimeter segments of vein, only 395 (21%) were narrowed 25% or less in cross-sectional area by plaque. Thus, in patients dying late after coronary bypass the atherosclerotic process continues in all segments of the saphenous veins used as aortocoronary conduits. Therapy after the operation must be directed toward prevention of progression of the atherosclerosis in the "new" coronary "arteries." (Am Heart J 1990;119:1164.)

Jay M. Kalan, MD,* and William C. Roberts, MD. *Bethesda, Md.*

Saphenous veins, when used as aortocoronary conduits, undergo changes in their intimal, medial, and adventitial layers.[1-15] The predominant late intimal change is a proliferation of fibrous tissue, a finding observed within 2 months after coronary artery bypass grafting. Other late changes in saphenous vein grafts include deposits of lipid, thrombus, and rarely aneurysm formation.[13, 16-18] Most previously published studies describing changes in saphenous veins used as bypass conduits involved few necropsy patients,[1-8] involved only operatively excised specimens,[9-15] or involved cases with relatively short intervals from coronary bypass to death or reoperation. We have studied at necropsy the hearts and grafts of 53 patients who lived longer than 1 year after coronary bypass. This article describes in a quantitative fashion the findings in 123 saphenous vein grafts and in 1865 five-millimeter segments of the grafts in these 53 patients, some of whom died of consequences of myocardial ischemia and some of whom died of noncardiac conditions.

From the Pathology Branch, National Heart, Lung, and Blood Institute, National Institutes of Health.

Received for publication Nov. 3, 1989; accepted Dec. 20, 1989.

Reprint requests: William C. Roberts, MD, Building 10, Room 2N258, NIH, Bethesda, MD 20892.

*Present address: Section of Cardiology, Department of Medicine, University Hospital, Boston University Medical Center, Boston, Mass.

4/1/19092

METHODS

Patient selection. The records in the Pathology Branch, National Heart, Lung, and Blood Institute, were reviewed in all patients having coronary bypass utilizing one or more saphenous vein grafts from March 1975 to June 1988. Of the 467 patients reviewed, 90 had cardiac valve replacement simultaneously with coronary bypass and they were excluded. Of the remaining 377 patients, 79 lived longer than 1 year after coronary bypass. The saphenous vein grafts or native coronary arteries were not available for reexamination in 26 of these patients, and they were excluded. The remaining 53 patients had both heart and by-

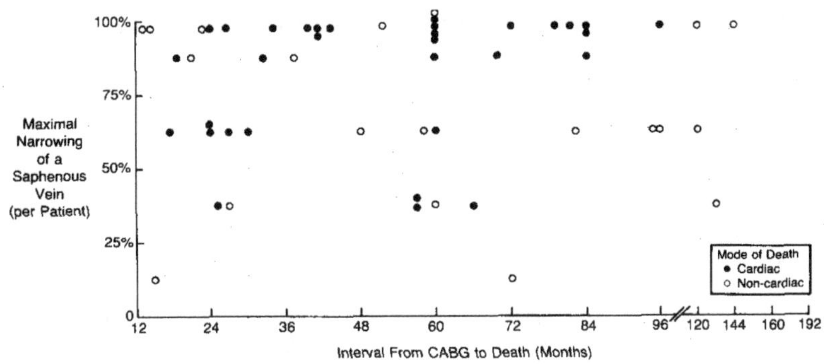

Fig. 1. Relation of maximal cross-sectional area narrowing of saphenous vein graft in each of 53 patients to interval (1 to 15 years [mean 5]) from coronary artery bypass grafting *(CABG)* to death.

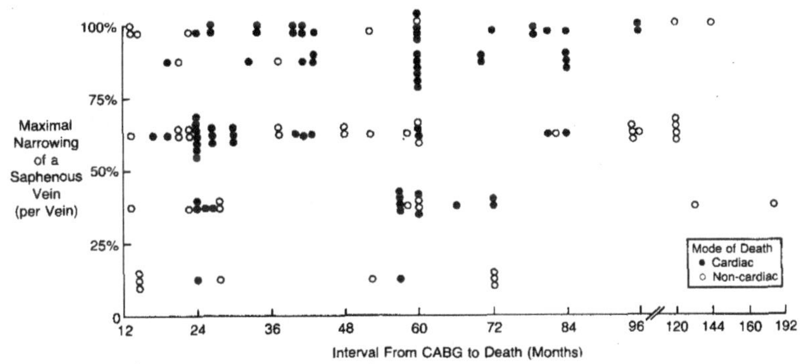

Fig. 2. Relation of maximal cross-sectional area narrowing of each of 123 saphenous vein grafts to interval (1 to 15 years [mean 5]) from coronary artery bypass grafting *(CABG)* to death.

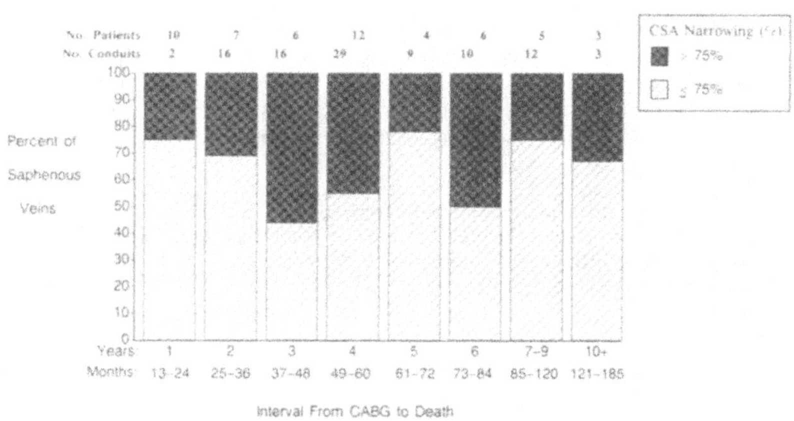

Fig. 3. Relation of percentage of 123 saphenous vein grafts narrowed more than and less than 75% in cross-sectional area *(CSA)* by plaque to interval from coronary artery bypass grafting *(CABG)* to death (1 to 15 years [mean 5]).

pass grafts available for study, and these 53 patients make up our study group.

Patient characteristics. Findings in the 53 patients are shown in detail in Table I and are summarized in Table II. The ages at death ranged from 39 to 82 years (mean 60); 43 (81%) were men and 10 (19%) were women. The interval from coronary artery bypass grafting to death ranged from 13 to 185 months (mean 58).

The 53 patients had a total of 127 grafts: 123 saphenous veins and four internal mammary arteries. All four patients with an internal mammary artery conduit also had one or more saphenous vein conduits. The number of grafts

Table I. Clinical and necropsy cardiac findings in 53 patients surviving more than 1 year after coronary artery bypass grafting

Patient No.	*Age at death (yr)*	*Sex*	*Interval CABG to death (mo)*	*SH*	*DM*	*After CABG* *AP*	*AMI*	*CHF*	*Mode of death*	*HW (gm)*	*Dilated LV*	*LV necrosis*	*LV fibrosis*
Cardiac death													
1	56	M	17	0	0	0	0	0	Sudden	475	0	0	+
2	54	M	19	+	+	0	0	+	CHF	510	+	0	+
3	64	F	24	+	+	+	0	+	CHF	490	+	0	+
4	60	M	24	0	0	0	0	+	CHF	540	+	0	+
5	70	F	24	0	0	0	0	+	CHF	500	+	0	+
6	51	M	25	0	0	0	0	0	Sudden	575	0	0	+
7	66	M	26	0	0	0	0	0	Sudden	460	0	0	+
8	44	F	26	+	0	0	0	+	Sudden	600	+	0	+
9	68	F	30	+	+	+	0	+	Sudden	550	+	0	0
10	47	M	32	0	+	+	0	0	AMI	390	0	+	0
11	69	M	34	0	0	+	+	0	Sudden	550	+	0	+
12	49	M	39	0	0	0	0	0	Sudden	370	0	0	0
13	54	M	41	0	0	0	0	0	Sudden	460	+	0	+
14	45	M	41	+	+	0	0	0	Sudden	520	0	0	+
15	44	F	43	0	+	+	+	+	CHF	498	+	0	+
16	71	M	57	+	0	0	0	+	CHF	550	+	0	+
17	54	M	57	+	0	+	0	0	Sudden	575	0	0	+
18	60	M	60	+	0	0	0	+	CHF	865	+	0	+
19	45	M	60	+	0	+	+	0	Sudden†	620	+	0	+
20	53	M	60	+	+	+	0	+	CHF	550	+	0	+
21	50	M	60	+	0	0	0	0	Sudden	580	+	0	+
22	47	M	60	+	0	+	0	+	CHF	580	+	+	+
23	51	M	60	0	+	+	+	0	Sudden	580	0	0	+
24	57	M	66	+	0	–	–	–	Sudden	660	+	0	+
25	68	F	70	+	+	0	0	+	Sudden	550	+	0	+
26	67	M	72	+	+	+	+	+	CHF	410	+	0	+
27	45	M	79	0	+	+	+	+	CHF	680	+	0	+
28	49	F	81	0	0	+	+	0	Sudden	640	+	0	+
29	39	M	84	0	0	+	+	0	AMI	400	0	+	+
30	57	M	84	+	+	+	0	0	Sudden	515	0	0	+
31	72	M	84	+	0	+	0	0	Sudden	590	0	0	+
32	49	M	96	0	0	+	0	+	CHF	520	+	0	+

AAA, Abdominal aortic aneurysm; AMI, acute myocardial infarction; AP, angina pectoris; CABG, coronary artery bypass grafting; CSA, cross-sectional area; DM, diabetes mellitus; HW, heart weight; LAD, left anterior descending; LV, left ventricle (ventricular); CHF, chronic congestive heart failure; COPD, chronic obstructive pulmonary disease; OM, obtuse marginal; SH, systemic hypertension by history.

*Widely patent internal mammary artery is also present.

†Immediately after cardiac catheterization.

‡Originating from saphenous vein anastomotic site.

§Result of mitral regurgitation.

||Multiple complications after CABG—never left hospital.

per patient ranged from one to four (mean 2.4). A saphenous vein with one aortic anastomosis and more than one coronary artery anastomosis was considered a single conduit.

Modes of death. Death was due to a *cardiac cause* in 32 patients (60%): sudden cardiac arrest in 18 patients (16 outside the hospital) without myocardial necrosis, chronic congestive heart failure in 12, and acute myocardial infarction in two. Death was attributed to a *noncardiac cause* in 21 patients (40%): a vascular condition in six patients (abdominal aortic aneurysm in two, stroke in two, aortic dissection in one, and complication of carotid endarterectomy in one), cancer in 10 (19%), and miscellaneous conditions in five (Parkinson's disease, chronic obstructive lung disease, pancreatitis, trauma, and infection).

Examination of hearts. The hearts were fixed in 10% formaldehyde and submitted to the Pathology Branch, National Heart, Lung, and Blood Institute, from 23 different hospitals. The aorta was cut transversely just cephalad to the saphenous vein anastomotic sites. After the parietal pericardium was excised, the hearts were weighed on a Mettler P1210 scale (Mettler Instrument Corp., Highstown, N.J.) and then examined grossly for the presence of fibrosis, necrosis, chamber dilatation, mural throm-

							Saphenous vein conduits	
	Number narrowed		Number of conduits containing:					
No. of conduits	<75%	>75%	Foam cells only	Extracellular lipid	Hemorrhage into plaque	Thrombus	Calcific deposits	No. of 5 mm segments
1	1*	0	1	0	0	0	0	15
2	1	1	0	0	0	0	0	37
3	3	0	0	0	0	0	0	58
4	3	1	3	0	1	0	0	47
3	3	0	1	0	0	0	0	54
1	1	0	0	0	0	0	0	9
3	3	0	2	0	0	0	0	50
3	1	2	0	0	0	0	0	48
3	3	0	0	0	0	0	0	37
1	0	1	0	1	1	1	0	9
2	0	2	0	2	2	2	1	52
3	1	2	0	3	3	0	0	33
2	0	2	1	1	2	0	0	35
2	1	1	0	0	0	0	0	32
4	1	3	0	3	1	0	0	53
3	3	0	0	0	0	0	0	43
2	2	0	1	0	1	0	0	21
3	0	3	1	2	2	1	1	59
2	0	2	0	1	0	0	0	28
2	1	1	0	1	1	1	0	12
3	3	0	1	2	0	0	0	51
1	0*	1	0	0	0	0	0	7
3	0	3	0	3	3	1	0	58
1	1	0	1	0	0	0	0	12
2	0	2	0	2	2	2	0	25
3	2	1	2	0	0	0	0	41
2	0	2	0	0	0	0	0	20
2	1	1	0	2	1	1	2	43
1	1	0	0	1	1	1	1	11
2	0	2	1	1	1	1	0	33
2	1	1	1	1	0	0	1	52
2	0	2	1	0	0	0	1	19

bus, and valvular abnormalities. Sections of left ventricular myocardium were available for review in 40 cases.

Examination of saphenous vein grafts. Saphenous vein bypass grafts were removed from the heart with the saphenous vein-coronary artery anastomoses intact. Each saphenous vein was cut transversely into 5 mm long segments. Each segment was processed in alcohol and xylene, embedded in paraffin, cut into 6 μm thick sections, and stained with Movat pentachrome.[19] A total of 1865 five-millimeter segments of saphenous vein graft (mean of 35 per patient) were studied. Luminal narrowing, measured as a decrease in the cross-sectional area enclosed by the intimal-medial border, was graded by visual inspection of the histologic sections at a magnification of 40 times. The amount of narrowing of each 5 mm long segment was categorized into five groups: 0% to 25%, 26% to 50%, 51% to 75%, 76% to 95%, and 96% to 100% of cross-sectional area.

Each component of tissue in the previous lumen of each segment of graft was determined by examination at higher magnifications by light microscopy (to ×430). *Fibrous tissue* was graded 1^+ to 4^+, with 1^+ indicating only a thin layer of fibrous tissue and 4^+ indicating complete or nearly complete occlusion by fibrous tissue. *Lipid*, both intracellular (foam cells) and extracellular (cholesterol clefts and pultaceous debris), and *calcium* were graded 0 (absent) to 3+, with 3+ corresponding to more than 50% of the luminal cross-sectional area narrowed by lipid or calcium. *Hemorrhage into plaque* indicated the presence of erythrocytes within lipid in the plaque, with or without histologic confirmation of plaque rupture. Antemortem *luminal thrombus* consisted of fibrin with or without erythrocytes or platelets within the lumen with attachment at some site to the wall bordering the lumen.

Examination of internal mammary artery grafts. The four internal mammary arteries were removed, sectioned, and examined by the same method as described above.

Table I. cont.

Patient No.	Age at death (yr)	Sex	Interval CABG to death (mo)	SH	DM	After CABG AP	AMI	CHF	Mode of death	HW (gm)	Dilated LV	LV necrosis	LV fibrosis
Noncardiac death—vascular													
33	65	M	14	0	0	0	0	0	AAA	430	0	0	+
34	76	M	23	0	0	+	0	+	Aortic dissection‡	670	0	0	0
35	60	M	95	+	+	0	0	0	Stroke	695	+	0	+
36	62	M	96	+	0	+	0	0	AAA	625	+	0	+
37	54	M	120	+	0	+	0	0	Carotid endarterectomy	560	0	0	+
38	82	M	132	+	0	0	0	0	Stroke	485	+§	0	0
Noncardiac death—cancer													
39	60	M	13	+	+	0	0	0	Cancer	520	0	0	0
40	67	M	21	+	0	0	0	0	Cancer	575	+	0	+
41	62	M	27	+	0	0	0	0	Cancer	450	0	0	0
42	78	F	37	+	0	0	0	0	Cancer	355	0	0	+
43	76	M	48	0	0	0	0	0	Cancer	395	0	0	+
44	70	M	58	+	0	0	0	0	Cancer	390	0	0	0
45	70	M	60	+	+	0	0	0	Cancer	480	0	0	0
46	59	F	72	0	0	0	0	0	Cancer	410	0	0	+
47	69	M	82	0	0	0	0	0	Cancer	440	0	0	0
48	63	M	144	0	0	0	0	0	Cancer	310	0	0	+
Noncardiac death—other													
49	59	M	14	0	0	0	0	0	Infection‖	710	0	0	+
50	58	M	52	+	+	+	0	0	Pancreatitis	340	0	0	0
51	73	M	60	+	0	0	0	0	COPD	540	0	0	+
52	74	F	120	0	0	0	0	0	Trauma	460	0	0	0
53	63	M	185	0	0	+	0	0	Parkinson's disease	345	0	0	0

Variable lengths of internal mammary arteries were studied, with the distal anastomoses intact in all specimens. The number of 5 mm segments studied per patient ranged from 4 to 20 (mean 10) (total 40).

Examination of native coronary arteries. The four major epicardial coronary arteries (left main, left anterior descending, left circumflex, and right) were removed from the heart in 51 of the 53 patients, divided into 5 mm segments, processed, and sectioned. In addition, the first diagonal and/or obtuse marginal coronary arteries were studied if a bypass graft was anastomosed to them. In the remaining two patients the proximal portions of the arteries were unavailable. A total of 2336 five-millimeter long coronary artery segments (mean 46 per patient) were studied. Arteries containing calcium were decalcified before processing. The degree of luminal narrowing, measured as a decrease in the cross-sectional area enclosed by the internal elastic membrane, was determined.

Statistical analyses. Statistical analyses of noncontinuous data was done by the chi-square method and of continuous data by the Student's t test. A probability <0.05 was considered significant.

RESULTS

Luminal narrowing of conduits

Saphenous vein narrowing (by number of patients). Of the 53 patients, 31 (58%) had at least one bypass graft maximally narrowed more than 75% in cross-sectional area at some point by fibromuscular tissue with or without lipid (Table I); 12 patients (23%) had maximal narrowing of a graft of 51% to 75%; eight patients (15%), 26% to 50%; and two patients (4%), 0% to 25%. The percentage of patients with a graft narrowed more than 75% was similar in men and women (26 of 43 [60%] versus 5 of 10 [50%]), in patients with and without a history of systemic hypertension (17 of 29 [59%]) versus 14 of 24 [58%]), and in patients with and without diabetes mellitus (12 of 16 [75%] versus 19 of 37 [51%]). The percentage of patients with a graft narrowed more than 75% at necropsy did not increase as the interval from bypass surgery to death increased (Fig. 1).

Saphenous vein narrowing (by number of veins). Of the 123 saphenous vein grafts, 47 (38%) were maximally narrowed more than 75% in cross-sectional area; 44 (36%), 51% to 75%; 22 (18%), 26% to 50%; and 10 (8%), 0% to 25%. Of the 47 grafts narrowed more than 75% in cross-sectional area, 29 actually were narrowed more than 95% in cross-sectional area by fibrous tissue. The percentage of saphenous veins narrowed more than 75% at necropsy

Saphenous vein conduits

No. of conduits	Number narrowed <75%	Number narrowed >75%	Number of conduits containing: Foam cells only	Extracellular lipid	Hemorrhage into plaque	Thrombus	Calcific deposits	No. of 5 mm segments
1	0	1	1	0	0	0	0	28
4	3	1	2	0	0	0	0	93
3	3	0	0	0	0	0	0	58
1	1*	0	0	1	0	0	0	12
2	1	1	2	0	0	0	0	21
1	1	0	0	1	0	1	1	12
4	2	2	0	0	0	0	0	55
3	2	1	3	0	0	0	0	63
3	3	0	2	0	0	0	0	29
3	2	1	1	1	1	1	0	33
2	2	0	0	0	0	0	0	62
2	2	0	0	1	0	0	2	16
3	2	1	1	1	1	1	1	38
3	3	0	1	0	0	0	1	32
1	1	0	0	0	0	0	0	12
1	0*	1	0	1	0	1	0	15
3	3	0	0	0	0	0	0	52
3	2	1	1	2	2	1	0	30
2	2	0	2	0	0	0	0	40
4	4	0	0	1	0	0	0	52
1	1	0	0	1	0	0	1	8

was not affected by sex (men 38%, women 36%), presence or absence of systemic hypertension (40% versus 33%), or presence or absence of diabetes mellitus (30% versus 48%). The percentage of grafts narrowed more than 75% in cross-sectional area did not correlate with the interval between bypass surgery and death (Figs. 2 and 3) or with the coronary artery to which the graft was connected (left anterior descending, 15 of 44 [34%]; first diagonal, 3 of 9 [33%]; obtuse marginal, 13 of 37 [35%]; and right, 14 of 33 [42%]).

The degree of narrowing of the saphenous vein graft was related to the degree of luminal narrowing of the native coronary artery at, or within 2 cm distal to, the saphenous vein-coronary artery anastomosis. Of the 49 grafts attached to a coronary artery that was narrowed more than 75% at or distal to the anastomosis, 33 (67%) were significantly narrowed; of the 74 grafts attached to a coronary artery narrowed less than 75% distal to the anastomotic site, 14 (19%) were severely narrowed ($p < 0.0001$) (Fig. 4).

Saphenous vein narrowing (by number of 5 mm segments). Analysis of the 1865 five-millimeter long saphenous vein segments disclosed that 209 segments (11%) were narrowed 96% to 100% in cross-sectional area; 172 (9%), 76% to 95%; 407 (22%), 51% to 75%; 685 (37%), 26% to 50%; and 392 (21%), 0% to 25% (Fig. 5). Similar percentages of segments were narrowed more than 75% in men and women (22% versus 15%), in patients with and without diabetes (18% versus 26%), and in patients with and without hypertension (21% versus 20%). Further, the interval from coronary bypass to death did not correlate with the percentage of segments severely narrowed (Fig. 5).

Although the percentage of saphenous vein segments narrowed more than 75% in cross-sectional area at necropsy did not correlate with the interval from bypass grafting to death, it did relate to the mode of death. Of the 32 patients dying of a cardiac cause, 295 (27%) of 1104 saphenous vein segments were narrowed more than 75%, whereas of the 21 patients dying of a noncardiac cause, 86 (11%) of 761 saphenous vein segments were so narrowed ($p < 0.01$) (Fig. 6). The percentage of segments of native coronary artery narrowed more than 75% was similar in patients with cardiac and noncardiac modes of death (673 of 1441 [47%] versus 333 of 895 [37%]) (Fig. 6).

Internal mammary artery as conduit. Each of the four internal mammary arteries was anastomosed to the left anterior descending coronary artery and each was widely patent. Of the 40 five-millimeter seg-

Table I. cont.

Patient No.	Age at death (yr)	Sex	Number (%) of 5 mm segments narrowed to various degrees in cross-sectional area by fibromuscular and/or lipid tissue: 0%-25%	26%-50%	51%-75%	76%-95%	96%-100%	Native coronary arteries: No. of 5 mm segments	No. (%) of segments narrowed >75% in CSA	Thrombus
Cardiac death										
1	56	M	0 (0)	4 (27)	11 (73)	0 (0)	0 (0)	38	11 (29)	0
2	54	M	2 (6)	13 (35)	16 (43)	6 (16)	0 (0)	38	9 (24)	OM
3	64	F	7 (12)	39 (67)	12 (21)	0 (0)	0 (0)	58	30 (52)	0
4	60	M	13 (28)	23 (48)	4 (9)	4 (0)	3 (6)	46	15 (33)	0
5	70	F	6 (11)	29 (54)	19 (35)	0 (0)	0 (0)	41	14 (34)	0
6	51	M	8 (89)	1 (11)	0 (0)	0 (0)	0 (0)	43	8 (19)	0
7	66	M	30 (60)	17 (34)	3 (6)	0 (0)	0 (0)	44	15 (34)	0
8	44	F	1 (2)	10 (21)	9 (19)	16 (33)	12 (25)	44	24 (55)	0
9	68	F	2 (5)	20 (54)	15 (41)	0 (0)	0 (0)	42	19 (45)	0
10	47	M	4 (44)	2 (22)	1 (12)	2 (22)	0 (0)	27	6 (22)	Right
11	69	M	2 (4)	16 (31)	13 (25)	13 (25)	8 (15)	49	36 (73)	LAD
12	49	M	1 (3)	18 (55)	5 (15)	7 (21)	2 (6)	53	27 (51)	0
13	54	M	0 (0)	5 (14)	13 (37)	4 (11)	13 (37)	46	26 (57)	0
14	45	M	0 (0)	14 (44)	2 (6)	0 (0)	16 (50)	51	17 (33)	Right
15	44	F	9 (17)	7 (13)	27 (51)	8 (15)	2 (4)	49	31 (63)	0
16	71	M	10 (23)	33 (77)	0 (0)	0 (0)	0 (0)	42	13 (31)	0
17	54	M	20 (95)	1 (5)	0 (0)	0 (0)	0 (0)	36	13 (36)	0
18	60	M	0 (0)	14 (24)	17 (29)	20 (34)	8 (14)	46	28 (61)	0
19	45	M	2 (8)	4 (14)	6 (21)	8 (29)	8 (29)	58	29 (50)	0
20	53	M	0 (0)	3 (25)	8 (67)	1 (8)	0 (0)	36	27 (75)	0
21	50	M	17 (33)	24 (45)	10 (22)	0 (0)	0 (0)	49	30 (61)	0
22	47	M	0 (0)	0 (0)	0 (0)	0 (0)	7 (100)	44	16 (36)	0
23	51	M	0 (0)	10 (18)	24 (41)	20 (34)	4 (7)	44	27 (61)	OM
24	57	M	0 (0)	12 (100)	0 (0)	0 (0)	0 (0)	40	5 (13)	0
25	68	F	0 (0)	12 (48)	9 (36)	4 (16)	0 (0)	36	16 (44)	0
26	67	M	22 (54)	5 (12)	0 (0)	0 (0)	14 (34)	37	12 (32)	0
27	45	M	0 (0)	0 (0)	0 (0)	5 (25)	15 (75)	73	44 (60)	OM
28	49	F	0 (0)	13 (30)	7 (17)	3 (7)	20 (47)	30	12 (40)	0
29	39	M	5 (45)	6 (55)	0 (0)	0 (0)	0 (0)	56	30 (54)	Right
30	57	M	15 (46)	13 (39)	2 (6)	1 (3)	2 (6)	45	23 (51)	0
31	72	M	6 (12)	16 (30)	13 (25)	6 (12)	11 (21)	52	37 (71)	0
32	49	M	0 (0)	1 (5)	0 (0)	11 (58)	7 (37)	48	29 (60)	0
Noncardiac death—vascular										
33	65	M	0 (0)	8 (29)	7 (25)	8 (29)	5 (18)	43	28 (65)	0
34	76	M	6 (7)	44 (47)	27 (29)	0 (0)	16 (17)	43	12 (28)	0
35	60	M	1 (2)	36 (62)	21 (36)	0 (0)	0 (0)	58	38 (66)	0
36	62	M	10 (83)	1 (8)	1 (8)	0 (0)	0 (0)	·	·	0
37	54	M	13 (62)	0 (0)	1 (5)	0 (0)	7 (33)	46	17 (37)	0
38	82	M	6 (50)	6 (50)	0 (0)	0 (0)	0 (0)	48	2 (4)	0
Noncardiac death—cancer										
39	60	M	4 (7)	18 (33)	10 (18)	0 (0)	23 (42)	64	12 (19)	0
40	67	M	0 (0)	15 (24)	44 (70)	4 (6)	0 (0)	46	32 (70)	0
41	62	M	26 (90)	3 (10)	0 (0)	0 (0)	0 (0)	42	11 (26)	0
42	78	F	6 (18)	13 (39)	12 (36)	2 (6)	0 (0)	53	13 (25)	0
43	76	M	2 (4)	53 (85)	7 (11)	0 (0)	0 (0)	49	26 (53)	0
44	70	M	0 (0)	14 (88)	2 (12)	0 (0)	0 (0)	40	9 (23)	0
45	70	M	0 (0)	10 (27)	13 (34)	13 (34)	2 (5)	74	12 (16)	0
46	59	F	32 (100)	0 (0)	0 (0)	0 (0)	0 (0)	46	12 (26)	0
47	69	M	1 (8)	9 (75)	2 (17)	0 (0)	0 (0)	·	·	0
48	63	M	5 (33)	6 (40)	1 (7)	1 (7)	2 (13)	40	26 (60)	Right
Noncardiac death—other										
49	59	M	52 (100)	0 (0)	0 (0)	0 (0)	0 (0)	51	25 (49)	0
50	58	M	14 (46)	11 (37)	2 (7)	1 (3)	2 (7)	27	10 (37)	0
51	73	M	24 (60)	16 (40)	0 (0)	0 (0)	0 (0)	32	8 (25)	LAD
52	74	F	6 (12)	38 (73)	8 (15)	0 (0)	0 (0)	56	23 (41)	Right
53	63	M	5 (62)	3 (38)	0 (0)	0 (0)	0 (0)	37	19 (51)	0

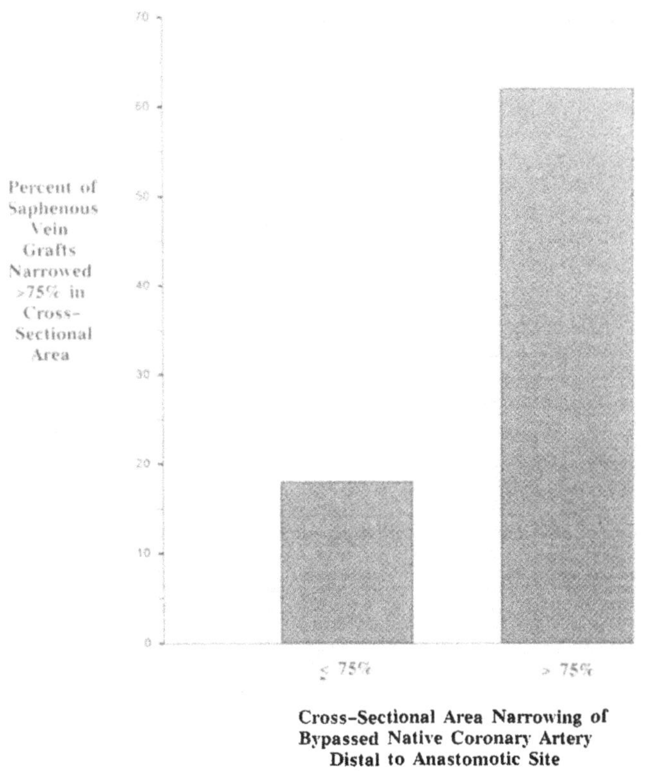

Fig. 4. Relation of percentage of 123 saphenous vein grafts narrowed >75% in cross-sectional area to presence or absence of >75% cross-sectional area narrowing of 123 native coronary arteries distal to coronary anastomotic site.

ments, one (2%) was narrowed 26% to 50%, and 39 (98%), 0% to 25%. No lipid deposits were present.

Composition of tissue causing luminal narrowing

General. Photomicrographs of saphenous veins in place from 13 to 144 months are shown in Figs. 7 to 22.

Lipid in saphenous vein conduits (by number of patients). Lipid was present in the wall of a graft in 39 patients (74%). Fifteen had intracellular lipid alone (foam cells), and 24 had both foam cells and extracellular lipid deposits (cholesterol clefts and pultaceous debris). Intracellular lipid was present in grafts from patients living from 14 months to 10 years after coronary bypass, and the frequency of its presence did not change as the interval from bypass surgery to death increased. Extracellular lipid was not found in a saphenous vein graft until 26 months after bypass (Figs. 11 to 15, 18, 19, and 22).

Lipid in saphenous vein conduits (by number of veins). Lipid was present in 69 of the 123 (56%) saphenous vein grafts from 39 patients. Intracellular lipid (foam cells) was present in all 69 grafts, either alone (33 grafts) or along with extracellular lipid (36 grafts). The amount of lipid present, as measured on a 0 to 3+ scale, appeared to increase as the interval from coronary bypass to death increased. Foam cells, in the absence of cholesterol clefts, were located on the luminal surfaces of the intimal fibrous tissue and did not appreciably narrow the saphenous vein lumen (Figs. 10, 16, and 19). Extracellular lipid deposits were located deeper in the plaque and never formed a portion of the border of the lumen. They were separated from the lumen by a layer of fibrous tissue. Larger deposits contributed significantly to luminal narrowing.

Hemorrhage into saphenous vein plaque (by patient and by vein). Hemorrhage into plaque was found in 26 (21%) saphenous vein grafts from 17 (32%) patients (Figs. 12, 13, 15, and 18). It occurred in a patient dying as early as 24 months after bypass and did not increase in frequency as the interval from bypass to death increased. The hemorrhage was into an area of extracellular lipid in 22 grafts and into an area of isolated foam cells in four grafts. Hemorrhage into fibrous tissue was not seen. Luminal narrowing greater than 75% in cross-sectional area was more common in grafts with plaque hemorrhage (16 of 26 [61%]) than in those without plaque hemorrhage (28 of 97 [29%]; $p < 0.004$).

Luminal thrombus in saphenous vein grafts (by patient and by vein). Luminal thrombus was present in 16 (13%) saphenous vein grafts from 14 (26%) patients (Figs. 12, 13, 18, and 22). Thrombus was not seen until 32 months after bypass, and its frequency did not increase as the interval from bypass to death increased. Typically a thin layer of fibrous tissue overlying a lipid deposit was disrupted, with either the lipid material exuded into the lumen with fresh thrombus attached to this material, or thrombus alone occluded the lumen, attached to both the lipid deposit and to the intimal fibrous tissue. Thrombus within the graft lumen was present in 16 of 69 grafts that had deposits of lipid in their walls and in none of 54 grafts devoid of lipid. In 14 of these 16 grafts, hemorrhage into plaque also was found. Thrombus occurred in the absence of identifiable plaque hemorrhage in two patients who died 132 and 144 months, respectively, after bypass. No thrombus was present in the 53 saphenous vein grafts devoid of lipid.

Calcific deposits in saphenous vein grafts (by patient and by vein). Calcific deposits were present in 13 (11%) of the 123 saphenous vein grafts from 11 patients, and they were first seen 34 months after coronary bypass (Figs. 14 and 19). All of the deposits were small ($1^+/3^+$), and they were present in 18 (1%) of the 1865 five-millimeter saphenous vein segments.

Luminal narrowing of native coronary arteries

Coronary artery narrowing. Of the 51 patients whose coronary arteries were available for analysis, all had at least one major epicardial coronary artery narrowed more than 75% in cross-sectional area by atherosclerotic plaque at some point: four arteries were so narrowed in 12 (24%) patients, three arte-

Table II. Summary of findings arranged according to mode of death in 53 patients surviving greater than 1 year after coronary artery bypass grafting

Mode of death	*No. of patients*	*M:F*	*Mean age at CABG (yr)*	*Mean age at death (yr)*	*Mean interval CABG to death (mo)*	*No. with SH*	*No. with DM*	*Mean HW (gm)*	*No. of SVs*	*No. (%) SVs >75% in CSA*	*No. of SVs narrowed*	
											76%-95%	*96%-100%*
Cardiac	32	25:7	52	56	51	17	12	542	73	37 (51)	15 (21)	22 (30)
Sudden	18	14:4	52	56	50	10	5	548	39	20 (51)	7 (18)	13 (33)
AMI	2	2:0	38	43	58	0	1	395	2	2	2	0
Chronic CHF	12	9:3	53	57	52	7	6	558	32	15 (47)	6 (19)	9 (28)
Noncardiac	21	18:3	61	67	69	12	4	485	50	10 (20)	3 (6)	7 (14)
Vascular	6	6:0	60	67	80	4	1	578	12	3 (25)	0	3 (25)
Cancer	10	8:2	62	67	56	6	2	432	25	6 (24)	3 (12)	3 (12)
Other	5	4:1	58	65	86	2	1	479	13	1 (8)	0	1 (8)
Totals	53	43:10	56	60	58	29	16	519	123	47	18	29

AMI, Acute myocardial infarction; CABG, coronary artery bypass grafting; CHF, congestive heart failure; CSA, cross-sectional area; DM, diabetes mellitus; FM, fibromuscular; HW, heart weight; SH, systemic hypertension by history; SV, saphenous vein.

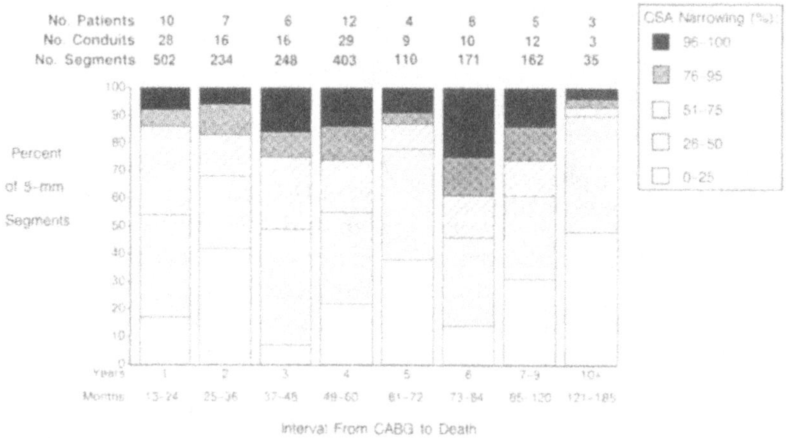

Fig. 5. Mean percentage of 5 mm segments of saphenous vein graft narrowed in cross-sectional area *(CSA)* to various degrees by plaque in patients surviving 1 to 15 years (mean 5) after coronary artery bypass grafting *(CABG)*.

ries in 30 (59%) patients, two arteries in five (10%) patients, and one artery in four (8%) patients. Of the 204 major epicardial coronary arteries, 151 (74%) were severely narrowed, a mean of 3.0/4 per patient: left main in 12 patients (24%), left anterior descending in 49 patients (96%), left circumflex in 44 patients (86%), and right in 46 patients (90%). The percentage of 5 mm segments of the four major native coronary arteries narrowed to the four categories of cross-sectional area narrowing are summarized in figure 23.

Comparison of bypassed versus nonbypassed native coronary arteries. The coronary arteries were divided into two groups: those bypassed and those not. In addition, among bypassed coronary arteries comparison was made between the segments proximal and distal to the anastomosis. Of the 51 patients, five arteries (four bypassed and one not) could not be included because of missing distal segments. Of the remaining 165 coronary arteries, 127 were bypassed and 38 were not. Of the 38 nonbypassed coronary arteries, 24 (63%) were maximally narrowed more than 75% in cross-sectional area by atherosclerotic plaque; of the 127 bypassed coronary arteries, 125 (98%) were severely narrowed ($p = 0.001$) (Fig. 24). Among the bypassed coronary arteries, the area proximal to

Thrombus		Hemorrhage into plaque		Lipid			Number (%) of 5 mm long SV segments narrowed to various degrees of CSA by FM and/or lipid tissue				
No. (%) of patients	No. (%) of SVs	No. (%) of patients	No. (%) of SVs	No. (%) of patients	No. (%) of SVs	No. of 5 mm SV segments	0%-25%	26%-50%	51%-75%	76%-95%	96%-100%
9 (28)	11 (15)	14 (44)	22 (30)	23 (72)	43 (59)	1104	182 (16)	385 (35)	246 (22)	139 (13)	152 (14)
5 (28)	7 (18)	8 (44)	15 (38)	14 (78)	27 (69)	634	104 (16)	210 (33)	142 (22)	82 (13)	96 (15)
2	2	2	2	2	2	20	9 (45)	8 (40)	1 (5)	2 (10)	0
2 (17)	2 (6)	4 (33)	5 (16)	7 (58)	14 (44)	450	69 (15)	167 (37)	103 (23)	55 (12)	56 (12)
5 (23)	5 (10)	3 (14)	4 (8)	16 (73)	26 (52)	761	213 (28)	304 (40)	158 (21)	29 (4)	57 (7)
0	1 (8)	0	0	5	7 (58)	224	36 (16)	95 (42)	57 (25)	8 (4)	28 (13)
3 (27)	3 (12)	2 (18)	2 (18)	7 (64)	12 (48)	355	76 (21)	141 (40)	91 (26)	20 (6)	27 (8)
1	1 (8)	2	2 (15)	4	7 (54)	182	101 (55)	68 (37)	10 (2)	1 (1)	2 (1)
14 (26)	16 (13)	17 (32)	26 (21)	39 (74)	69 (56)	1865	395 (21)	689 (37)	404 (22)	168 (9)	209 (11)

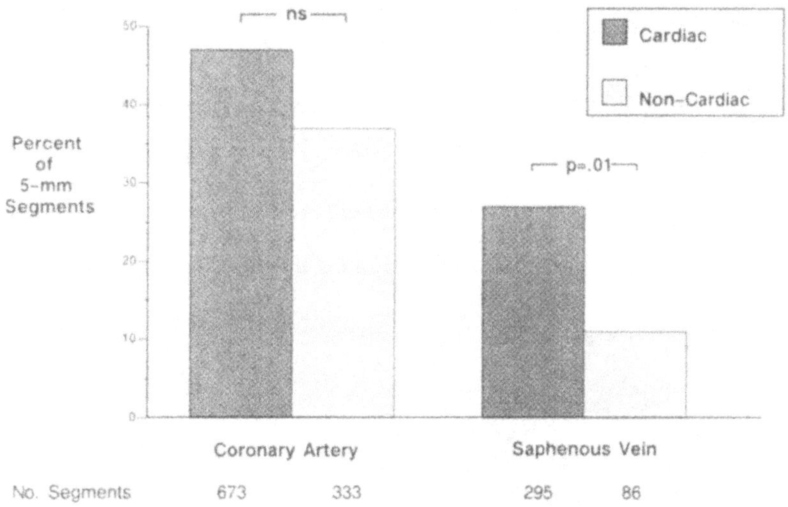

Fig. 6. Comparison of percentage of 5 mm segments of bypassed native coronary arteries and of saphenous vein grafts narrowed more than 75% in cross-sectional area in 32 patients with cardiac modes of death and in 21 patients with noncardiac modes of death (1 to 15 years [mean 5]).

the anastomosis was maximally narrowed more than 75% in cross-sectional area in 125 coronary arteries (98%), and the lumen distal to the graft anastomosis was severely narrowed in 49 arteries (39%).

Amount of narrowing (by number of segments). Of the 2336 five-millimeter segments of coronary artery, 1277 were from the area proximal to a bypass graft anastomosis. Of these, 739 (58%) were narrowed more than 75% in cross-sectional area (Fig. 25). Of the 538 five-millimeter segments from the area distal to an anastomosis, 89 (17%) were so narrowed ($p = 0.001$) (Fig. 25). Of the 491 segments of nonbypassed coronary arteries, 163 (33%) were narrowed more than 75%, less than the percentage of narrowed segments of preanastomosis coronary arteries ($p = 0.001$) and more than the postanastomotic coronary segments ($p = 0.001$) (Fig. 25).

DISCUSSION

The aforementioned data indicate that virtually all saphenous veins used as aortocoronary conduits for longer than a year develop atherosclerotic plaques in each 5 mm segment of their entire lengths. Of the 1865 five-millimeter segments of saphenous vein conduit studied, only 392 (21%) were narrowed 25% or less in cross-sectional area, and none was entire-

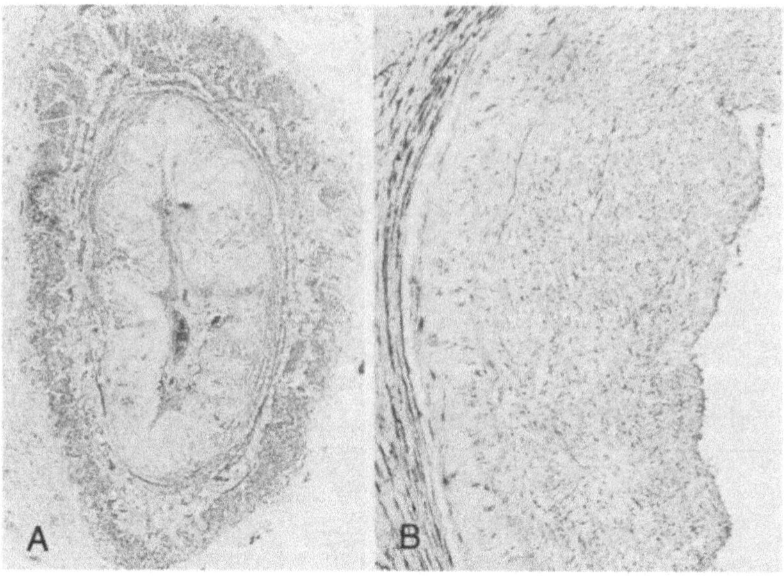

Fig. 7. Patient 39, Table I. Saphenous veins to left anterior descending **(A)** and right coronary artery **(B)** in a 60-year-old man (GT No. 76A-224) who died of pancreatic cancer 13 months after insertion of four saphenous vein conduits for unstable angina pectoris. He never had evidence of myocardial ischemia postoperatively, but at necropsy two of the four saphenous vein conduits were occluded except for recanalized channels. **A,** Occluded graft (except for recanalized channels) to left anterior descending artery. Original smooth muscle of saphenous vein is well preserved. (Movat stain. ×40). **B,** Portion of wall of patient graft to right coronary artery showing considerable intimal thickening by fibromuscular tissue. (Movat stain. 126×.)

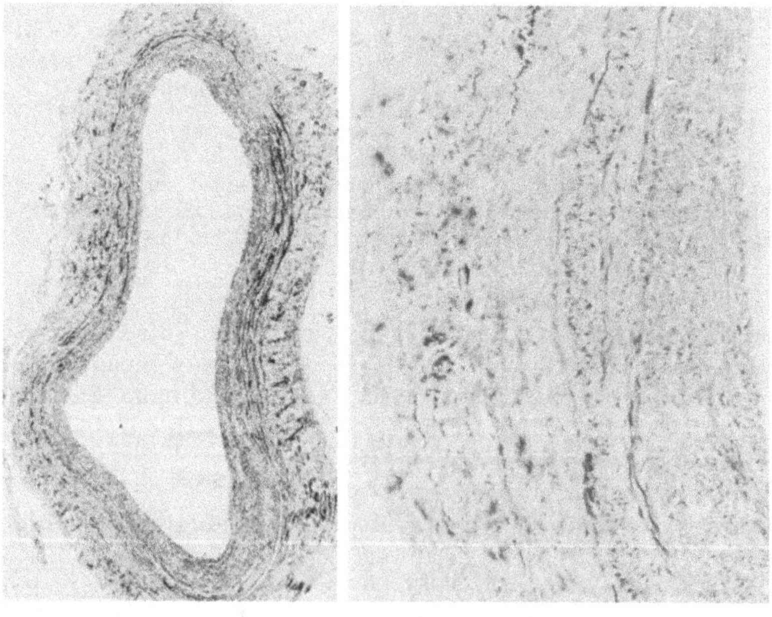

Fig. 8. Patient 49, Table I. Saphenous vein to first diagonal *(left)* and close-up of its wall *(right)* in a 59-year-old man (NIH No. A85-93) who died of infection 13 months after insertion of three saphenous vein conduits, all of which were wide open postoperatively. He never had evidence of myocardial ischemia postoperatively. Relatively few smooth muscle fibers remain in the medial wall of the saphenous vein. Intimal thickening is due to a combination of smooth muscle cell plus fibrous tissue proliferation. (Movat stains. 27× *[left]* and 126× *[right]*.)

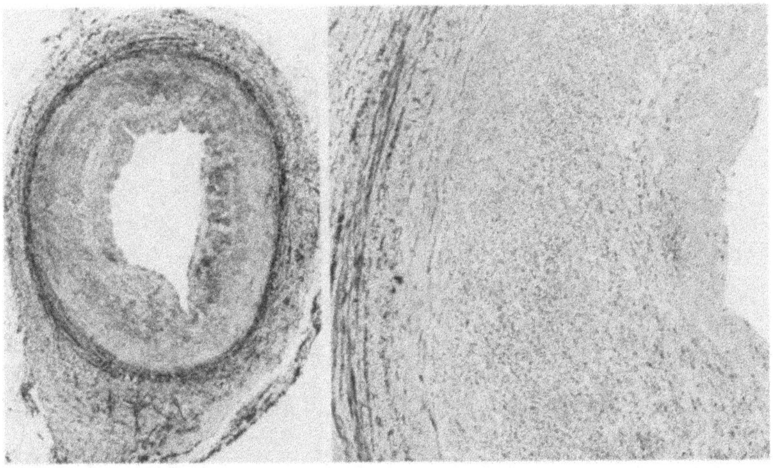

Fig. 9. Patient 2, Table I. Saphenous vein conduit *(left)* to left anterior descending coronary artery and close-up of a portion of its wall *(right)* in a 54-year-old man (GT No. A83-104) who died 19 months after coronary bypass with grafts to two arteries, one of which was severely narrowed at necropsy. Luminal narrowing is by fibromuscular tissue. (Movat stains. 20× *[left]* and 80× *[right]*.)

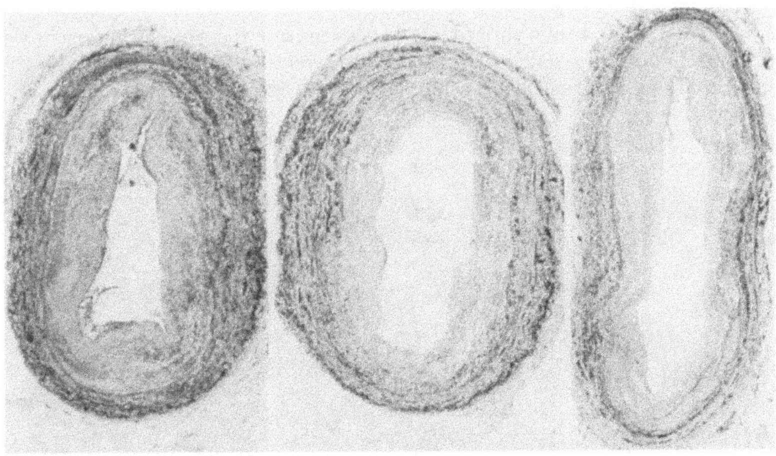

Fig. 10. Patient 40, Table I. Saphenous veins to right *(left)*, left anterior descending *(center)*, and left obtuse marginal *(right)* coronary arteries in a 67-year-old man (DCVAH No. 84-A-149) who lived 21 months after coronary bypass. All lumens are adequate in each of the sites shown in these photomicrographs; at another site one of the three conduits was severely narrowed. Intimal tissue consists primarily of collagen and smooth muscle cells. (Movat stains. Each ×20.)

ly normal. Therefore, 1473 five-millimeter segments (79%) were narrowed more than 25% in cross-sectional area. Of the latter 1473 segments, 209 (11% of total) were virtually totally occluded (>95% narrowed in cross-sectional area), and 172 segments (9% of total) were narrowed 76% to 95% in cross-sectional area. Thus, the atherosclerotic plaquing late in saphenous veins used as aortocoronary conduits is diffuse, just as it is in native coronary arteries in patients with fatal myocardial ischemia.[20]

The amount of luminal narrowing in the saphenous veins used as aortocoronary conduits was significantly ($p < 0.01$) greater in those patients who died of a cardiac cause compared to those who died of a noncardiac cause. Of the 73 saphenous venous conduits in the 32 patients dying of a cardiac cause, 37

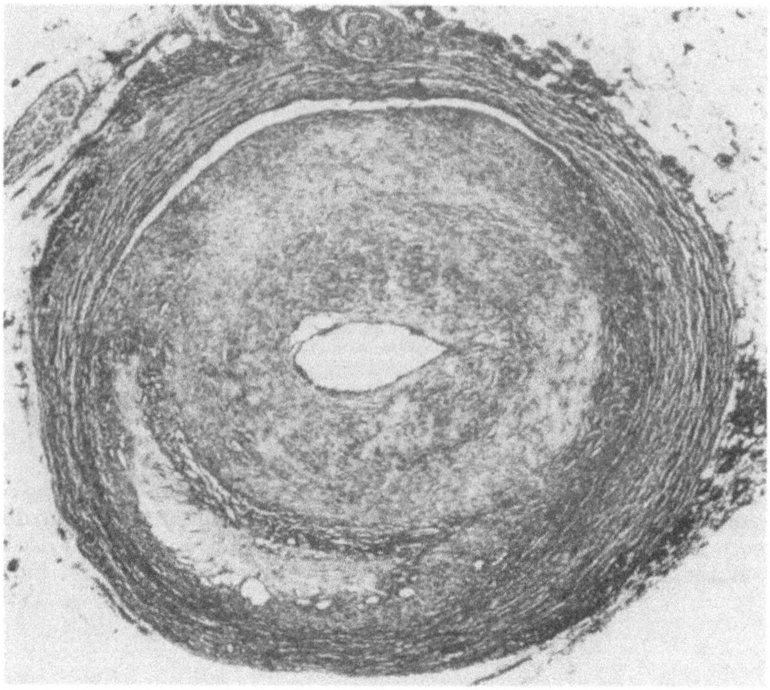

Fig. 11. Patient 8, Table I. Saphenous vein to left obtuse marginal coronary artery in a 44-year-old woman (GW No. 7983) who died suddenly 26 months after three-vessel bypass. Two of the three grafts were severely narrowed primarily by fibrous tissue as shown here. (Movat stain. 34×.)

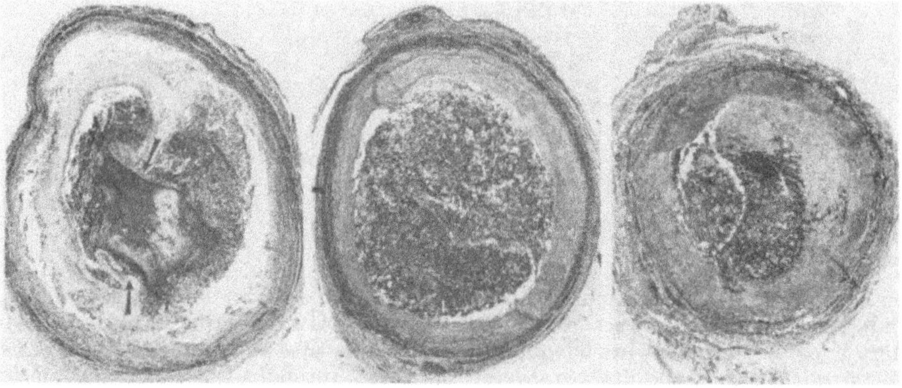

Fig. 12. Patient 11, Table I. Saphenous vein to left anterior descending coronary artery in a 69-year-old man (NNMC No. A84-122) who died of acute myocardial infarction 34 months after three-vessel bypass. Two of the three conduits, one of which is shown here, were severely narrowed. **Left,** In the section shown here fibrous capsule over extracellular lipid has ruptured *(between arrows)* with thrombus in residual lumen and hemorrhage into pultaceous debris. **Center,** Lumen at this site is occluded by organizing fibrous tissue and hemorrhage into pultaceous debris. **Right,** At this level there is fibrous tissue, organizing thrombus, and hemorrhage into plaque. Each 5 mm segment of the saphenous vein conduits is different. (Movat stains. Each 20×.)

(51%) were narrowed more than 75% in cross-sectional area, and 295 (27%) of the 1104 five-millimeter segments of saphenous vein were narrowed to this extent; in contrast, of the 50 saphenous venous conduits in the 21 patients dying of a noncardiac cause, 10 (20%) were narrowed more than 75%, and 86 (11%) of the 761 five-millimeter segments of vein were narrowed to this degree. Additionally, the per-

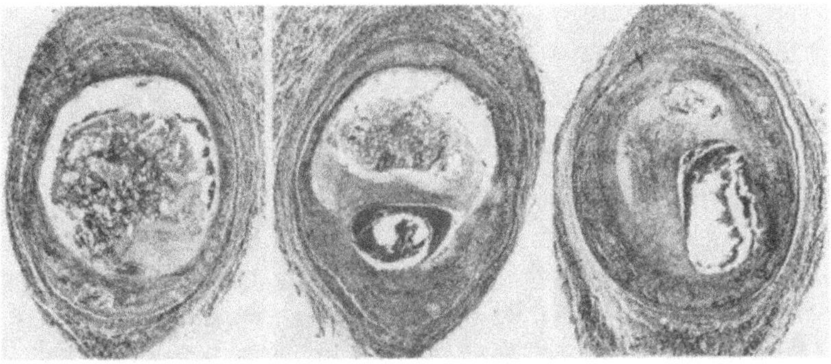

Fig. 13. Patient 15, Table I. Saphenous vein to right coronary artery in a 44-year-old woman (NNMC No. A83-104) who died of chronic congestive heart failure 43 months after four-vessel bypass. Graft was the only graft severely narrowed. **Left,** At this site graft is totally occluded by combination of fibrous tissue and pultaceous debris that contains both extravasated erythrocytes and fibrin. Open space in this section is an artifact of sectioning. **Center,** Narrowing at this site is due primarily to extracellular lipid. **Right,** Narrowing at this site is due mainly to fibrous tissue. Residual lumen *(middle* and *right)* contain postmortem clot. (Movat stains. Each 20×.)

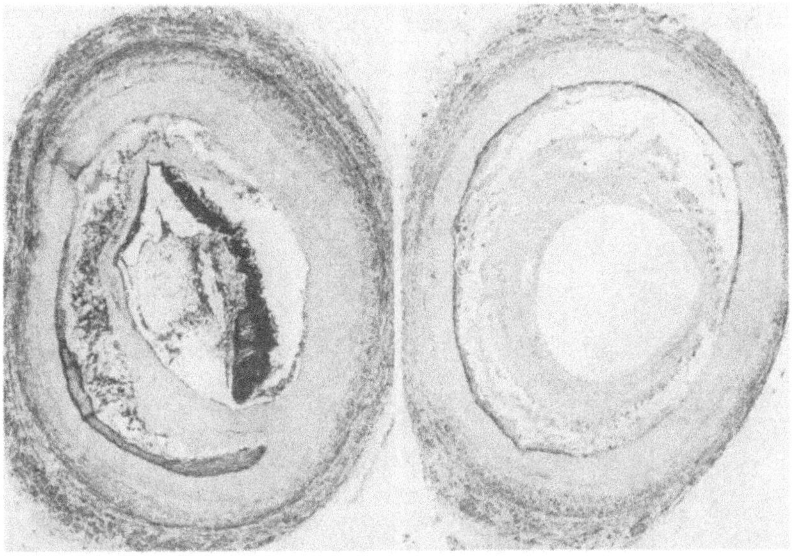

Fig. 14. Patient 45, Table I. Saphenous vein to left obtuse marginal coronary artery in a 70-year-old man (NNMC No. A84-62) who died of acute leukemia 60 months after three-vessel bypass. One of the three conduits was severely narrowed at necropsy. **Left** and **Right,** Graft to obtuse marginal artery at two different sites. In addition to fibrous and lipid components of the plaques, there is a large deposit of calcium. (Movat stains. Each 20×.)

centage of vein conduits and the percentage of 5 mm segments of the vein conduits totally occluded or nearly so (>95% in cross-sectional area) were significantly greater in the patients dying of a cardiac cause compared with those dying of a noncardiac cause (22 [30%] of 73 veins versus 7 [14%] of 50 veins, and 152 of [14%] of 1104 segments versus 57 [27%] of 213 segments).

Surprisingly, the interval from coronary bypass to death did not correlate with either the percentage of vein conduits or the percentage of 5 mm segments of vein conduit narrowed more than 75% in cross-sectional area by plaque. The percentage of venous conduits narrowed severely (>75%), for example, was similar in the 18 conduits (seven patients) in place from 13 to 24 months and in the nine conduits (five patients) in place for longer than 10 years. Moreover, the percentage of 5 mm segments of saphenous vein

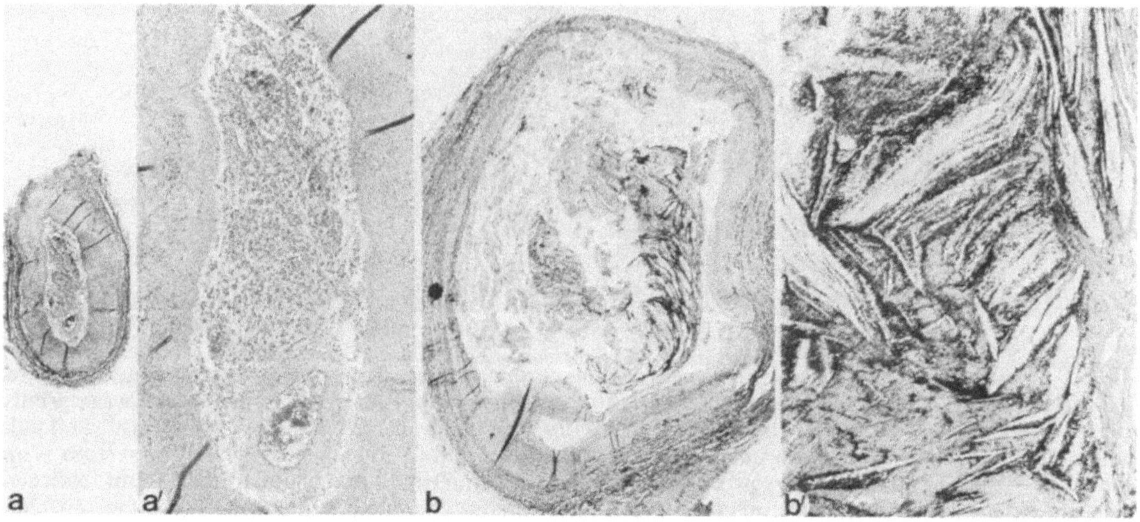

Fig. 15. Patient 18, Table I. Saphenous vein grafts to right (a, a^1) and left anterior descending (b, b^1) coronary arteries in a 60-year-old man (GT No. 84A-33) who died of chronic congestive heart failure 60 months after three-vessel bypass. At necropsy all three grafts were occluded. **a,** Graft is occluded except for recanalized channels. **b,** Graft at this site is severely narrowed primarily by pultaceous debris. **b¹**, Close-up of area of cholesterol clefts. (Movat stains. 20× (*a* and *b*), 80× (a^1), and 200× (b^1).

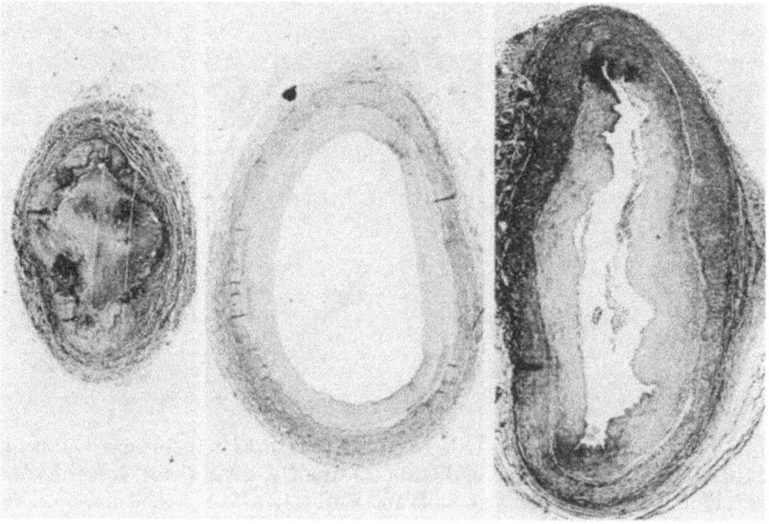

Fig. 16. Patient 26, Table I. Saphenous vein grafts to right *(left)*, left anterior descending *(center)*, and left obtuse marginal *(right)* coronary arteries in a 67-year-old man (SJH No. A78-14) who died of chronic congestive heart failure 72 months after three-vessel bypass. (Movat stains. Each 20×.)

conduit severely narrowed was similar in the 35 patients surviving up to 5 years compared to the 18 patients surviving more than 5 years (268 [19%] of 1387 segments versus 113 [24%] of 478 segments).

Why some saphenous vein conduits became severely narrowed or occluded or nearly so and others did not may be related more to the status of the native coronary artery containing the graft than to the graft itself. Of the 123 native coronary arteries containing a saphenous vein conduit, 49 (40%) of the arteries distal to the anastomotic site were narrowed more than 75% in cross-sectional area by plaque, and

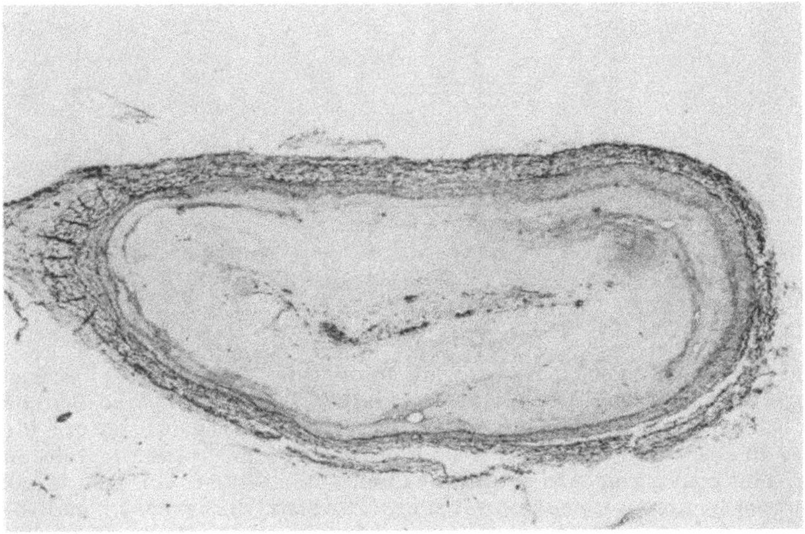

Fig. 17. Patient 28, Table I. Occluded saphenous vein to posterior descending coronary artery in a 49-year-old woman (FH No. 78A-27) who died suddenly 72 months after two-vessel bypass. One conduit was occluded by fibrous tissue and the other conduit was adequately patent. (Movat stain. 20×.)

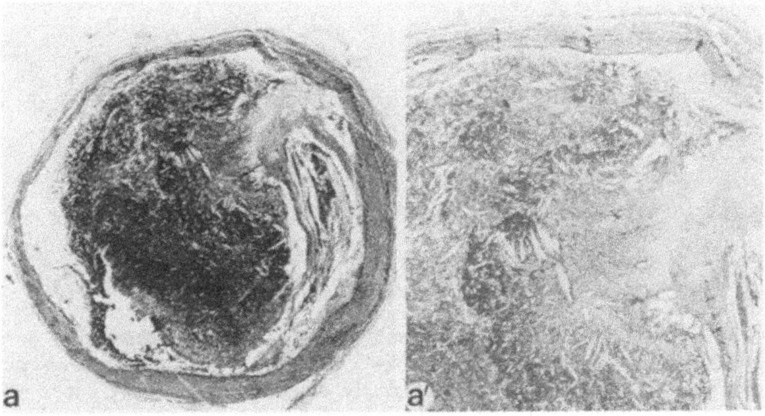

Fig. 18. Patient 29, Table I. Totally occluded saphenous vein graft to left anterior descending coronary artery in a 39-year-old man (GW No. 79A-99) who had a fatal acute myocardial infarction 84 months after single bypass. **Left,** Vein graft has hemorrhage into plaque consisting almost entirely of pultaceous debris. Fibrous capsule over plaque is ruptured and thrombus is present in residual lumen. **Right,** Close-up of pultaceous debris containing numerous cholesterol clefts. (Hematoxylin & eosin stains. ×10 *[left]* and ×80 *[right]*.)

the anastomosed saphenous vein was severely narrowed in 33 (67%) of them. In contrast, of the 74 native coronary arteries narrowed less than 75% distal to the anastomotic site, the attached saphenous vein was severely narrowed in only 14 (19%) ($p < 0.001$). Thus, the amount of narrowing in the native coronary artery distal to the anastomotic site plays a major determining role in the fate of the attached saphenous vein.

The composition of the plaques in the saphenous venous conduits is similar to that in the native coronary arteries. Fibrous tissue or fibromuscular tissue was the dominant component of the plaques in the saphenous vein conduits just as it is the dominant component of plaques in the native coronary arteries in patients with fatal coronary artery disease without coronary bypass.[21] Lipid was present in plaques in saphenous veins in much smaller amounts than was

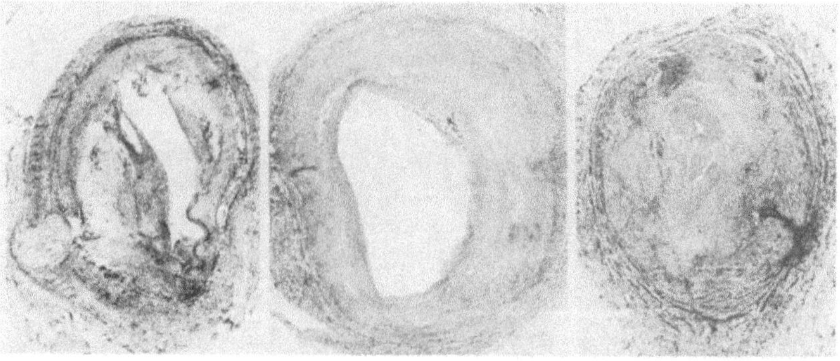

Fig. 19. Patient 31, Table I. Saphenous vein grafts to right *(left),* left anterior descending *(center),* and first diagonal *(right)* coronary arteries in a 72-year-old man (GT No. 87A-64) who died suddenly 84 months after two-vessel bypass. Anastomosis to left anterior descending was side to side and it continued to first diagonal with end-to-side anastomosis. **Left,** This graft contains some calcific deposits and extensive lipid deposits. **Center,** This graft is narrowed entirely by fibrous tissue. **Right,** This graft is occluded (except for recanalized channels) by fibrous tissue. (Movat stains. 20× *[left],* 31× *[center],* and 40× *[right].*)

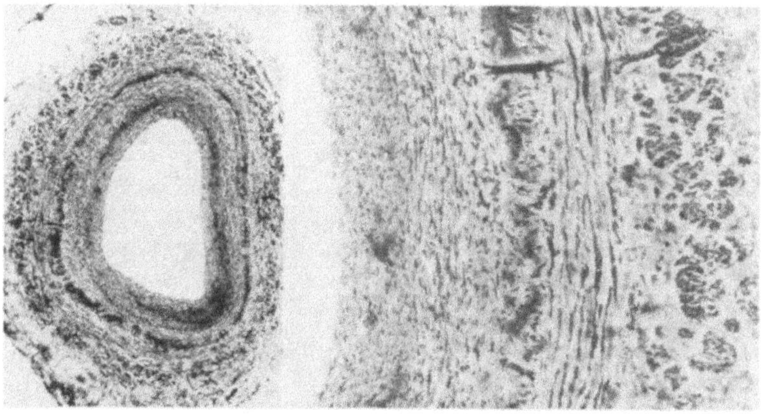

Fig. 20. Patient 35, Table I. Saphenous vein graft to left anterior descending coronary artery in a 60-year-old man (SH No. A87-25) who died of a stroke 95 months after three-vessel bypass. All three grafts were wide open. **Left,** Smooth muscle in vein wall is fairly well preserved. **Right,** Close-up of vein wall. (Movat stain. 20× *[left]* and 126× *[right].*)

fibrous tissue. Intracellular lipid was found in a saphenous vein as early as 14 months after coronary bypass, and it did not increase in either frequency or amount as the interval from bypass to death increased. Extracellular lipid was first seen at 26 months after bypass, and it did not appear to increase thereafter as the interval from bypass increased. Hemorrhage into plaque, which occurred almost entirely into extracellular lipid deposits (containing cholesterol clefts within pultaceous debris), was first seen at 32 months after bypass. Intraluminal thrombus was found in saphenous veins in 14 patients (26%) and was first observed at 32 months. Thrombus was always superimposed on underlying lipid plaque. Calcific deposits were found in saphenous vein conduits in 11 patients (21%), they were first noted at 34 months after bypass, and they did increase in frequency with time.

The frequency of the various modes of death among the patients dying late after coronary bypass is a bit different from that of patients with symptomatic myocardial ischemia without coronary bypass.[22] Of the 53 coronary bypass patients studied, only 32 (60%) died of a cardiac cause and therefore 21 (40%) died of a noncardiac cause. Among patients with symptomatic myocardial ischemia who do not

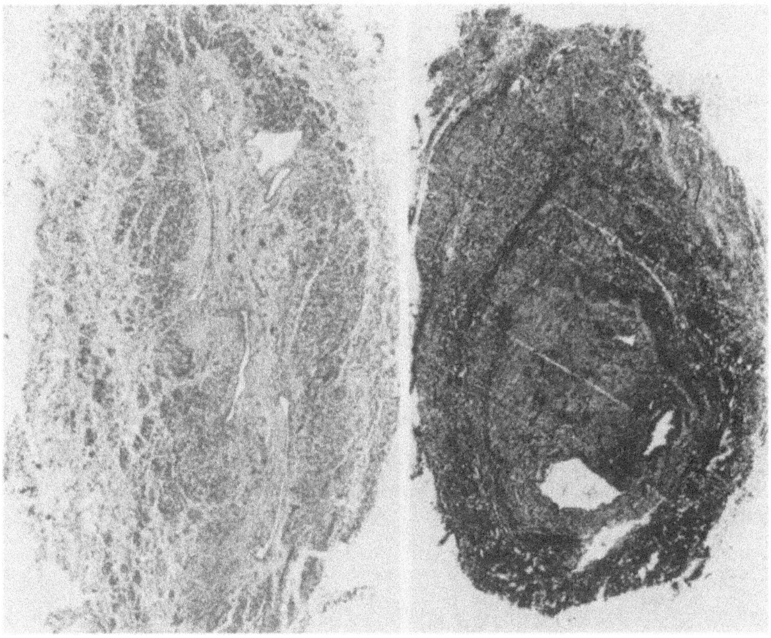

Fig. 21. Patient 32, Table I. Saphenous veins to left anterior descending *(left)* and left obtuse marginal *(right)* coronary arteries in a 49-year-old man (GT No. 85A-52) who died of chronic congestive heart failure 96 months after two-vessel bypass. These grafts are occluded by fibrous tissue except for recanalized channels. (Movat stains. 40× *[left]* and 20× *[right]*.)

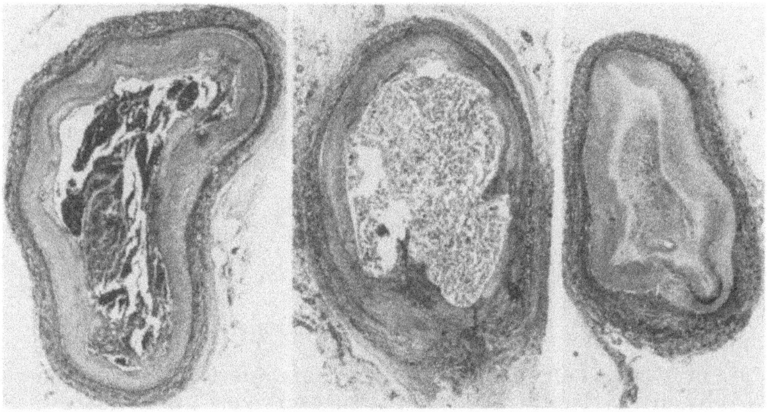

Fig. 22. Patient 48, Table I. Saphenous vein graft to right coronary artery at three different sites in a 63-year-old man (GT No. 84A-137) who died of cancer (malignant mesothelioma) 144 months after insertion of saphenous vein graft to right coronary artery and internal mammary artery to left anterior descending coronary artery. He never had evidence of myocardial ischemia postoperatively. Saphenous vein graft was occluded and internal mammary artery graft was wide open. **Left,** At this site thrombus is present in the graft. **Center,** At this site lumen is obliterated, mainly by pultaceous debris. **Right,** At this site graft is occluded by fibrous tissue except for a few revascularized channels. (Movat stains. Each 20×.)

have coronary bypass, approximately 95% die of a cardiac cause, and therefore only about 5% die of a noncardiac cause. The fact that 40% of the bypass cases studied died of a noncardiac cause supports the view that the bypass operation in many patients prolongs life long enough in many for various fatal noncardiac conditions to develop. Of our 53 bypass patients, 10 (19%) died of cancer, a percentage far

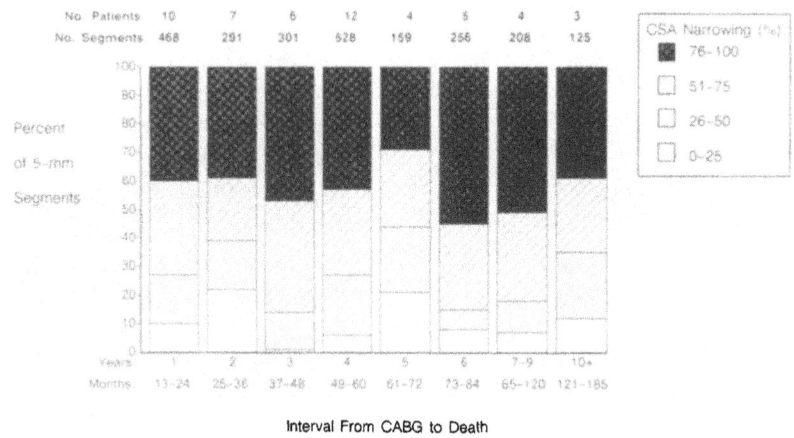

Fig. 23. Mean percentage of 5 mm segments of four major native coronary arteries narrowed in cross-sectional area *(CSA)* to various degrees by plaque in patients surviving 1 to 15 years (mean 5) after coronary artery bypass grafting *(CABG)*.

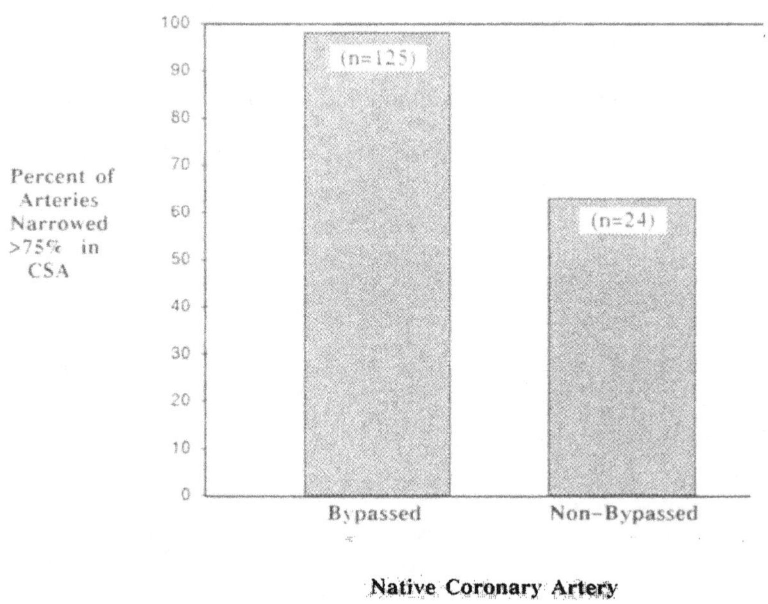

Fig. 24. Percentage of bypassed and nonbypassed coronary arteries narrowed more than 75% in cross-sectional area (*CSA*) by atherosclerotic plaque in patients surviving 1 to 15 years (mean 5) after coronary artery bypass grafting (51 patients).

higher than patients with symptomatic myocardial ischemia not having coronary surgery.

The present study is not the first to examine saphenous veins used as aortocoronary conduits. Most previously published necropsy studies describing various morphologic findings in saphenous veins used as aortocoronary conduits concerned patients who died within 1 year of the bypass operation, and few necropsy studies have included more than 10 patients who survived more than a year after the bypass operation.[1-8] Studies of operatively excised saphenous veins used as aortocoronary conduits are of course quite different from the present study, became most of the operatively excised conduits were totally occluded or nearly so.[2, 6, 9-15] The one previously published report with which our report potentially can be compared is that of Atkinson et al.,[8] who described changes in 117 saphenous veins used as aortocoronary conduits from 12 to 168 months (mean 63) in 56 patients. These authors described three morphologic features observed in the bypass conduits: (1) "atherosclerosis" in 25 grafts; (2) "fibrointimal pro-

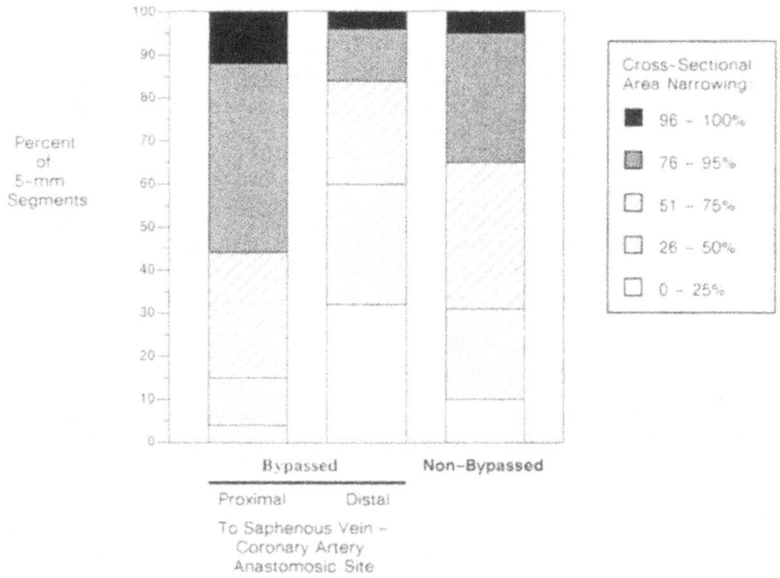

Fig. 25. Percentage of 5 mm segments of bypassed and nonbypassed native coronary arteries narrowed to various degrees by atherosclerotic plaque in patients surviving 1 to 15 years (mean 5) after coronary artery bypass grafting.

liferation" in 66 grafts, and (3) grafts which were "... fibrotic with total occlusion." These authors suggested that the "fibrointimal proliferation" (undefined) was the consequence of associated systemic hypertension and that the "atherosclerosis" (undefined) lesion was the consequence of associated hypercholesterolemia. Of their 56 patients, 43 (78%) died of cardiac causes and 13 (22%) died of noncardiac causes. These authors studied only random sections of the saphenous vein conduits, and therefore quantitation of the amounts of narrowing throughout the conduits was not possible. The predominately "atherosclerotic grafts" were in place longer than either the predominately "fibrointimal proliferation grafts" or the "fibrotic grafts" (76 versus 57 or 57 months).

The present study reemphasizes that coronary bypass is useful but that it does not deter progression of the underlying atherosclerotic process. In a slight way the bypass operation might even cause acceleration of the atherosclerotic process because in about 25% of persons having coronary bypass the serum total cholesterol increases and the body weight increases substantially during the first year after operation. Because lowering the serum (or plasma) total cholesterol level (and specifically the low-density lipoprotein cholesterol) causes some portion of atherosclerotic plaques to regress and the chances of a fatal or nonfatal subsequent atherosclerotic event to decrease, a strong case can be advanced for combined simultaneous initiation of both low-fat, low-cholesterol diet therapy and lipid-lowering drug therapy as soon as is reasonably feasible after a coronary bypass operation.[23]

REFERENCES

1. Vlodaver Z, Edwards JE. Pathologic changes in aortic coronary arterial saphenous vein grafts. Circulation 1971;64:719-28.
2. Barboriak JJ, Pintar K, Korns ME. Atherosclerosis in aortocoronary vein grafts. Lancet 1974;2:621-4.
3. Bulkley BH, Hutchins GM. Accelerated "atherosclerosis." A morphologic study of 97 saphenous vein coronary artery bypass grafts. Circulation 1977;55:163-9.
4. Spray TL, Roberts WC. Changes in saphenous veins used as aortocoronary bypass grafts. AM HEART J 1977;94:500-16.
5. Lie JT, Lawrie GM, Morris Jr GC. Aortocoronary bypass saphenous vein graft atherosclerosis. Anatomic study of 99 vein grafts from normal and hyperlipoproteinemic patients up to 75 months postoperatively. Am J Cardiol 1977;40:906-13.
6. Barboriak JJ, Pintar K, Van Horn DL, Batayias GE, Korns ME. Pathologic findings in the aortocoronary vein grafts. A scanning electron microscope study. Atherosclerosis 1978; 29:69-80.
7. Smith SH, Geer JC. Morphology of saphenous vein-coronary artery bypass grafts. Seven to 116 months after surgery. Arch Pathol Lab Med 1983;107:13-18.
8. Atkinson JB, Forman MB, Vaughan WK, Robinowitz M, McAllister HA, Virmani R. Morphologic changes in long-term saphenous vein bypass grafts. Chest 1985;88:341-8.
9. Kern WH, Wells WJ, Meyer BW. The pathology of surgically excised aortocoronary saphenous vein bypass grafts. Am J Surg Pathol 1981;5:491-6.
10. Walts AE, Fishbein MC, Sustaita H, Matloff JM. Ruptured atheromatous plaques in saphenous vein coronary artery bypass grafts. A mechanism of acute, thrombotic, late graft occlusion. Circulation 1982;65:197-201.
11. Neitzel GF, Barboriak JJ, Pintar K, Qureshi I. Atheroscle-

sis in aortocoronary bypass grafts. Morphologic study and risk factor analysis 6 to 12 years after surgery. Arteriosclerosis 1986;6:594-600.
12. Walts AE, Fishbein MC, Matloff JM. Thrombosed, ruptured atheromatous plaques in saphenous vein coronary artery bypass grafts. Ten years experience. AM HEART J 1987;114:718-23.
13. Liang BT, Antman EM, Taus R, Collins Jr JJ, Schoen FJ. Atherosclerotic aneurysms of aortocoronary vein grafts. Am J Cardiol 1988;61:185-8.
14. Solymoss BC, Nadeau P, Millette D, Campeau L. Late thrombosis of saphenous vein coronary bypass grafts related to risk factors. Circulation 1988;78:I-140-3.
15. Ratliff NB, Myles JL. Rapidly progressive atherosclerosis in aortocoronary saphenous vein grafts. Possible immune-mediated disease. Arch Pathol Lab Med 1989;113:772-6.
16. Riahi M, Vasu CM, Tomatis LA, Schlasser RJ, Zimmerman G. Aneurysm of saphenous vein bypass graft to coronary artery. J Thorac Cardiovasc Surg 1975;70:358-9.
17. Benchimol A, Harris CL, Desser KB, Fleming H. Aneurysms of an aorta-coronary artery saphenous vein bypass graft—a case report. Vasc Surg 1975;9:261-4.
18. Teja K, Dillingham R, Mentzer RM. Saphenous vein aneurysms after aortocoronary bypass grafting. Post-operative interval and hyperlipidemia as determining factors. AM HEART J 1987;113:1527-9.
19. Movat MZ. Demonstration of all connective tissue elements in a single section. Pentachrome stains. Arch Pathol 1985;60:289-95.
20. Roberts WC. Qualitative and quantitative comparison of amounts of narrowing by atherosclerotic plaques in the major epicardial coronary arteries at necropsy in sudden coronary death, transmural acute myocardial infarction, transmural healed myocardial infarction and unstable angina pectoris. Am J Cardiol 1989;64:324-8.
21. Kragel AH, Reddy SG, Wittes JT, Roberts WC. Morphometric analysis of the composition of atherosclerotic plaques in the four major epicardial coronary arteries in acute myocardial infarction and in sudden coronary death. Circulation 1989; 80:1747-56.
22. Roberts WC, Potkin BN, Solus DE, Reddy SG. Mode of death, frequency of healed and acute myocardial infarction, number of major epicardial coronary arteries severely narrowed by atherosclerotic plaque, and heart weight in fatal atherosclerotic coronary artery disease: analysis of 889 patients studied at necropsy. J Am Coll Cardiol 1990;15:196-203.
23. Roberts WC. Lipid-lowering therapy after an atherosclerotic event. Am J Cardiol 1989;64:693-5.

Changes in Venous Autografts Used as Aortocoronary Conduits

William C. Roberts
Baylor University Medical Center, Dallas, Texas

Since its introduction 30 years ago, numerous patients have benefited from coronary artery bypass grafting. Despite its benefits to most patients, coronary bypass is not free of complications. Stenosis or complete occlusion of venous grafts used as aortocoronary conduits still occurs. While all venous grafts develop some morphologic changes, the degree and functional significance of the changes vary widely. This chapter describes structural changes observed early and late in saphenous veins used as aortocoronary conduits.

I. DEGREES OF NARROWING OF THE NATIVE EPICARDIAL CORONARY ARTERIES IN SYMPTOMATIC MYOCARDIAL ISCHEMIA

Before focusing on the changes in saphenous veins used as aortocoronary conduits, a brief discussion on the status of the native epicardial coronary arteries in patients likely to undergo aortocoronary bypass grafting appears appropriate. Examination at necropsy or examination of coronary endarterectomy specimens during life of the four major (right, left main, left anterior descending, and left circumflex) epicardial coronary arteries in patients over 30 years of age with symptomatic myocardial ischemia and angiographic narrowing >50% in diameter of one or more major coronary arteries discloses that atherosclerotic plaques are present in virtually every 5-mm segment of the entire lengths of the arteries [1,2]. In patients with angiographically so-called "single-vessel disease," approximately 40% of the lumen of each 5-mm segment of the four major arteries (average of 54 segments per patient) is obliterated by plaque; in patients with angiographically "double-vessel disease," approximately 50% of the total lumen is obliterated by plaque; in patients with "triple-vessel disease," approximately 60% of the total lumen is filled with plaque; and in patients with "quadruple-vessel disease," approximately 70% of the total lumen is filled with plaque. Thus, the greater the number of major coronary arteries significantly narrowed at angiography, the greater the total amount of atherosclerotic plaque in the major epicardial coronary arteries.

II. THE NORMAL SAPHENOUS VEIN

The normal human saphenous vein contains a thin *intima* consisting of relatively acellular fibrous tissue covered by a single layer of endothelial cells separated from the media by a rudimentary internal elastic membrane. The *media* consists of multiple layers of smooth muscle cells separated by bundles of collagen, ground substance, and occasional short elastic fibers. Most medial smooth muscle layers have a circular orientation; in areas near the venous valves, however, the middle circular layers have a more longitudinal arrangement. Frequently, longitudinally oriented smooth muscle fascicles make up the innermost layers of the media. The *adventitia* is composed of bundles of collagen with scattered fascicles of longitudinally oriented smooth muscle cells. Broad, loose bands of elastic fibers are present in abundance. Vasa vasorum are present and may extend into the outermost portion of the media.

III. FINDINGS IN REMNANT SAPHENOUS VEINS EXCISED FOR AORTOCORONARY CONDUITS BUT NEVER USED

Some degree of intimal fibrous thickening occurs commonly in saphenous veins excised for aortocoronary bypass but never used. Waller and Roberts [3] examined nearly 3,500 cm of unused but excised saphenous vein from 402 patients having coronary bypass surgery. The length of the unused saphenous veins ranged from 0.5 to 52 cm per patient (mean 8.5). A histologic section was examined from each of the 6,788 5-mm-long segments: The lumen in 0.4% of the sections was narrowed 76–100% in cross-sectional area by fibrous tissue; 0.6% were narrowed 51–75% in cross-sectional area; 12% were narrowed 26–50%; and 87% were narrowed 25% or more in cross-sectional area. The percentage of 5-mm segments of unused vein narrowed more than 75% in cross-sectional area was similar in men and women, and it was similar in each of five decades (31–40, 41–50, 51–60, 61–70, and 71–80 years). Thus, approximately 1% of saphenous veins excised for coronary bypass are narrowed more than 50% in cross-sectional area by fibrous tissue before they are used as aortocoronary conduits.

IV. NUMBER OF AORTIC ANASTOMOTIC SITES, NUMBERS OF CONDUITS, AND NUMBERS OF CORONARY ANASTOMOTIC SITES

I doubt if any two surgeons perform the bypass operation in quite the same manner, and such individual variations may affect patient outcome and graft outcome. The phrases "two bypasses" and "three bypasses" and "four bypasses" are commonly used, but their meaning is not always precise. I suspect that most users of the phrase "three bypasses" are referring to the number of coronary anastomoses. A patient may have three coronary anastomotic sites and only one conduit ("round-the-world" bypass) or two conduits or three conduits with similar numbers of aortic anastomotic sites. To prevent confusion, it might be best always to state the number of aortic anastomosis sites, the number of conduits, and the number of coronary anastomotic sites. To me it seems most reasonable for each of these three to be the same: If a patient is to have three coronary anastomotic sites, it might be ideal to have three conduits and three separate aortic anastomitic sites. If only one conduit is used with a single aortic anastomotic site and the single conduit is anastomosed to seven different coronary arteries, the outcome is not ideal if the single aortic anastomosis closes or the single conduit closes proximally. With similar numbers of aortic anastomotic sites, conduits, and coronary anastomotic sites, this circumstance is less likely to occur.

The location of the coronary anastomotic site appears to be relatively similar with most surgeons. The distal 1 cm of the right coronary artery is probably ideal, because the most severe narrowing of this artery tends to be its distal third rather than the proximal or middle third [4]. The most common anastomotic site of the left anterior descending artery is probably about two-thirds down its length, and this location, of course, is logical, because this artery tends to be more severely narrowed in its proximal third than in either its middle or its distal third [4]. The same situation also appears reasonable for the first diagonal artery. Anastomoses in the obtuse marginal arteries are usually within 3 cm of their origin from the left circumflex.

Tension on the conduit is one of the various technical factors that can affect flow in aortocoronary conduits [5]. Abnormal tension is indicated by grooving or indentation into the right atrial wall or right atrioventricular sulcus or by flattening of the graft passing anterior to the pulmonary trunk. If the graft is under tension, leakage at the bypass anastomosis is probably more likely than without tension. *Twisting of a conduit* may prevent successful bypass grafting [6].

V. EARLY CHANGES IN SAPHENOUS VEINS USED AS AORTOCORONARY CONDUITS

In 1906, Carrel and Guthrie [7] described intimal thickening of veins implanted into the arterial system in dogs, and concluded that veins placed in the arterial circulation had a strong tendency to assume the character of an artery. In further vein transplantation experiments in 1908, Carrel [8] described four characteristic changes in veins used as arteries in the peripheral circulation: (a) intimal thickening, (b) adventitial thickening (from fibrosis), (c) loss of the inner one-third of the media, and (d) loss of elastic fibers producing a fibrous tube. In addition, medial hypertrophy was observed in some grafts. These changes have subsequently been confirmed in humans in saphenous veins used for femoral–popliteal and aortocoronary bypass.

Spray and Roberts [9,10] studied a large number of saphenous vein grafts from patients dying within a year after aortocoronary bypass. Vein grafts from patients dying intraoperatively showed minimal medial edema (clear spaces between layers of smooth muscle) and disrupted adventitia (occurring during excision of the vein before grafting). By two weeks, mural edema was more pronounced, some medial smooth muscle cells were necrotic, and inflammatory infiltrates were present. The endothelium often was disrupted, and the intimal surface usually was covered, either partially or completely, by fibrin. By three weeks, cells with characteristics of smooth muscle appeared in the subendothelial portion of the intima. The cells generally were oriented such that their longest diameter was parallel to the direction of blood flow. Thereafter, the subendothelial intimal lesions became more generalized, less cellular ground substance appeared in abundance, and short elastic fibers and vascular channels occasionally were present. The smooth muscle fibers of the media gradually diminished in number and were replaced, in part or in whole, by fibrous tissue. Fibrous tissue also increased in the adventitia, and its elastic fibers became severely disrupted or disappeared completely. Organizing fibrin on the external surface of the grafts probably contributed to the adventitial fibrosis. Capillaries were present in the adventitia, and they often extended into the fibrotic media. Thus, the saphenous vein used as an artery becomes a fibrous-tissue conduit.

VI. LATE CHANGES IN SAPHENOUS VEINS USED AS AORTOCORONARY CONDUITS

Kalan and Roberts [11] described at necropsy findings in 123 saphenous vein grafts and in 1,865 5-mm segments of the grafts in 53 patients who had had a single aortocoronary bypass operation 13–185 months (mean 58) before death. Of the 53 patients, 32 (60%) died from a cardiac cause, and of their 73 saphenous vein aortocoronary conduits, 36 (49%) were narrowed at some point more than 75% in cross-sectional area by atherosclerotic plaque. The remaining 21 patients (40%) died from a noncardiac cause, and of their 50 saphenous vein conduits, 10 (20%) were narrowed at some point more than 75% in cross-sectional area by plaque. Of the 53 patients, 31 (58%) had at least one bypass graft maximally narrowed greater than 75% in cross-sectional area at some point by fibromuscular tissue with or without lipid; 12 patients (23%) had maximal graft narrowing of 51–75%; 8 patients (15%), 26–50%; and 2 patients (4%), 0–25%. The percentage of patients with a graft narrowed over 75% at necropsy did not increase as the interval from bypass surgery to death increased.

Of the 123 saphenous vein grafts, 47 (38%) were maximally narrowed greater than 75% in cross-sectional area; 44 (36%), 51–75%; 22 (18%), 26–50%; and 10 (8%), 0–25%. Of the 47 grafts narrowed over 75% in cross-sectional area, 29 actually were narrowed greater than 95% in cross-sectional area by fibrous tissue. The percentage of saphenous veins narrowed greater than 75% at necropsy was not affected by gender (men 38%, women 36%), presence or absence of systemic hypertension (40% vs. 33%), or presence or absence of diabetes mellitus (30% vs. 48%). The percentage of grafts narrowed over 75% in cross-sectional area did not correlate with the interval between bypass surgery and death or with the coronary artery to which the graft was connected.

The degree of narrowing of the saphenous vein graft was related to the degree of luminal narrowing of the native coronary artery at, or within 2 cm distal to, the saphenous vein–coronary artery anastomosis. Of the 49 grafts attached to a coronary artery that was narrowed greater than 75% at or distal to the anastomosis, 33 (67%) were significantly narrowed; of the 74 grafts attached to a coronary artery narrowed less than 75% distal to the anastomotic site, 14 (19%) were severely narrowed.

Analysis of the 1,865 5-mm-long saphenous vein segments disclosed that 209 segments (11%) were narrowed 96–100% in cross-sectional area; 172 (5%), 76–95%; 407 (22%), 51–675%; 685 (37%), 26–50%; and 392 (21%), 0–25%. Similar percentages of segments were narrowed greater than 75% in men and women (22% vs. 15%); in diabetics and nondiabetics (18% vs. 26%), and in hypertensives and nonhypertensives (21% vs. 20%). Further, the interval from coronary bypass to death did not correlate with the percentage of segments severely narrowed.

Although the percentage of saphenous vein segments narrowed greater than 75% in cross-sectional area at necropsy did not correlate with the interval from bypass grafting to death, it did relate to the mode of death. Of the 32 patients dying from a cardiac cause, 295 (27%) of 1,104 saphenous vein segments were narrowed greater than 75%, whereas of the 21 patients dying from a noncardiac cause, 86 (11%) of 761 saphenous vein segments were so narrowed. The percentage of segments of native coronary artery narrowed greater than 75% was similar in patients with cardiac and noncardiac modes of death [673 of 1,441 (47%) vs. 333 of 895 (37%)].

VII. COMPOSITION OF TISSUE CAUSING LUMINAL NARROWING LATE IN THE SAPHENOUS VEINS USED AS AORTOCORONARY CONDUITS

Lipid was present in the wall of a graft (Figure 1) in 39 of the 53 patients (74%). Fifteen had intracellular lipid alone (foam cells), and 24 had both foam cells and extracellular lipid. Extracellular lipid was not found in a saphenous vein graft until 26 months after bypass. Lipid was present in 69 (56%) of the 123 saphenous vein grafts from the 39 patients. Intracellular lipid was present in all 69 grafts, either alone (33 grafts) or along with extracellular lipid (36 grafts). The amount of lipid present appeared to increase as the interval from coronary bypass to death increased. Foam cells were located near the luminal surfaces of the intimal fibrous tissue, and they did not narrow the lumen appreciably. Extracellular lipid deposits were located deeper in the plaque, separated from the lumen by a layer of fibrous tissue, and they often contributed significantly to luminal narrowing.

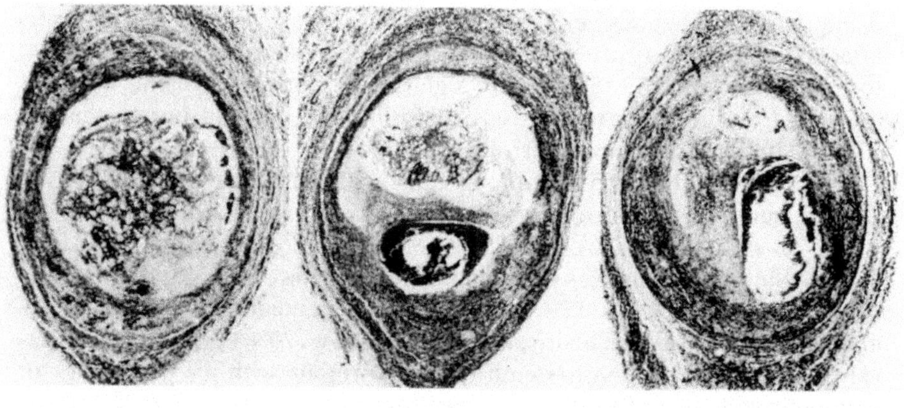

Figure 1 Saphenous vein to right coronary artery in a 44-year-old woman (NNMC No. A83-104) who died of chronic congestive heart failure 43 months after four-vessel bypass. This graft was the only graft severely narrowed. Left, at this site, graft is totally occluded by combination of fibrous tissue and pultaceous debris that contains both extravasated erythrocytes and fibrin. Open space in this section is an artifact of sectioning. Center, narrowing at this site is due primarily to extracellular lipid. Right, narrowing at this site is due mainly to fibrous tissue. Residual lumen (middle and right) contain postmortem clot. (Movat stains. Each 20×.) (From Ref. 27.)

Hemorrhage into plaque (into the lipid portion only) was found in 26 (21%) of the saphenous vein grafts from 17 (32%) of the patients (Figure 2). It was seen as early as 24 months after bypass, and it did not increase in frequency thereafter as the interval from bypass to death increased. Luminal narrowing greater than 75% in cross-sectional area was significantly more common in grafts with plaque hemorrhage than in those without.

Luminal thrombus was present in 16 (13%) of the saphenous vein grafts from 14 (26%) of the patients. Thrombus was not seen until 32 months after bypass, and its frequency did not increase thereafter as the interval from bypass to death increased. Thrombus within the graft lumen was present in 16 of 69 grafts that had deposits of lipid in their walls (Figure 3), and was present in none of 54 grafts devoid of lipid. In 14 of these 16 grafts, hemorrhage into plaque also was found.

Calcific deposits were present in 13 (11%) of the 123 saphenous vein grafts from 11 patients, and they were first seen 34 months after coronary bypass. All the deposits were small. They were present in 18 (1%) of the 1,865 5-mm saphenous vein segments.

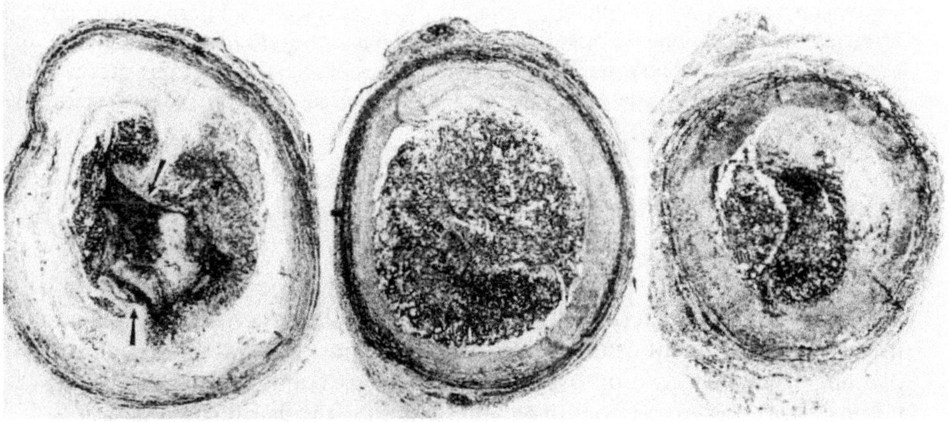

Figure 2 Saphenous vein to left anterior descending coronary artery in a 69-year-old man (NNMC No. A84-122) who died of acute myocardial infarction 34 months after three-vessel bypass. Two of the three conduits, one of which is shown here, were severely narrowed. Left, in the section shown here, fibrous capsule over extracellular lipid has ruptured (between arrows) with thrombus in residual lumen and hemorrhage into pultaceous debris. Center, lumen at this site is occluded by organizing fibrous tissue and hemorrhage into pultaceous debris. Right, at this level there is fibrous tissue, organizing thrombus, and hemorrhage into plaque. Each 5-mm segment of the saphenous vein conduits is different. (Movat stains. Each 20×.) (From Ref. 27.)

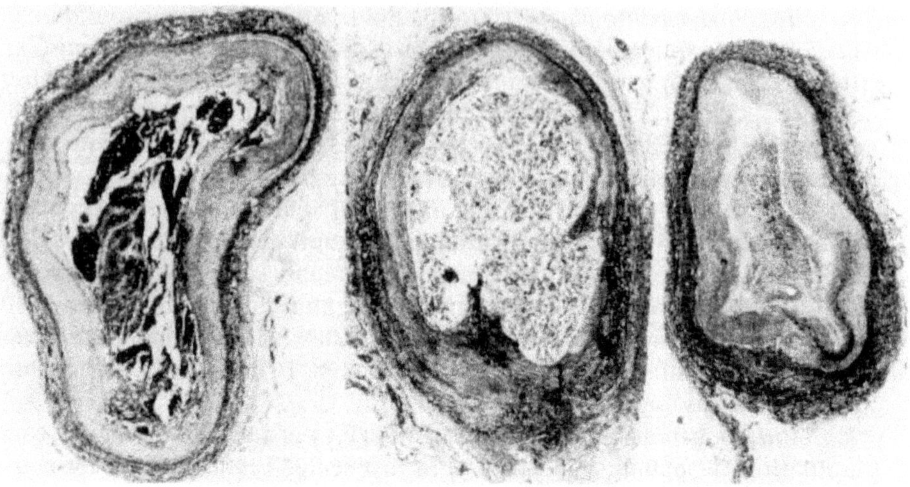

Figure 3 Saphenous vein graft to right coronary artery at three different sites in a 63-year-old man (GT No. 84A-137) who died of cancer (malignant mesothelioma) 144 months after insertion of saphenous vein graft coronary artery and internal mammary artery to left anterior descending coronary artery. He never had evidence of myocardial ischemia postoperatively. Saphenous vein graft was occluded and internal mammary artery graft was wide open. Left, at this site, thrombus is present in the graft. Center, at this site, lumen is obliterated, mainly by pultaceous debris. Right, at this site, graft is occluded by fibrous tissue except for a few revascularized channels. (Movat stains. Each 20×.) (From Ref. 27.)

The aforementioned data indicate that virtually all saphenous veins used as aortocoronary conduits for longer than a year develop atherosclerotic plaques in each 5-mm segment of their entire lengths. Thus, the late atherosclerotic plaquing in saphenous veins used as aortocoronary conduits is diffuse, just as it is in native coronary arteries in patients with fatal myocardial ischemia [1,2]. The amounts of luminal narrowing in the saphenous veins used as aortocoronary conduits were significantly greater in those patients who died from a cardiac cause than in those who died from a noncardiac cause. Surprisingly, the interval from coronary bypass to death did not correlate with either the percentage of vein conduits or the percentage of 5-mm segments of vein conduit narrowed over 75% in cross-sectional area by plaque. Moreover, the percentage of 5-mm segments of saphenous vein conduit severely narrowed was similar in the 35 patients surviving up to 5 years compared to the 18 patients surviving over 5 years.

The composition of the plaques in the saphenous vein conduits is similar to that in the native coronary arteries. Fibrous tissue or fibromuscular tissue was the dominant component of the plaques in the saphenous vein conduits, just as it is the dominant component of plaques in the native coronary arteries in patients with fatal coronary artery disease without coronary bypass [12,13].

The frequency of the various modes of death among the patients dying late after coronary bypass is a bit different from that of patients with symptomatic myocardial ischemia without coronary bypass [14]. Of the 53 coronary bypass patients studied, only 32 (60%) died from a cardiac cause; therefore, 21 (40%) died from a noncardiac cause. Among patients with symptomatic myocardial ischemia who do not have coronary bypass, approximately 95% die from a cardiac cause. The fact that 40% of the bypass cases studied died from a noncardiac cause supports the view that the bypass operation in many patients prolongs life, long enough in many to develop various fatal noncardiac conditions. Of the 53 bypass patients reported by Kalan and Roberts [11], 10 (19%) died from cancer, a percentage far higher than for patients with symptomatic myocardial ischemia not having coronary surgery.

The study by Kalan and Roberts [11] reemphasizes that coronary bypass is useful but that it does not deter progression of the underlying atherosclerotic process. In a slight way, the bypass operation might even cause acceleration of the atherosclerotic process, because in about 25% of persons having coronary bypass the serum total cholesterol increases and the body weight increases substantially during the first year after operation. Because lowering the serum (or plasma) total cholesterol level (and specifically the low-density lipoprotein [LDL] cholesterol) decreases the chances of "heart attack" and may cause some portion of atherosclerotic plaques to regress and other portions to at least not progress, a strong case can be advanced for combined simultaneous initiation of both low-fat, low-cholesterol diet therapy and lipid-lowering drug therapy as soon as is reasonably feasible after a coronary bypass operation [15].

In January 1997, the Post Coronary Artery Bypass Graft Trial Investigators [16] reported results of studying 1,351 patients who had undergone aortocoronary bypass grafting 1–11 years earlier and who had LDL cholesterol levels between 130 and 175 mg/dL, triglyceride levels <300 mg/dL, and at least one patent vein graft on coronary angiography. The study divided the patients into those in whom an "aggressive" treatment plan was employed, with the goal of lowering LDL cholesterol to 60–85 mg/dL, and those in whom a "moderate" treatment plan was employed, with the goal of lowering LDL cholesterol to 130–140 mg/dL. In the aggressive treatment group a mean of 76 ± 13 mg of lovastatin was employed, and 30% also received 8 g/day of cholestyramine; in the moderate treatment group a mean of 4 ± 1 mg of lovastatin was employed, and 5% also received 8 g/day of cholestyramine. Coronary angiography was repeated an average of 4.3 years after the baseline angiogram. The primary angiographic outcome was the mean percentage per patient of grafts with a decrease of 0.6 mm or more in lumen diameter. As measured annually during the study, the mean LDL cholesterol level of patients who received aggressive treatment ranged from 93 to 97 mg/dL; with moderate treatment, the range was from 132 to 136 mg/dL. The mean percentage of grafts with progression of atherosclerosis was 27% for patients whose LDL cholesterol level was lowered with aggressive treatment and 39% for those who received moderate treatment. There was no significant difference in angiographic outcome between the patients receiving warfarin and those who did not receive warfarin. The rate of revascularization over the four years of study was 29% lower in the group whose LDL cholesterol level was lowered aggressively compared to the group receiving moderate treatment (6.5% vs. 9.2%). Thus, aggressive lowering of LDL cholesterol levels to <100 mg/dL reduced the progression of atherosclerosis in aortocoronary bypass grafts. This recent study, therefore, gives strong support to the use of lipid-lowering agents, particularly the statin drugs, after aortocoronary bypass operations to lower the LDL cholesterol to <100 mg/dL.

VIII. CAUSES OF MORPHOLOGIC CHANGES IN SAPHENOUS VEINS USED AS AORTOCORONARY CONDUITS

Although the causes of the changes in saphenous vein grafts are in many ways similar to the causes leading to atherosclerotic plaques in native coronary arteries [17], additional mechanisms almost surely play a role when a vein is switched to an arterial location. The early changes in the saphenous veins are similar to the phlebosclerotic lesions in venous varicosities, changes presumably caused by the response of the vein to increases in hydrostatic pressure. Arteriovenous shunts of any origin (congenital, traumatic, or iatrogenic) show intimal thickening, presumably the result of increased pressure and flow. Subendothelial proliferative lesions in the pulmonary arteries of patients with pulmonary hypertension and in vena cava and portal veins in patients with chronic right-sided congestive cardiac failure or portal hypertension also are seen in the saphenous veins transferred to the aortocoronary position. Brody and colleagues [18,19] attempted to differentiate the effects of pressure and ischemia on femoral vein grafts in dogs. Vein segments were either left intact or dissected free from their adventitia, thereby severing the vasa vasora and producing medial ischemia. Next, the vein segments either were left in the venous system or were arterialized by creation of an arteriovenous fistula. The presence of medial ischemia in the absence of elevated pressure and flow produced medial fibrosis in the vein without subendothelial intimal proliferative lesions. Elevated intravascular pressure alone, however, without alterations in blood supply to the media by the vasa vasorum produced intimal lesions without evidence of medial fibrosis. The combination of elevated intraluminal pressure and medial ischemia resulted in medial and intimal changes similar to the changes seen in human saphenous veins used as aortocoronary conduits.

The intimal process in saphenous veins, and specifically the degree of luminal narrowing in saphenous veins in the aortocoronary position, is almost certainly accelerated when flow through the conduit is relatively poor. The major cause of poor flow is severe narrowing in the native coronary artery (to which the vein is attached) at or just distal to the site of anastomosis [9–11,20]. The smaller the native coronary arteries to which the graft is to be connected, the less the amount of atherosclerotic plaque necessary to cause significant luminal narrowing. Smaller-sized hearts have smaller coronary arteries than larger-sized hearts [21]. Small patients tend to have smaller hearts than larger patients. Thus, similar amounts of plaque cause more luminal narrowing in small patients than in large patients. Women, on average, are smaller than men, and, therefore, on average they have smaller hearts and smaller coronary arteries. Coronary bypass might be expected therefore to have poorer results in women than in men because the smaller arteries might cause poor flow through the conduits by plaque in the native coronary arteries.

Kalan and Roberts [22] found this very scenario to be probably the case. Their 121 necropsy patients dying within 60 days of a coronary bypass operation had significantly lower mean heart weights than did the 90 patients dying late, and this fact held true for both sexes. Most patients with normal-sized hearts were in the early-death group; conversely, most patients in the late-death group had hearts of increased weight. These findings suggest that patients with normal- or near-normal-sized hearts have a higher early mortality after coronary bypass than do persons with hearts of increased weight. Furthermore, more changes leading to luminal narrowing of bypass conduits might be expected in persons with small native coronary arteries (small hearts), because the runoff through the graft may not be as good as in patients with larger native coronary arteries (larger hearts).

IX. COMPARISON OF MORPHOLOGIC CHANGES IN SAPHENOUS VEINS TO THOSE IN INTERNAL MAMMARY ARTERIES USED AS AORTOCORONARY CONDUITS

For practical purposes, none of the aforedescribed changes in saphenous veins used as aortocoronary conduits are found in internal mammary arteries used in the coronary position. As pointed out by others clinically [23,24], the patency rate both early and late is splendid with the mammary artery but much less with the saphenous vein. Although the internal mammary artery late after bypass remains much smaller than the saphenous vein when each is utilized in the same patient, the internal mammary artery remains virtually devoid of intimal deposits, whereas the saphenous vain (in the same patient), although much larger, may develop severe atherosclerotic plaque in its lumen [25,26].

REFERENCES

1. Roberts WC. Qualitative and quantitative comparison of amounts of narrowing by atherosclerotic plaques in the major epicardial coronary arteries at necropsy in sudden coronary death, transmural acute myocardial infarction, transmural healed myocardial infarction and unstable angina pectoris. Am J Cardiol 1989; 64: 324–328.
2. Roberts WC. Coronary "lesion," coronary "disease," "single-vessel disease," "two-vessel disease": word and phrase misnomers providing false impressions of the extent of coronary atherosclerosis in symptomatic myocardial ischemia. Am J Cardiol 1990; 66:
3. Waller BF, Roberts WC. Remnant saphenous veins after aortocoronary bypass grafting: analysis of 3,394 centimeters of unused vein from 402 patients. Am J Cardiol 1985; 55:65–71.
4. Vlodaver Z, Edwards JE. Pathology of coronary atherosclerosis. Progr Cardiovasc Dis 1971; 14:256–274.
5. Spray TL, Roberts WC. Tension on coronary bypass conduits. A neglected cause of real or potential obstruction of saphenous vein grafts. J Thorac Cardiovasc Surg 1976; 72:282–287.
6. Roberts WC, Lachman AS, Virmani R. Twisting of an aortocoronary bypass conduit. A complication of coronary surgery. J Thorac Cardiovasc Surg 1978; 75: 772–776.
7. Carrel A, Guthrie CC. Results of biterminal transplantation of veins. Am J Med Sci 1906; 132:415–422.
8. Carrel A. Results of transplantation of blood vessels, organs, and limbs. JAMA 1908; 51:1662–1667.
9. Spray TL, Roberts WC. Status of the grafts and the native coronary arteries proximal and distal to coronary anastomotic sites of aortocoronary bypass grafts. Circulation 1977; 55:741–749.
10. Spray TL, Roberts WC. Changes in saphenous veins used as aortocoronary bypass grafts. Am Heart J 1977; 94:500–516.
11. Kalan JM, Roberts WC. Morphologic findings in saphenous veins used as coronary arterial bypass conduits for longer than 1 year: necropsy analysis of 53 patients, 123 saphenous veins, and 1,865 five-millimeter segments of veins. Am Heart J 1990; 119:1164–1184.
12. Kragel AH, Reddy SG, Wittes JT, Roberts WC. Morphometric analysis of the composition of atherosclerotic plaques in the four major epicardial coronary arteries in acute myocardial infarction and in sudden coronary death. Circulation 1989; 80:1747–1756.

13. Kragel AH, Reddy SG, Wittes JT, Roberts WC. Morphometric analysis of the composition of coronary arterial plaques in isolated unstable angina pectoris with pain at rest. Am J Cardiol 1990; 66:
14. Roberts WC, Potkin BN, Solus DE, Reddy SG. Mode of death, frequency of healed and acute myocardial infarction, number of major epicardial coronary arteries severely narrowed by atherosclerotic plaque, and heart weight in fatal atherosclerotic coronary artery disease: analysis of 889 patients studied at necropsy. J Am Coll Cardiol 1990; 15:196–203.
15. Roberts WC. Lipid-lowering after an atherosclerotic event. Am J Cardiol 1989; 64:693–695.
16. The Post Coronary Artery Bypass Graft Trial Investigators. The effect of aggressive lowering of low-density lipoprotein cholesterol levels and low-dose anticoagulation on obstructive changes in saphenous-vein coronary-artery bypass grafts. N Engl J Med 1997; 336(3):153–162.
17. Roberts WC. Preventing and arresting coronary atherosclerosis. Am Heart J 1995; 130:580–600.
18. Brody WR, Kosek JC, Angell WW. Changes in vein grafts following aortocoronary bypass induced by pressure and ischemia. J Thorac Cardiovasc Surg 1972; 64: 847–854.
19. Brody WR, Angell WW, Kosek JC. Histologic fate of the venous coronary artery bypass in dogs. Am J Pathol 1972; 66:111–130.
20. Waller BF, Roberts WC. Amount of narrowing by atherosclerotic plaque in 44 nonbypassed and 52 bypassed major epicardial coronary arteries in 32 necropsy patients who died within 1 month of aortocoronary bypass grafting. Am J Cardiol 1980; 46:956–962.
21. Roberts CS, Roberts WC. Cross-sectional area of the proximal portions of the three major epicardial coronary arteries in 98 necropsy patients with different coronary events. Relationship to heart weight, age, and sex. Circulation 1980; 62: 953–959.
22. Kalan JM, Roberts WC. Significance of cardiac weight in patients having coronary artery bypass grafting for angina pectoris. Am J Cardiol 1988; 62:36–40.
23. Grondin CM, Campeau L, Lesperance J, Enjalbert M, Bourassa MG. Comparison of late changes in internal mammary artery and saphenous vein grafts in two consecutive series of patients 10 years after operation. Circulation 1984; 70(suppl I): I-208–I-212.
24. Loop FD, Lytle BW, Cosgrove DM, Stewart RW, Goormastic M, Williams GW, Golding LAR, Gill CC, Taylor PC, Sheldon WC, Proudfit WL. Influence of the internal-mammary-artery graft on 10-year survival and other cardiac events. N Engl J Med 1986; 314:1–6.
25. Barbour DJ, Roberts WC. Additional evidence for relative resistance to atherosclerosis of the internal mammary artery compared to saphenous vein when used to increase myocardial blood flow. Am J Cardiol 1985; 56:488.
26. Kalan JM, Roberts WC. Comparison of morphologic changes and luminal sizes of saphenous vein and internal mammary artery after simultaneous implantation for coronary arterial bypass grafting. Am J Cardiol 1987; 60:193–196.

Comparison of Composition of Atherosclerotic Plaques in Saphenous Veins Used as Aortocoronary Bypass Conduits with Plaques in Native Coronary Arteries in the Same Men

Susanne L. Mautner, MD, Gisela C. Mautner, MD,
Sally A. Hunsberger, PhD, and William C. Roberts, MD

This study describes quantitatively the components of atherosclerotic plaques in saphenous vein grafts used for aortocoronary bypass and compares the findings with the plaques in the native coronary arteries in the same men. A total of 607 five-mm segments of saphenous veins and 797 five-mm segments of native coronary arteries were examined by computerized planimetric technique in 19 men, aged 39 to 82 years (mean 61), who had survived bypass operation for >1 year. Comparison of the mean percentages of the plaque components in saphenous vein grafts in place for 14 to 26 months with those of the native coronary arteries revealed significant differences: *cellular* fibrous tissue, 86 vs 7%; *dense* fibrous tissue, 13 vs 82%; p <0.05. As survival time after the bypass operation increased, composition of the plaques in the saphenous veins changed so that by approximately 80 months the amounts of cellular and dense fibrous tissue in both saphenous vein grafts and native coronary arteries were similar: 10 vs 16%, and 75 vs 71%; p = not significant. Thus, by about 7 years after a coronary bypass operation the composition of plaques in saphenous vein grafts is similar to that in the native coronary arteries of the same patients.

(Am J Cardiol 1992;70:1380–1387)

From the Pathology and Biostatistics Research Branches, National Heart, Lung, and Blood Institute, National Institutes of Health, Bethesda, Maryland. Manuscript received June 16, 1992; revised manuscript received and accepted July 15, 1992.

Address for reprints: Susanne L. Mautner, MD, National Heart, Lung, and Blood Institute, National Institutes of Health, Building 10, Room 2N258, 9000 Rockville Pike, Bethesda, Maryland 20892.

Morphologic changes in saphenous veins that had been inserted into the aortocoronary position as bypass conduits have been described previously.[1–11] No studies, however, have examined the composition of the developing atherosclerotic plaques of saphenous vein bypass grafts in a detailed quantitative fashion including a comparison with the atherosclerotic plaques of the native coronary arteries of the same patients. Such is the purpose of this report.

METHODS

Patients: Cases selected were limited to men in whom the heart, the native coronary arteries, and the saphenous venous bypass grafts were available for study, and in whom the saphenous veins had been in the aortocoronary position for >1 year.[12]

Patient characteristics: Clinical features of the 19 men are listed in Table I. Their ages at death ranged from 39 to 82 years (mean 61). The interval from the coronary artery bypass grafting to death ranged from 14 to 185 months (mean 69). The 19 men had a total of 41 saphenous venous grafts; the number of grafts per patient ranged from 1 to 4 (mean 2.2). A saphenous vein having 1 aortic anastomosis and either 1 or >1 coronary arterial anastomosis was considered a single conduit.

Death was due to a cardiac cause in 9 patients (47%): sudden cardiac arrest in 4 patients without myocardial necrosis, chronic congestive heart failure in 3, and acute myocardial infarction in 2. Death was attributed to a noncardiac cause in 10 patients (53%): a vascular condition in 2 patients, cancer in 4, and miscellaneous conditions in 4 (Parkinson's disease, chronic obstructive lung disease, pancreatitis and infection).

Method of examination of saphenous vein grafts and native coronary arteries: The saphenous vein grafts and native coronary arteries were studied in a similar fashion. The hearts were fixed in formalin. The saphenous vein bypass grafts and the 4 major epicardial coronary arteries (left main, left anterior descending, left circumflex, and right) were removed from the heart intact and cut transversely into 5-mm-long intervals. (In 3 patients the left main coronary artery was not available for examination.) The segments were labeled sequentially from their origin. Each segment was processed in alcohol and xylene, embedded in paraffin, cut into 6 μm thick sections and stained by the Movat method.[13] Of 1,470 sections initially examined, 66 were excluded be-

TABLE I Clinical and Necropsy Findings in 19 Men Surviving More Than One Year After Coronary Bypass Grafting

Case	Age (years) at Death	Interval CABG–Death (months)	SH	DM	After CABG AP	AMI	CHF	Mode of Death	HW (g)	Dilated LV	LV Necrosis	LV Fibrosis
1	59	14	0	0	0	0	0	Infection*	710	0	0	+
2	54	19	+	+	0	0	+	CHF	510	+	0	+
3	60	24	0	0	0	0	+	CHF	540	+	0	+
4	66	26	0	0	0	0	0	Sudden	460	0	0	+
5	62	27	+	0	0	0	0	Cancer	450	0	0	0
6	47	32	0	+	+	0	0	AMI	390	0	+	0
7	69	34	0	0	+	+	0	Sudden	550	+	0	+
8	49	39	0	0	0	0	0	Sudden	370	0	0	0
9	76	48	0	0	0	0	0	Cancer	395	0	0	+
10	58	52	+	+	+	0	0	Pancreatitis	340	0	0	0
11	73	60	+	0	0	0	0	COPD	540	0	0	+
12	69	82	0	0	0	0	0	Cancer	440	0	0	0
13	39	84	0	0	+	+	0	AMI	400	0	+	+
14	57	84	+	+	+	0	0	Sudden	515	0	0	+
15	49	96	0	0	+	0	+	CHF	520	+	0	+
16	54	120	+	0	+	0	0	Carotid operation	560	0	0	+
17	82	132	+	0	0	0	0	Stroke	485	+†	0	0
18	63	144	0	0	0	0	0	Cancer	310	0	0	+
19	63	185	0	0	+	0	0	Parkinsonism	345	0	0	0
Total or mean	61	69	7	4	8	2	3		465	5	2	12

*Multiple complications after CABG—never left hospital.
†Result of mitral regurgitation.
AMI = acute myocardial infarction; AP = angina pectoris; CABG = coronary artery bypass grafting; CHF = chronic congestive heart failure; COPD = chronic obstructive pulmonary disease; DM = diabetes mellitus; HW = heart weight; LV = left ventricle (ventricular); SH = systemic hypertension by history.

cause of sectioning artifacts. Thus, a total of 607 segments of saphenous vein grafts (mean 32/patient) and 797 five-mm segments of native coronary arteries (mean 42/patient) were studied. Evaluation of plaque composition was performed by planimetry: Movat-stained sections were placed on the stage of a projection light microscope enlarging the image approximately 150 times. A tracing of the artery was made using a GTCO micro Digi-Pad (GTCO Corp, Columbia, Maryland); the area was calculated using MacMeasure,[14] which is a morphometric software package used in conjunction with a Macintosh SE computer. The following areas were outlined: potential lumen (total area enclosed by the internal elastic membrane), residual lumen (potential lumen minus area of atherosclerotic plaque), and the components of the plaque separated into dense fibrous tissue, cellular fibrous tissue, calcific deposits, pultaceous debris (extracellular lipid), foam cells (intracellular lipid) with and without lymphocytes, and inflammatory infiltrates without significant numbers of foam cells. Analysis of components was performed in each of the 4 major epicardial coronary arteries and saphenous venous bypass grafts in every patient.

Dense fibrous tissue consisted of nearly acellular relatively homogeneous fibrous tissue staining yellow or yellow-brown by the Movat stain. *Cellular fibrous tissue* contained numerous spindle cells resembling myofibroblasts, smooth muscle cells, or fibroblasts admixed with fibrous tissue and often elastic fibers. *Calcific deposits* were detected by blackish, brownish or purple collections of granular staining areas in Movat-stained sections. *Pultaceous debris* (presumably rich in extracellular lipid) consisted of collections of amorphous pale-staining material with abundant cholesterol clefts. *Foam cell aggregates* were composed of plump, rounded, finely vacuolated cells. *Foam cells and lymphocytes* were areas containing round cells with finely granular or vacuolated cytoplasm admixed with lymphocytes. *Inflammatory infiltrates without foams cells* were isolated aggregates of lymphocytes and other inflammatory cells that were almost always seen surrounding small vascular channels. The defined areas were recognized using the projection microscope and were confirmed by standard light microscopy. The area of each component of plaque was then converted to a percentage of the total plaque area. For each patient a mean percentage of each plaque component was determined by calculating the mean of all 5-mm segments of the grafts of each patient and the native coronary arteries, respectively. The total mean was calculated based on the means of the 19 men (Tables II and III).

The presence of *intraluminal thrombus, intraplaque hemorrhage, and intraplaque multiluminal channels* also was recorded in each 5-mm segment. Since intraplaque hemorrhage occupies part of the plaque area it was outlined in the same fashion as previously described and substracted from the total plaque area. The extent of hemorrhagic areas was highly variable, from <1% to as much as 37% in 1 patient. The lumina of the multiluminal channels also were outlined, added up and subtracted from the total plaque area. They were not added to the total luminal area and were usually <1% of the total plaque area. The total mean percentages of plaque components for each patient in Tables II and III therefore do not add up to 100% in patients in whom intraplaque hemorrhage or multiluminal channels were present. Intraluminal thrombus, intraplaque hemorrhage and multiluminal channels were listed based on their

TABLE II Degree of Narrowing and Composition of Atherosclerotic Plaques in the Saphenous Vein Grafts

Case	No. of 5-mm Segments	No. and Percent of 5-mm Segments Narrowed to 5 Categories of CSA by Plaque 0–25%	26–50%	51–75%	76–95%	96–100%	Percent of Plaques Consisting of* DFT	CFT	CD	PD	FC	FC + L	ICWFC
1	53	52 (98)	1 (2)	0 (0)	0 (0)	0 (0)	0.6	99.4	0.0	0.0	0.0	0.0	0.0
2	42	8 (19)	15 (36)	10 (24)	9 (21)	0 (0)	1.3	98.5	0.0	0.0	0.1	0.0	0.0
3	48	0 (0)	39 (81)	1 (2)	2 (4)	6 (13)	30.8	67.8	0.0	0.0	0.0	0.0	0.0
4	51	27 (53)	23 (45)	1 (2)	0 (0)	0 (0)	21.1	78.0	0.0	0.0	0.9	0.0	0.0
5	30	13 (43)	16 (53)	1 (3)	0 (0)	0 (0)	94.9	3.5	0.0	0.8	0.5	0.3	0.0
6	9	2 (22)	4 (44)	2 (22)	1 (11)	0 (0)	50.4	0.0	0.0	13.5	10.1	0.0	0.0
7	45	8 (18)	8 (18)	7 (16)	14 (31)	8 (18)	81.7	6.3	1.3	8.5	0.8	1.2	0.2
8	27	0 (0)	4 (15)	8 (30)	15 (56)	0 (0)	79.6	2.4	0.3	9.3	1.8	1.0	0.3
9	62	36 (58)	23 (37)	3 (5)	0 (0)	0 (0)	0.0	100.0	0.0	0.0	0.0	0.0	0.0
10	32	9 (28)	13 (41)	4 (13)	3 (9)	3 (9)	78.6	15.7	1.8	3.0	0.1	0.03	0.8
11	38	29 (76)	9 (24)	0 (0)	0 (0)	0 (0)	69.0	30.9	0.1	0.1	0.04	0.0	0.0
12	55	3 (5)	22 (40)	22 (40)	8 (15)	0 (0)	96.9	3.1	0.0	0.0	0.0	0.0	0.0
13	10	0 (0)	3 (30)	2 (20)	5 (50)	0 (0)	48.3	0.5	1.2	10.8	0.5	1.0	0.3
14	30	13 (43)	11 (37)	3 (10)	1 (3)	2 (7)	94.2	4.6	0.0	0.5	0.6	0.0	0.0
15	19	0 (0)	2 (11)	1 (5)	5 (26)	11 (58)	29.9	61.3	5.6	2.5	0.1	0.02	0.6
16	21	13 (62)	0 (0)	0 (0)	1 (5)	7 (33)	98.8	0.0	0.7	0.4	0.0	0.0	0.01
17	12	8 (67)	3 (25)	0 (0)	1 (8)	0 (0)	93.4	1.5	0.3	3.9	0.4	0.5	0.1
18	15	0 (0)	0 (0)	0 (0)	1 (7)	14 (93)	49.9	7.2	0.1	20.0	0.0	0.0	0.7
19	8	2 (25)	6 (75)	0 (0)	0 (0)	0 (0)	91.3	0.0	3.4	1.3	1.6	2.4	0.0
Total	607	223 (37)	202 (33)	65 (11)	66 (11)	51 (8)	58.4	30.6	0.8	3.9	0.9	0.3	0.2

*Intraplaque hemorrhage and multiluminal channels are not listed; therefore numbers may not add up to 100% in each patient.
CD = calcific deposits; CFT = cellular fibrous tissue; CSA = cross-sectional area; DFT = dense fibrous tissue; FC = foam cells; FC + L = foam cells plus lymphocytes; ICWFC = inflammatory cells without foam cells; PD = pultaceous debris.

TABLE III Degree of Narrowing and Composition of Atherosclerotic Plaques in the (native) Coronary Arteries

Case	No. of 5-mm Segments	No. and Percent of 5-mm Segments Narrowed to 5 Categories of CSA by Plaque 0–25%	26–50%	51–75%	76–95%	96–100%	Percent of Plaques Consisting of* DFT	CFT	CD	PD	FC	FC + L	ICWFC
1	51	5 (10)	6 (12)	9 (18)	21 (41)	10 (20)	60.1	17.9	19.5	1.5	0.01	0.03	0.2
2	37	0 (0)	19 (51)	10 (27)	2 (5)	6 (16)	81.3	4.3	2.2	10.7	1.2	0.2	0.3
3	45	13 (29)	8 (18)	13 (29)	11 (24)	0 (0)	93.5	0.0	3.5	1.7	0.2	0.2	0.0
4	40	10 (25)	7 (18)	11 (28)	11 (28)	1 (3)	93.7	4.5	1.8	0.0	0.0	0.0	0.1
5	39	9 (23)	7 (18)	5 (13)	12 (31)	6 (15)	86.5	0.6	11.0	1.7	0.0	0.2	0.0
6	30	16 (53)	8 (27)	0 (0)	5 (17)	1 (3)	96.6	1.4	1.4	0.0	0.5	0.0	0.1
7	49	5 (10)	5 (10)	2 (4)	24 (49)	13 (27)	69.5	15.8	13.4	0.2	0.01	0.0	0.04
8	47	2 (4)	5 (11)	12 (26)	17 (36)	11 (23)	89.1	0.5	4.9	4.6	0.2	0.2	0.5
9	48	0 (0)	1 (2)	6 (13)	34 (71)	7 (15)	78.1	6.5	12.0	3.1	0.0	0.0	0.01
10	25	1 (4)	2 (8)	5 (20)	14 (56)	3 (12)	78.1	12.8	3.5	4.8	0.1	0.1	0.04
11	29	2 (7)	5 (17)	9 (31)	8 (28)	5 (17)	61.6	12.7	18.1	5.5	0.04	0.0	0.01
12	56	0 (0)	5 (9)	5 (9)	20 (36)	26 (46)	92.9	2.0	4.1	0.5	0.1	0.0	0.01
13	55	6 (11)	3 (5)	9 (16)	27 (49)	10 (18)	33.9	58.0	2.5	5.2	0.02	0.2	0.2
14	44	0 (0)	2 (5)	6 (14)	26 (59)	10 (23)	90.9	1.9	4.0	2.5	0.3	0.1	0.2
15	47	7 (15)	6 (13)	4 (9)	8 (17)	22 (47)	44.2	41.7	10.5	3.1	0.0	0.0	0.1
16	44	6 (14)	1 (2)	5 (11)	20 (45)	12 (27)	87.3	0.0	4.0	8.0	0.1	0.0	0.6
17	37	9 (24)	5 (14)	11 (30)	12 (32)	0 (0)	76.8	0.0	21.8	0.7	0.2	0.1	0.0
18	40	10 (25)	4 (10)	2 (5)	10 (25)	14 (35)	60.9	26.5	8.9	1.5	0.0	0.0	0.2
19	34	3 (9)	1 (3)	4 (12)	24 (71)	2 (6)	84.8	0.0	14.8	0.4	0.1	0.0	0.0
Total	797	104 (13)	100 (13)	128 (16)	306 (38)	159 (20)	76.8	10.9	8.5	2.9	0.2	0.1	0.1

*Intraplaque hemorrhage and multiluminal channels are not listed; therefore numbers may not add up to 100% in each patient.
Abbreviations as in Table II.

TABLE IV Frequency of Coronary Intraluminal Thrombus, Intraplaque Hemorrhage, and Intraplaque Multiluminal Channels at Necropsy in the 19 Men Surviving Coronary Bypass More than One Year

	Saphenous Vein Grafts Thrombus	Plaque Hemorrhage	Multiluminal Channels	Native Coronary Arteries Thrombus	Plaque Hemorrhage	Multiluminal Channels
Patients	6/19 (32%)	5/19 (26%)	6/19 (32%)*	7/19 (37%)	9/19 (47%)	14/19 (74%)*
Vessels	6/41 (15%)	7/41 (17%)	7/41 (17%)	8/73 (11%)	15/73 (21%)	23/73 (32%)
Five-mm segments	40/607 (7%)†	34/607 (6%)‡	25/607 (4%)§	12/797 (2%)†	21/797 (3%)‡	72/797 (9%)§

*p <0.05; †p <0.001; ‡p <0.05; §p <0.001.

frequency in patients, vessels and 5-mm segments (Table IV).

Luminal narrowing, measured as a decrease in the cross-sectional area enclosed by the border of the internal elastic membrane, was graded by visual inspection of the histologic sections at a magnification of ×40. The amount of narrowing of each 5-mm segment was categorized into 5 groups: 0 to 25, 26 to 50, 51 to 75, 76 to 95 and 96 to 100%.

Statistical analysis: To analyze the plaque components a linear regression model was used. First, a test was performed on whether the slopes of the different plaque components in the saphenous vein grafts and native coronary arteries were the same, i.e., whether the components increased, decreased or remained constant over time. If the slopes were the same, a further examination was conducted to determine if the amount of each component differed in the veins compared with the native coronary arteries and whether there was a change over time. If the slopes for the saphenous vein grafts and native coronary arteries were not the same, then the components of the saphenous vein grafts and native coronary arteries only were compared at specific times. Because the measurements are percentages the values were transformed using a logit transformation, $\log[\%/(100 - \%)]$. As some percentages were 0, a constant (0.1667) was added so that the logit transformation could be applied. It was assumed that the components of the saphenous vein grafts are uncorrelated with those of the native coronary arteries. This assumption was examined and found to be valid. Figure 1 shows the regression curves plotted for cellular and dense fibrous tissue based on the actual data using the linear regression model.

Statistical comparisons of the frequencies of intraluminal thrombi, hemorrhage into plaques, and multiluminal channels in the vein grafts and the native coronary arteries were performed by chi-square tests. A p value <0.05 was considered significant (Table IV).

RESULTS

Cross-sectional area narrowing: The results are summarized in Tables II and III. Thirteen of the 19 men had 1 or more saphenous vein conduits narrowed by atherosclerotic plaque >75% in cross-sectional area. Of the 607 five-mm saphenous vein segments examined, 117 (19%) were narrowed >75% in cross-sectional area by plaque (Table II). In all 19 men, 1 or more epicardial coronary arteries were narrowed by atherosclerotic plaque >75% in cross-sectional area. Of the 797 five-mm native coronary segments examined, 465 (58%) were narrowed >75% in cross-sectional area by plaque (Table III). In the saphenous vein grafts and native coronary arteries in all 5 categories of cross-sectional area narrowing there was no significant change noted across time, i.e., from bypass operation to death. Comparing patients *with* symptoms of myocardial ischemia such as angina pectoris or acute myocardial infarct late (>1 year) after bypass operation to those patients *without* symptoms disclosed no difference in the number of 5-mm segments narrowed significantly, i.e., >75% narrowing of cross-sectional area, in the saphenous veins (35 vs 13%; p = not significant) and native coronary arteries (67 vs 52%; p = not significant).

Plaque composition: The results are summarized in Tables II and III, and in Figure 2.

FIBROUS TISSUE: The mean percentage of fibrous tissue in all plaques of the saphenous vein grafts and native coronary arteries was 89 and 88%, respectively. Fibrous tissue decreased as the degree of cross-sectional area narrowing increased, both in the saphenous vein grafts and in the native coronary arteries, which mainly

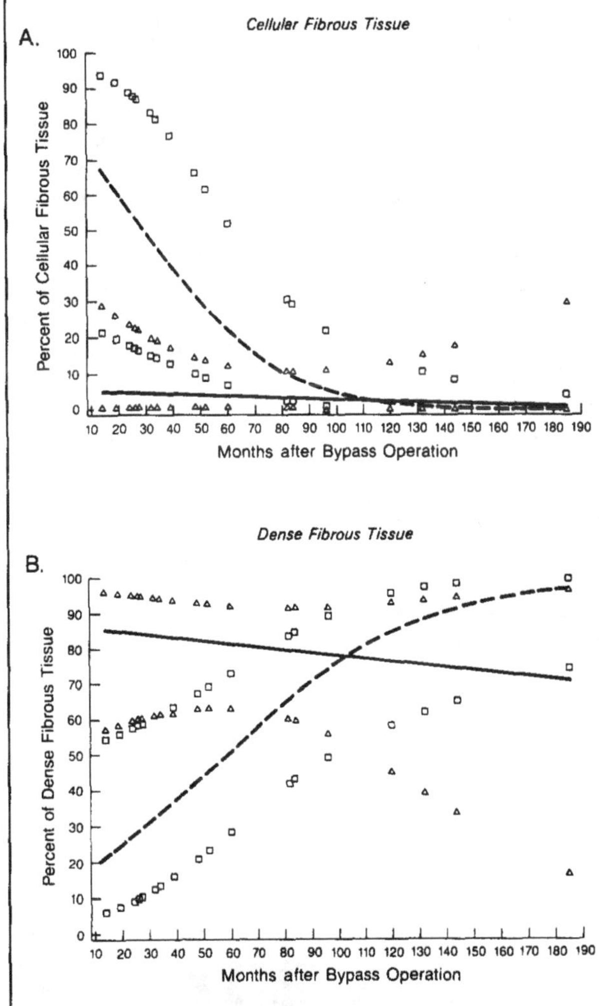

FIGURE 1. Graph showing development of fibrous tissue in plaques over time. As the time interval from bypass operation was short, the mean percentage of cellular *(A)* and dense *(B)* fibrous tissue in the plaques of the saphenous vein grafts was significantly different compared with that of the native coronary arteries. As the time interval increased, the mean percentage of cellular fibrous tissue decreased and that of dense fibrous tissue increased and at ≥82 months reached the 95% confidence interval of that of the native coronary arteries. The mean percentage of cellular and dense fibrous tissue in the native coronary arteries remained constant over time. Thus after 82 months plaque composition of the plaques in the saphenous vein grafts and native coronary arteries have become similar. *Broken line,* regression curve for the plaques of the saphenous vein grafts; *solid line,* regression curve for the plaques of the native coronary arteries; *boxes,* 95% pointwise confidence interval of the regression curve of the saphenous vein grafts; *triangles,* 95% pointwise confidence interval of the regression curve of the native coronary arteries.

was due to a decrease in *cellular* fibrous tissue (Figure 2).

CALCIFIC DEPOSITS: The mean percentage of calcific deposits in all plaques of the saphenous veins was <1%, and in the native coronary arteries, 8.5%. The mean percentage of calcific deposits in both increased as the degree of cross-sectional area narrowing increased.

PULTACEOUS DEBRIS (EXTRACELLULAR LIPID): In the saphenous vein grafts pultaceous debris was found in the plaques in 13 of the 19 men. In these 13 men, the mean percentage of pultaceous debris in all plaques of the saphenous vein grafts was 6%. Extracellular lipid was not found in a saphenous vein graft in any of the 4 patients in whom the graft had been in place for ≤26 months. In the coronary arteries pultaceous debris was present in the plaques in 17 of the 19 patients. In these 17 patients, the mean percentage of pultaceous debris in all plaques of the coronary arteries was 3%. The mean percentage of pultaceous debris increased as the degree of cross-sectional area narrowing increased.

FOAM CELLS (INTRACELLULAR LIPID), FOAM CELLS WITH LYMPHOCYTES AND INFLAMMATORY INFILTRATES WITHOUT FOAM CELLS: The mean percentage of foam cells in all plaques of the saphenous vein grafts and native coronary arteries was 0.9 and 0.2%, respectively. Usually they were located on or near the borders of the lumen. The mean percentage of foam cells with lymphocytes was 0.3% in all plaques of the saphenous vein grafts and 0.1% in those of the native coronary arteries; the mean percentage of pure inflammatory cells was 0.2% in all plaques of the grafts and 0.1% in those of the native coronary arteries.

Development of plaque composition over time: The results are summarized in Table IV, and in Figures 1 to 3. The plots in Figure 1 give the predicted mean response for cellular and dense fibrous tissue at specified times after bypass operation along with the pointwise 95% confidence intervals. One year after bypass operation cellular fibrous tissue comprised a higher percentage of the plaques in the saphenous vein grafts compared with the plaques in the native coronary arteries ($p < 0.05$); dense fibrous tissue comprised a lower percentage of the plaques in the saphenous vein grafts compared with the plaques in the native coronary arteries ($p < 0.05$). With time, the mean percentage of cellular fibrous tissue in the grafts decreased, and that of dense fibrous tissue increased. At 82 months (about 7 years) after the bypass operation, the mean percentage of cellular and dense fibrous tissue in the plaques of the saphenous vein grafts was within the confidence interval of the mean percentage of the native coronary arteries (p = not significant). The mean percentage of cellular and dense fibrous tissue in the plaques of the native coronary arteries remained constant over the time interval from bypass operation to death. If divided into groups according to the time of survival after the bypass operation (Figure 3), in patients surviving 14 to 26 months, the mean percentage of cellular fibrous tissue in all venous plaques was 86% and that of dense fibrous tissue, 13%; in contrast, in patients surviving 82 to 185 months the mean percentage of cellular fibrous tissue in all venous plaques was 10% and that of dense fibrous tissue 75%. In the native coronary arteries the mean percentage of cellular fibrous tissue in all plaques in patients surviving 14 to 26 months was 7% and that of dense fibrous tissue 82%; in patients surviving 82 to 185 months the mean percentage of cellular fibrous tissue in all native coronary artery plaques was 16% and that of

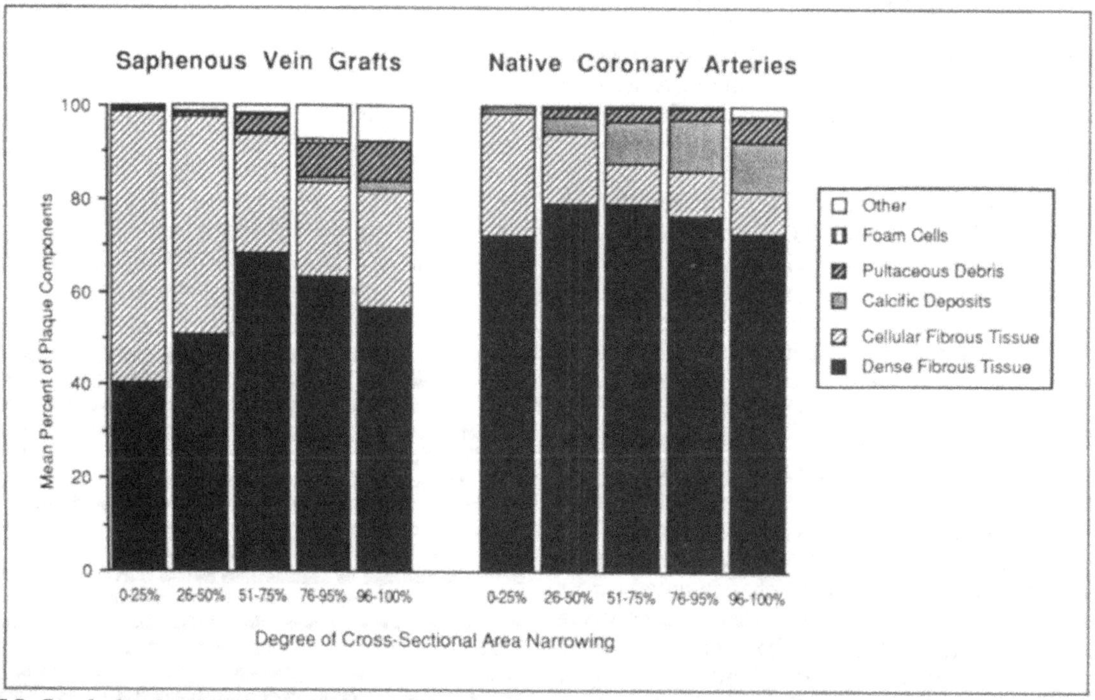

FIGURE 2. Graph showing the relation of plaque composition in the saphenous vein grafts and native coronary arteries according to the degrees of cross-sectional area narrowing. The mean percentage of fibrous tissue decreased, and that of calcific deposits and pultaceous debris increased as luminal narrowing increased both in the plaques of the saphenous vein grafts and of the native coronary arteries. The category "Other" includes foam cells plus lymphocytes and pure inflammatory infiltration.

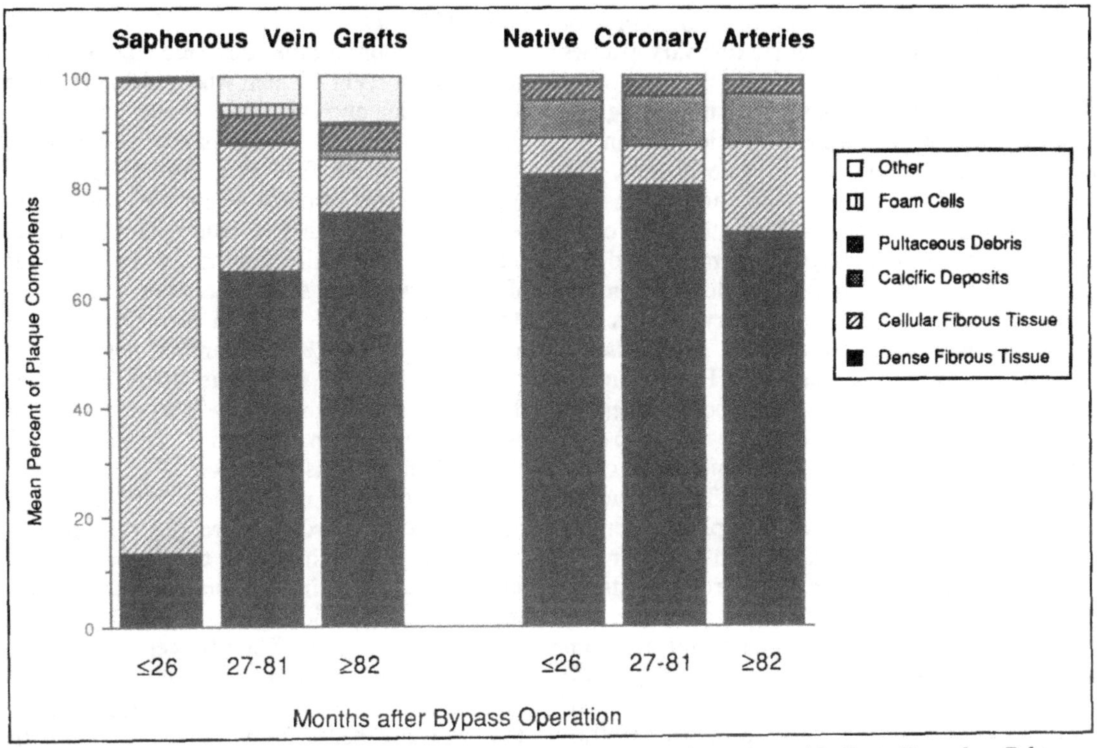

FIGURE 3. Graph showing the relation of plaque composition in saphenous vein grafts and in the native epicardial coronary arteries according to the time interval from bypass operation to death. In patients surviving ≤26 months cellular fibrous tissue was the dominant component in the plaques of the saphenous vein grafts. After ≥82 months the plaques of the saphenous vein grafts consisted predominantly of dense fibrous tissue, similar to the plaque composition in the native coronary arteries. The composition of the plaques in the native coronary arteries remained constant after bypass operation. The category "Other" includes foam cells plus lymphocytes and pure inflammatory infiltration.

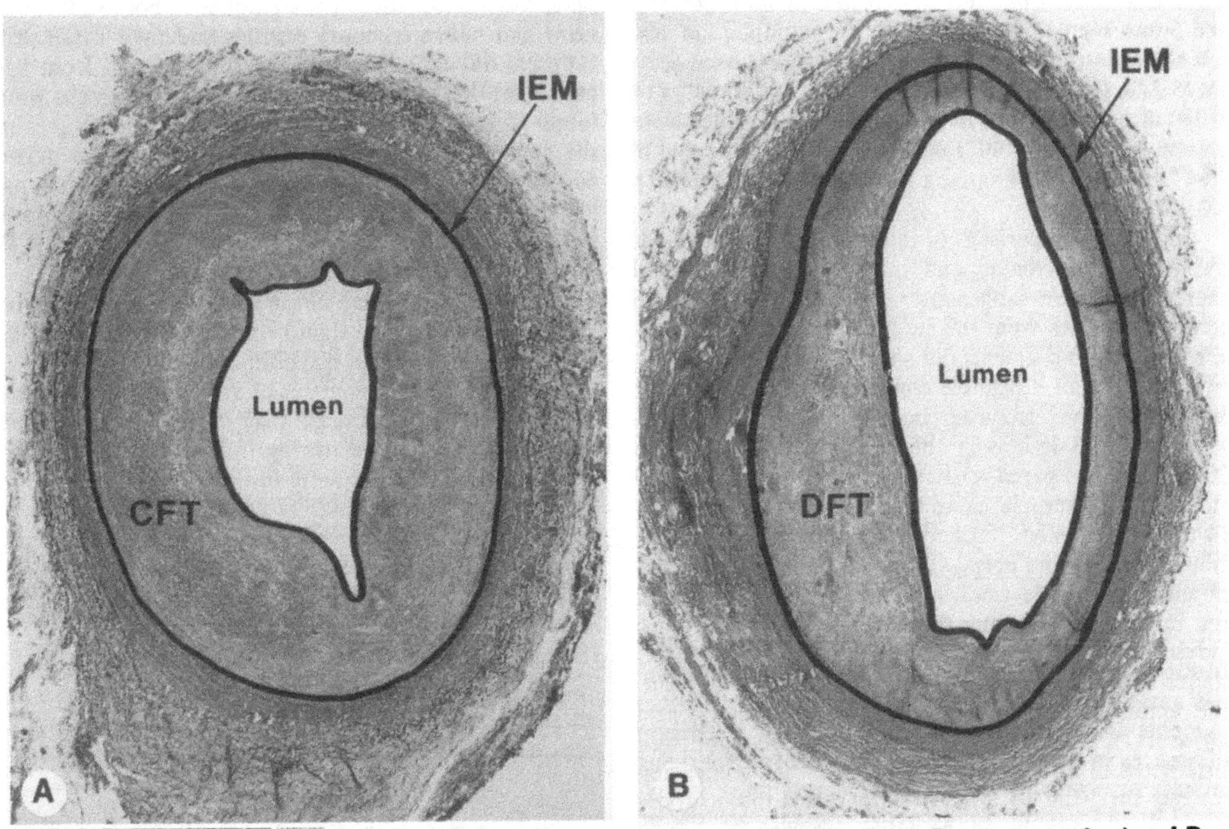

FIGURE 4. Patient 2, Table I. *A*, example of a saphenous vein graft (to the left anterior descending coronary artery), and *B*, a native coronary artery (left circumflex) of a patient surviving 19 months after coronary bypass surgery. The saphenous vein graft consists primarily of cellular fibrous tissue (CFT), whereas the dominant component in the native coronary artery is dense fibrous tissue (DFT). IEM = internal elastic membrane *(arrow)*. (Movat stains: *A*, ×25; and *B*, ×34).

dense fibrous tissue 71%, demonstrating no change of those plaque components in the native coronary arteries after bypass operation.

The mean percentage of calcific deposits was significantly higher in the native coronary arteries than in the vein grafts. This relation did not change over time. The mean percentages of pultaceous debris and foam cells remained constant in the grafts and in the native coronary arteries from the time of bypass operation to death and did not appear to be significantly different in the venous grafts compared with the coronary arteries.

Intraluminal thrombus, intraplaque hemorrhage, and intraplaque multiluminal channels: The frequency of these 3 lesions in patients, in vessels (both saphenous vein grafts and native coronary arteries) and in 5-mm segments of both saphenous vein grafts and native coronary arteries is summarized in Table IV. The frequency of intraluminal thrombus and of intraplaque hemorrhage was similar in both saphenous vein grafts and in native coronary arteries when analyzed from the standpoint of both patients and vessels, but was significantly different when examined from the standpoint of 5-mm segments. Thrombus was present, for example, in 7% (40 of 607) of all venous segments and in 2% (12 of 797) of all native coronary artery segments ($p < 0.001$); intraplaque hemorrhage was present in 6% (34 of 607) of venous segments and in 3% (21 of 797) of native coronary artery segments ($p < 0.05$). Intraplaque multiluminal channels were significantly less frequent in saphenous vein grafts than in native coronary arteries when examined from the standpoints of both patients and 5-mm segments but not from the standpoint of vessels alone. Intraplaque multiluminal channels were present in 32% (6 of 19) of grafts in patients and in 74% (14 of 19) of native arteries in patients ($p < 0.05$); they were present in 4% (25 of 607) of all venous segments and in 9% (72 of 797) of all native coronary artery segments ($p < 0.001$).

Although comparisons of intraluminal thrombus, intraplaque hemorrhage, and intraplaque multiluminal channels between saphenous venous grafts and native coronary arteries from the standpoints of patients, vessels, and 5-mm segments did show some significant differences (in 4 of 9 possible comparisons, Table IV), all differences were produced because of the virtual absence of the 3 lesions in the patients surviving 14 to 26 months compared with those surviving 27 to 185 months. For example, none of the 4 patients surviving 14 to 26 months had intracoronary thrombi or multiluminal channels and only 1 of these 4 patients had intraplaque hemorrhage (in 1 of 12 saphenous vein grafts and in 3 of 194 five-mm segments of saphenous vein). Indeed, comparison of intraluminal thrombus, intraplaque hemorrhage, and intraplaque multiluminal channels among patients, saphenous vein grafts and 5-mm segments of saphenous vein grafts disclosed significant differences in all 9 comparative areas when comparing patients surviving 14 to 26 months versus those surviving 27 to 185 months. In the native coronary arteries no differences in frequency of these 3 lesions were found irrespective of which time period was analyzed.

DISCUSSION

Composition of atherosclerotic plaques in the saphenous vein grafts of 19 men who underwent coronary bypass operation and survived >1 year was examined and compared with that in the native coronary arteries in the same patients. The data indicate that virtually all saphenous veins in place as aortocoronary conduits for >1 year develop atherosclerotic plaques in each 5-mm segment of their entire lengths. Furthermore, the degree of narrowing in the saphenous veins of our 19 men was striking: of the 607 five-mm segments of the 41 veins examined, 117 (19%) had luminal narrowing >75% in cross-sectional area by plaque alone. No differences in the amounts of significant (>75%) narrowing in the saphenous veins or in the native coronary arteries were observed in patients *with* compared to those *without* symptoms of myocardial ischemia (either angina pectoris or acute myocardial infarction) postoperatively.

The length of time that the saphenous vein grafts had been in place in the aortocoronary position influenced the composition of the atherosclerotic plaques in these venous conduits. The younger plaques in the veins consisted predominantly of cellular fibrous tissue, whereas the older plaques in the veins consisted predominantly of dense fibrous tissue. In the native coronary arteries the plaques consisted mainly of dense fibrous tissue and remained constant throughout the time periods studied (Figure 4). Thus, the plaques in the saphenous vein grafts became similar to those of the native coronary arteries over time. Intra- and extracellular lipids were infrequent in the plaques in both saphenous veins and native coronary arteries and their mean percentages did not change as the time interval from bypass operation to death increased. Calcific deposits were found at least 10 times less frequently in the plaques of the saphenous vein grafts than in those of the native coronary arteries. Intraluminal thrombus, intraplaque hemorrhage, and intraplaque multiluminal channels were found mainly in patients who had survived >26 months after bypass operation.

In summary, the amount of cross-sectional area narrowing did not change significantly after the saphenous vein grafts had been in place for >1 year. Therefore, it appears that the development of atherosclerotic plaques was a relatively fast process that within 1 year resulted in extensive luminal narrowing. Thereafter, the plaques did not increase significantly in size, but their structure changed, from predominantly *cellular* fibrous tissue to predominantly *dense* fibrous tissue. Because cellular fibrous tissue has some reversible characteristics, as opposed to dense fibrous tissue,[15] plaques in vein grafts may have the potential for reversal during the first 7 years after bypass surgery.

Acknowledgment: We thank Vivian E. Norman for her secretarial assistance, and Ricardo V. Dreyfuss and Christopher R. Dame for their photographic expertise.

REFERENCES

1. Vlodaver Z, Edwards JE. Pathologic changes in aortic coronary arterial saphenous vein grafts. *Circulation* 1971;64:719–728.

2. Barboriak JJ, Pintar K, Korns ME. Atherosclerosis in aortocoronary vein grafts. *Lancet* 1974;2:621–624.
3. Spray TL, Roberts WC. Changes in saphenous veins used as aortocoronary bypass grafts. *Am Heart J* 1977;94:500–516.
4. Smith SH, Geer JC. Morphology of saphenous vein-coronary artery bypass grafts. Seven to 116 months after surgery. *Arch Pathol Lab Med* 1983;107:13–18.
5. Atkinson JB, Forman MB, Vaughan WK, Robinowitz M, McAllister HA, Virmani R. Morphologic changes in long-term saphenous vein bypass grafts. *Chest* 1985;88:341–348.
6. Kern WH, Wells WJ, Meyer BW. The pathology of surgically excised aortocoronary saphenous vein bypass grafts. *Am J Surg Pathol* 1981;5:491–496.
7. Neitzel GF, Barboriak JJ, Pintar K, Qureshi I. Atherosclerosis in aortocoronary bypass grafts. Morphologic study and risk factor analysis 6 to 12 years after surgery. *Arteriosclerosis* 1986;6:594–600.
8. Ratliff NB, Myles JL. Rapidly progressive atherosclerosis in aortocoronary saphenous vein grafts. Possible immune-mediated disease. *Arch Pathol Lab Med* 1989;113:772–776.
9. Campeau L, Lespérance J, Corbara F, Hermann J, Grondin CM, Bourassa MG. Aortocoronary saphenous vein bypass graft changes 5 to 7 years after surgery. *Circulation* 1978;58(suppl I):I-170–I-175.
10. Walts AE, Fishbein MC, Matloff JM. Thrombosed, ruptured atheromatous plaques in saphenous vein coronary artery bypass grafts. Ten years experience. *Am Heart J* 1987;114:718–723.
11. Solymoss BC, Nadeau P, Millette D, Campeau L. Late thrombosis of saphenous vein coronary bypass grafts related to risk factors. *Circulation* 1988;78(suppl I):I-140–I-143.
12. Kalan JM, Roberts WC. Morphologic findings in saphenous veins used as coronary arterial bypass conduits for longer than 1 year: necropsy analysis of 53 patients, 123 saphenous veins and 1865 five-millimeter segments of veins. *Am Heart J* 1990;119:1164–1184.
13. Movat HZ. Demonstration of all connective tissue elements in a single section. *Arch Pathol* 1955;60:289–295.
14. Hook GR, Rasband W. Macmeasure: a low-cost, easy to operate quantitative morphometrics system for the Macintosh computer. In: Baily GW, ed. Proceedings of the 45th Annual Meeting of the Electron Microscopy Society of America. San Francisco, CA: San Francisco Press, 1987:920–921.
15. Armstrong ML, Megan MB. Lipid depletion in atheromatous coronary arteries in rhesus monkeys after regression diets. *Circ Res* 1972;30:675–680.

Comparison in Women Versus Men of Composition of Atherosclerotic Plaques in Native Coronary Arteries and in Saphenous Veins Used as Aortocoronary Conduits

SUSANNE L. MAUTNER, MD, FENGRU LIN, MD, GISELA C. MAUTNER, MD,
WILLIAM C. ROBERTS, MD, FACC

Bethesda, Maryland

Objectives. This study quantifies and compares the components of atherosclerotic plaques in native coronary arteries and in saphenous vein grafts used for aortocoronary bypass surgery in women versus those in men.

Background. Plaque composition has been described in various manifestations of fatal coronary artery disease and after the bypass operation, but no reports have investigated this composition according to gender.

Methods. A total of 979 5-mm segments of native coronary arteries and 842 5-mm segments of saphenous vein grafts were examined by computerized planimetric technique in 11 women and 11 men who were matched for survival time after the bypass operation.

Results. Comparison of the plaque components revealed that atherosclerotic plaques in women, compared with those in men, contained significantly more cellular fibrous tissue, both in native coronary arteries (mean 38% vs. 4%, $p < 0.001$) and in saphenous vein grafts (mean 70% vs. 36%, $p < 0.05$). In contrast, the proportion of dense fibrous tissue was significantly less in the atherosclerotic plaques of women than in those of men, both in native coronary arteries (mean 50% vs. 85%, $p < 0.001$) and in saphenous vein grafts (mean 25% vs. 57%, $p < 0.05$).

Conclusions. Cellular fibrous tissue is often found at an early stage of plaque development, whereas dense fibrous tissue is a major component in later stages. Thus, the plaque composition of the native coronary arteries and saphenous venous conduits differed in men and women, with the plaques of the women appearing younger than those of the men.

(J Am Coll Cardiol 1993;21:1312–8)

Although several studies have described the composition of atherosclerotic plaques in patients with various manifestations of coronary artery disease (1–5) and in patients who underwent aortocoronary bypass surgery (6–12), none have compared the composition of atherosclerotic plaques in women and men.

Accordingly, we examined in detail plaque composition in 11 women and 11 men, matched for survival time after an aortocoronary bypass operation performed >1 year earlier. Both the native coronary arteries and the saphenous veins used as aortocoronary conduits were studied.

Methods

Study patients. We limited our study to women and men in whom the heart, the native coronary arteries and the saphenous vein bypass grafts were available for examination and whose saphenous veins had been in the aortocoronary position for >1 year. Because a previous study (13) had shown that the duration of saphenous vein placement in the aortocoronary position was the most important determinant of plaque composition, we selected pairs of women and men with a similar time interval from bypass operation to death. Of 19 women and 53 men who met the aforementioned criteria, 11 pairs were matched according to survival time after an aortocoronary bypass operation. In all three tables in this study, patients are listed by survival time (from the shortest to the longest); Patient 1 of the women matches to Patient 1 of the men, and so forth. The interval from the bypass operation to death ranged from 22 to 120 months (mean 45) in the 11 women and from 19 to 120 months (mean 46) in the 11 men. The age of the women ranged from 44 to 78 years (mean 63), that of the men ranged from 47 to 76 years (mean 62). The women had a total of 35 saphenous vein conduits, the men had 25; the number of grafts per patient ranged from one to four (mean 3.2 in women and 2.3 in men). A saphenous vein having one aortic anastomosis and one or more coronary artery anastomoses was considered a single conduit. Clinical features of the 22 patients are shown in Table 1. Death had a *cardiac cause* in seven women (64%) and six men (55%): sudden cardiac arrest without myocardial necrosis in four women and three men, chronic congestive heart failure in three women and two men

From the Pathology Branch, National Heart, Lung, and Blood Institute, National Institutes of Health, Bethesda, Maryland.

Manuscript received July 8, 1992; revised manuscript received October 23, 1992, accepted October 28, 1992.

Address for correspondence: Susanne L. Mautner, MD, NHLBI-NIH, Building 10, Room 2N258, 9000 Rockville Pike, Bethesda, Maryland 20892.

Table 1. Clinical and Necropsy Findings in 11 Women and 11 Men Surviving 1 Year After Coronary Artery Bypass Grafting

Case No.	Age at Death (yr)	Interval From CABG to Death (mo)	Htn	DM	After CABG: AP	After CABG: AMI	After CABG: CHF	Mode of Death	Heart Weight (g)	Dilated LV	LV Necrosis	LV Fibrosis
A. Women												
1	65	22	+	+	0	+	0	Sudden	565	+	+	+
2	64	24	+	+	+	0	+	CHF	490	+	0	+
3	70	24	0	0	0	0	+	CHF	500	+	0	+
4	44	26	+	0	0	0	+	Sudden	600	+	0	+
5	68	30	+	+	+	0	+	Sudden	550	+	0	0
6	61	31	+	+	0	0	0	GI bleeding	440	+	0	+
7	78	37	+	0	0	0	0	Cancer	355	0	0	+
8	44	43	0	+	+	+	+	CHF	498	+	0	+
9	68	70	+	+	0	0	+	Sudden	550	+	0	+
10	59	72	0	0	0	0	0	Cancer	480	0	0	0
11	74	120	0	0	0	0	0	Trauma	466	0	0	0
Total* or mean	63	45	7*	6*	3*	2*	6*		499	8*	1*	8*
B. Men												
1	54	19	+	+	0	0	+	CHF	510	+	0	+
2	60	24	0	0	0	0	+	CHF	540	+	0	+
3	66	26	0	0	0	0	0	Sudden	460	0	0	+
4	62	27	+	0	0	0	0	Cancer	450	0	0	0
5	47	32	0	+	+	0	0	AMI	390	0	+	0
6	69	34	0	0	+	+	0	Sudden	550	+	0	+
7	49	39	0	0	0	0	0	Sudden	370	0	0	0
8	76	48	0	0	0	0	0	Cancer	395	0	0	+
9	73	60	+	0	0	0	0	COPD	540	0	0	+
10	69	82	0	0	0	0	0	Cancer	440	0	0	0
11	54	120	+	0	+	0	0	Carotid operation	560	0	0	+
Total* or mean	62	46	4*	2*	3*	1*	2*		473	3*	1*	7*

AMI = acute myocardial infarction; AP = angina pectoris; CABG = coronary artery bypass grafting; CHF = chronic congestive heart failure; COPD = chronic obstructive pulmonary disease; DM = diabetes mellitus; GI = gastrointestinal; Htn = systemic hypertension by history; LV = left ventricle (ventricular); + = present; 0 = absent.

and acute myocardial infarction in one man. Death was attributed to a *non-cardiac cause* in four women (36%) and five men (45%): cancer in two women and three men and miscellaneous conditions in the other patients (gastrointestinal bleeding, trauma, chronic obstructive pulmonary disease and carotid operation).

Method of examination of native coronary arteries and saphenous vein grafts. The native coronary arteries and saphenous vein grafts were studied in a similar fashion. The hearts were fixed in formalin. The four major epicardial coronary arteries (left main, left anterior descending, left circumflex and right) and the saphenous vein bypass grafts were removed from the heart intact and cut transversely at 5-mm intervals. In one woman and one man the left main coronary artery was not available for examination. Except for the segments adjacent to anastomoses, the entire lengths of the native coronary arteries and vein conduits were available for examination. The segments were labeled sequentially from their origin. Each segment was processed in alcohol and xylene, embedded in paraffin, cut into sections 6 μm thick and stained by the Movat method (14). Of 1,918 sections initially examined, 97 were excluded because of sectioning artifacts. Thus, a total of 979 5-mm segments of native coronary arteries (mean 45/patient) and 842 segments of saphenous vein grafts (mean 38/patient) were studied. Plaque composition was assessed by planimetry: Movat-stained sections were placed on the stage of a projection light microscope, enlarging the image approximately 150 times. A tracing of the artery was made using a GTCO micro Digi-Pad. The area was calculated using Macmeasure (15), a morphometric software package used in conjunction with a Macintosh computer. The following areas were outlined: potential lumen (total area enclosed by the internal elastic membrane); residual lumen (potential lumen minus area of atherosclerotic plaque), and the components of the plaque separated into dense fibrous tissue, cellular fibrous tissue, calcific deposits, pultaceous debris (extracellular lipid), foam cells (intracellular lipid) with and without lymphocytes and inflammatory infiltrates without significant numbers of foam cells. Analysis of components was performed in all 5-mm segments in each of the four major epicardial coronary arteries and all saphenous venous bypass grafts in every patient.

Dense fibrous tissue consisted of nearly acellular, relatively homogeneous fibrous tissue staining yellow or yellow-brown by the Movat stain. *Cellular fibrous tissue* contained numerous spindle cells resembling myofibroblasts, smooth muscle cells or fibroblasts admixed with fibrous tissue and often elastic fibers. *Calcific deposits* were detected by blackish, brownish or purple collections of granular staining areas in Movat-stained sections. *Pultaceous debris* (presumably rich in extracellular lipid) consisted of collections of amorphous pale-staining material with abundant cholesterol clefts. *Foam cell aggregates* were composed of plump, rounded, finely vacuolated cells. *Foam cells and lymphocytes* were areas containing round cells with finely granular or vacuolated cytoplasm admixed with lymphocytes. *Inflammatory infiltrates without foams cells* were isolated aggregates of lymphocytes and other inflammatory cells that were almost always seen surrounding small vascular channels. The defined areas were recognized using the projection microscope and were confirmed by standard light microscopy.

After outlining and measuring the area of the plaque components, the area of each plaque component was converted to a percentage of the total plaque area. Other findings, such as hemorrhage into plaques and multilumen channels, were recorded but were not part of the analysis because they were considered to be a result of complications such as rupture of a plaque or total occlusion of the lumen by plaque.

Lumen narrowing, measured as a decrease in the cross-sectional area enclosed by the border of the internal elastic membrane, was graded by visual inspection of the histologic sections at a magnification of ×40. The amount of narrowing of each 5-mm segment was categorized into five groups: 0% to 25%, 26% to 50%, 51% to 75%, 76% to 95% and 96% to 100%.

Statistical analysis. For each patient a mean percentage of segments narrowed in each category of cross-sectional area narrowing was determined. Based on the mean for each patient, the total mean ± SD for the women and men was calculated for each category of narrowing.

The area of each plaque component was converted to a percentage of the total plaque area. For each patient the average plaque composition in the native coronary arteries was determined by calculating the mean of all 5-mm segments of the four coronary arteries of each individual patient. On the basis of the mean value for each patient, the

Table 2. Degree of Narrowing and Composition of Atherosclerotic Plaques in the Native Coronary Arteries in Women Compared With Men

Case No.	5-mm Segments (no.)	5-mm Segments With CSA Plaque Narrowing (no. [%]) 0% to 25%	26% to 50%	51% to 75%	76% to 95%	96% to 100%	Plaque Composition* DFT (%)	CFT (%)	CD (%)	PD (%)	FC (%)	FC+L (%)	ICWFC (%)
A. Women													
1	64	34 [53]	15 [23]	10 [16]	4 [6]	1 [2]	34.1	58.7	0.8	5.9	0.1	0.2	0.1
2	50	4 [8]	4 [8]	11 [22]	22 [44]	9 [18]	61.9	14.5	21.1	0.7	0.1	0.4	0.2
3	42	15 [36]	4 [10]	10 [24]	13 [31]	0 [0]	52.9	38.6	7.9	0.5	0.1	0.0	0.1
4	46	7 [15]	4 [9]	7 [15]	20 [43]	8 [17]	49.4	39.4	6.1	2.4	1.8	0.1	0.2
5	35	1 [3]	3 [9]	11 [31]	16 [46]	4 [11]	84.5	8.9	3.2	3.0	0.1	0.0	0.0
6	49	4 [8]	5 [10]	29 [59]	11 [22]	0 [0]	26.9	63.9	6.9	1.1	0.6	0.5	0.1
7	51	12 [24]	15 [29]	15 [29]	7 [14]	2 [4]	30.2	61.4	5.0	2.9	0.2	0.3	0.0
8	48	3 [6]	6 [13]	11 [23]	16 [32]	12 [25]	51.6	26.8	19.8	1.4	0.0	0.1	0.4
9	36	4 [11]	2 [6]	11 [31]	16 [44]	3 [8]	69.6	21.3	0.0	7.9	0.1	0.0	1.1
10	40	8 [20]	7 [18]	12 [30]	10 [25]	3 [8]	20.7	62.0	17.2	0.1	0.0	0.0	0.0
11	54	12 [22]	10 [19]	11 [20]	10 [19]	11 [20]	63.3	24.4	7.6	3.9	0.0	0.0	0.0
Mean	47	9 [19]	7 [15]	13 [28]	13 [28]	5 [10]	49.6	38.2	8.7	2.7	0.3	0.1	0.2
B. Men													
1	37	0 [0]	19 [51]	10 [27]	2 [5]	6 [16]	81.3	4.3	2.2	10.7	1.2	0.2	0.3
2	45	13 [29]	8 [18]	13 [29]	11 [24]	0 [0]	93.5	0.0	3.5	1.7	0.2	0.2	0.0
3	40	10 [25]	7 [18]	11 [28]	11 [28]	1 [3]	93.7	4.5	1.8	0.0	0.0	0.0	0.1
4	39	9 [23]	7 [18]	5 [13]	12 [31]	6 [15]	86.5	0.6	11.0	1.7	0.0	0.2	0.0
5	30	16 [53]	8 [27]	0 [0]	5 [17]	1 [3]	96.6	1.4	1.4	0.0	0.5	0.0	0.1
6	49	5 [10]	5 [10]	2 [4]	24 [49]	13 [27]	69.5	15.8	13.4	0.2	0.0	0.0	0.0
7	47	2 [4]	5 [11]	12 [26]	17 [36]	11 [23]	89.1	0.5	4.9	4.6	0.2	0.2	0.5
8	48	0 [0]	1 [2]	6 [13]	34 [71]	7 [15]	78.1	6.5	12.0	3.1	0.0	0.0	0.0
9	29	2 [7]	5 [17]	9 [31]	8 [28]	5 [17]	61.6	12.7	18.1	5.5	0.0	0.0	0.0
10	56	0 [0]	5 [9]	5 [9]	20 [36]	26 [46]	92.9	2.0	4.1	0.5	0.1	0.0	0.0
11	44	6 [14]	1 [2]	5 [11]	20 [45]	12 [27]	87.3	0.0	4.0	8.0	0.1	0.0	0.6
Mean	42	6 [14]	6 [14]	7 [17]	15 [36]	8 [19]	84.5	4.4	6.9	3.3	0.2	0.1	0.1

*Hemorrhage into plaques or multilumen channels are not listed; therefore, numbers do not add up to 100% in each patient. CD = calcific deposits; CFT = cellular fibrous tissue; CSA = cross-sectional area; DFT = dense fibrous tissue; FC = foam cells; FC+L = foam cells plus lymphocytes; ICWFC = inflammatory cells without foam cells; PD = pultaceous debris.

Table 3. Degree of Narrowing and Composition of Atherosclerotic Plaques in the Saphenous Vein Grafts in Women Compared With Men

Case No.	5-mm Segments (no.)	5-mm Segments With CSA Plaque Narrowing (no. [%]) 0% to 25%	26% to 50%	51% to 75%	76% to 95%	96% to 100%	Plaque Composition* DFT (%)	CFT (%)	CD (%)	PD (%)	FC (%)	FC+L (%)	ICWFC (%)
A. Women													
1	15	0 [0]	0 [0]	0 [0]	1 [7]	14 [93]	1.1	87.0	0.0	0.0	0.0	0.0	0.0
2	58	24 [41]	31 [53]	3 [5]	0 [0]	0 [0]	2.7	95.0	0.0	0.0	0.0	0.0	0.0
3	54	8 [15]	37 [69]	9 [17]	0 [0]	0 [0]	0.9	99.0	0.1	0.0	0.0	0.0	0.0
4	33	1 [3]	7 [21]	7 [21]	4 [12]	14 [42]	37.6	59.2	0.0	0.0	0.0	0.0	0.0
5	34	6 [18]	28 [82]	0 [0]	0 [0]	0 [0]	0.0	99.8	0.0	0.0	0.2	0.0	0.0
6	46	0 [0]	0 [0]	0 [0]	19 [41]	27 [59]	3.5	96.2	0.2	0.0	0.0	0.0	0.0
7	31	5 [16]	13 [42]	11 [35]	2 [6]	0 [0]	10.0	86.7	0.0	0.3	0.1	0.1	0.0
8	41	0 [0]	7 [17]	17 [41]	15 [37]	2 [5]	56.6	31.2	0.0	5.6	0.6	0.1	0.3
9	25	1 [4]	9 [36]	2 [8]	7 [28]	6 [24]	28.7	49.9	0.0	19.4	0.7	0.2	0.1
10	26	6 [23]	20 [77]	0 [0]	0 [0]	0 [0]	42.8	56.7	0.3	0.0	0.2	0.0	0.0
11	51	25 [49]	24 [47]	2 [4]	0 [0]	0 [0]	89.7	9.1	0.0	0.9	0.1	0.04	0.1
Mean	38	7 [18]	16 [42]	5 [13]	4 [11]	6 [16]	24.9	70.0	0.1	2.4	0.2	0.04	0.04
B. Men													
1	42	8 [19]	15 [36]	10 [24]	9 [21]	0 [0]	1.3	98.5	0.0	0.0	0.1	0.0	0.0
2	48	0 [0]	39 [81]	1 [2]	2 [4]	6 [13]	30.8	67.8	0.0	0.0	0.0	0.0	0.0
3	51	27 [53]	23 [45]	1 [2]	0 [0]	0 [0]	21.1	78.0	0.0	0.0	0.9	0.0	0.0
4	30	13 [43]	16 [53]	1 [3]	0 [0]	0 [0]	94.9	3.5	0.0	0.8	0.5	0.3	0.0
5	9	2 [22]	4 [44]	2 [22]	1 [11]	0 [0]	55.4	0.0	0.0	13.5	10.1	0.0	0.0
6	45	8 [18]	8 [18]	7 [16]	14 [31]	8 [18]	81.7	6.3	1.3	8.5	0.8	1.2	0.2
7	27	0 [0]	4 [15]	8 [30]	15 [56]	0 [0]	79.6	2.4	0.3	9.3	1.8	1.0	0.3
8	62	36 [58]	23 [37]	3 [5]	0 [0]	0 [0]	0.0	100.0	0.0	0.0	0.0	0.0	0.0
9	38	29 [76]	9 [24]	0 [0]	0 [0]	0 [0]	69.0	30.9	0.1	0.1	0.04	0.0	0.0
10	55	3 [5]	22 [40]	22 [40]	8 [15]	0 [0]	96.9	3.1	0.0	0.0	0.0	0.0	0.0
11	21	13 [62]	0 [0]	0 [0]	1 [5]	7 [33]	98.8	0.0	0.7	0.4	0.0	0.0	0.01
Mean	39	13 [33]	15 [38]	5 [13]	5 [13]	2 [5]	57.2	35.5	0.2	3.0	1.3	0.2	0.04

*Hemorrhage into plaques or multilumen channels are not listed; therefore, numbers do not add up to 100% in each patient. Abbreviations as in Table 2.

total mean value ± SD for the women and men was calculated for the native coronary arteries. In the same fashion, the total plaque composition of the saphenous vein grafts was determined.

For statistical evaluation, the mean percentages for each patient were used. The unit of comparison was the pairs of women and men matched by survival time after bypass operation. A paired *t* test was performed with a probability of < 0.05 (two-tailed) considered to be significant.

Results

Cross-sectional area narrowing. The results are summarized in Tables 2 and 3. In all 22 patients, one or more epicardial coronary arteries were narrowed significantly (>75% in cross-sectional area) by atherosclerotic plaque; an average of 38 ± 19% of coronary artery segments in the women and 55 ± 25% of segments in the men were narrowed to this degree. Six of the 11 women and 7 of the 11 men had one or more saphenous vein conduits narrowed by atherosclerotic plaque >75% in cross-sectional area; an average of 27 ± 40% of saphenous vein segments in the women and 18 ± 20% in the men were narrowed to this degree. Statistical comparison based on the pairs of women and men matched according to time interval from bypass operation to death did not reveal any difference between women and men with respect to narrowing in cross-sectional area in the native coronary arteries and in the saphenous vein grafts.

Plaque composition. The results are summarized in Tables 2 and 3 and Figures 1 and 2.

Fibrous tissue. The mean percentage of fibrous tissue in all plaques of the native coronary arteries was 88 ± 6% in women and 89 ± 7% in men; in the saphenous vein grafts it was 95 ± 7% and 93 ± 14%, respectively (paired *t* test: p = NS).

Analysis of the subtypes of fibrous tissue revealed that the mean percentage of *cellular* fibrous tissue in the plaques of the native coronary arteries was 38 ± 21% in women and 4 ± 5% in men ($p < 0.001$); in the plaques of the saphenous vein grafts it was 70 ± 31% and 36 ± 42%, respectively ($p < 0.05$). The mean percentage of *dense* fibrous tissue in the plaques of the native coronary arteries was 50 ± 20% in women and 85 ± 11% in men ($p < 0.001$); in the plaques of the saphenous vein grafts it was 25 ± 29% and 57 ± 38%, respectively ($p < 0.05$).

Calcific deposits. Calcific deposits were present in the plaques of the native coronary arteries in all patients except one woman. The mean percentage was 9 ± 7% in women and

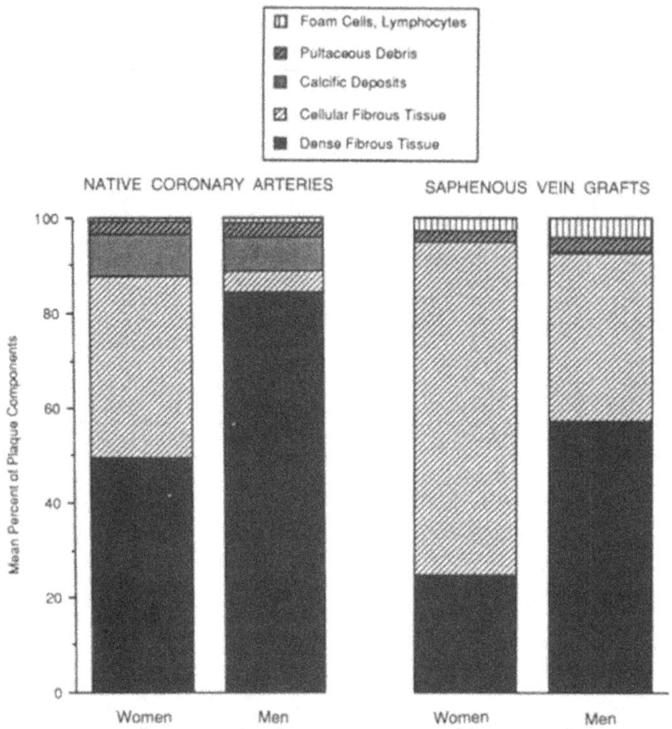

Figure 1. Graph comparing the mean composition of the plaques in the native coronary arteries and saphenous vein grafts of women and men. The plaques in women had a higher percentage of cellular fibrous tissue than did those in men. This difference was observed in the saphenous vein grafts and was even more pronounced in the native coronary arteries. In both men and women, calcific deposits were found mainly in native coronary arteries.

7 ± 6% in men. In the saphenous veins, calcific deposits were present in the plaques of three women and four men. The mean percentage was <1% in both groups. Statistically, the percentage of calcific deposits in the plaques did not differ between women and men in either the native coronary arteries or the vein grafts (p = NS).

Pultaceous debris (extracellular lipid). In the native coronary arteries, pultaceous debris was present in the plaques in 20 of the 22 patients. The mean percentage of pultaceous debris in all plaques of the coronary arteries was 2.7 ± 2.4% in women and 3.3 ± 3.6% in men (p = NS). In the saphenous vein grafts, pultaceous debris was found in the plaques in 4 of the 11 women and 6 of the 11 men. The mean percentage of pultaceous debris in all plaques of the saphenous vein grafts was 2.4 ± 5.9% in women and 3.0 ± 5.0% in men (p = NS).

Foam cells (intracellular lipid), foam cells with lymphocytes and inflammatory infiltrates without foam cells. The mean percentage of foam cells in all plaques of the native coronary arteries was 0.3 ± 0.5% in women and 0.2 ± 0.3% in men, and in the saphenous vein grafts it was 0.2 ± 0.2% in women and 1.3 ± 3.0% in men. Usually these cells were located on or near the borders of the lumen. The mean percentage of foam cells with lymphocytes and pure inflammatory cells was <1% in all plaques of both the native coronary arteries and the saphenous vein grafts in women as well as in men. Statistically, the percentage of foam cells, foam cells with lymphocytes, and inflammatory infiltrates without foam cells in the plaques did not differ between women and men in the native coronary arteries or the saphenous vein grafts (p = NS for all comparisons).

Figure 2 (opposite page). Photomicrographs of sections of native coronary arteries and saphenous vein grafts. **Left panels (A to D),** From a woman who survived 26 months after a coronary bypass operation (Case 4, Table 1A). **Right panels (E to H),** From a man who survived 27 months after a coronary bypass operation (Case 4, Table 1B). **A,** Section of a native coronary artery from a woman (Case 4). **B,** Higher magnification of the section in A. The plaque consists of 68% dense and 32% cellular fibrous tissue. **C and D,** The saphenous vein graft in this patient consists mostly of cellular fibrous tissue (90%). **E, F,** Example of a native coronary artery of a man (Case 4, Table 1B), revealing as main plaque component dense fibrous tissue (95%). A small area of calcific deposit is also present. **G, H,** In the plaque of the saphenous vein graft in this patient, dense fibrous tissue (89%) is the predominant component, whereas only a small amount (11%) of cellular fibrous tissue is present. CA = native coronary artery; SVG = saphenous vein graft; B, D, F, H are each higher magnifications of the area indicated by the rectangle in the section above. Movat stains: A ×34; C ×16; E ×34; G ×22; B, D, F, H ×200, all reduced by 22%.

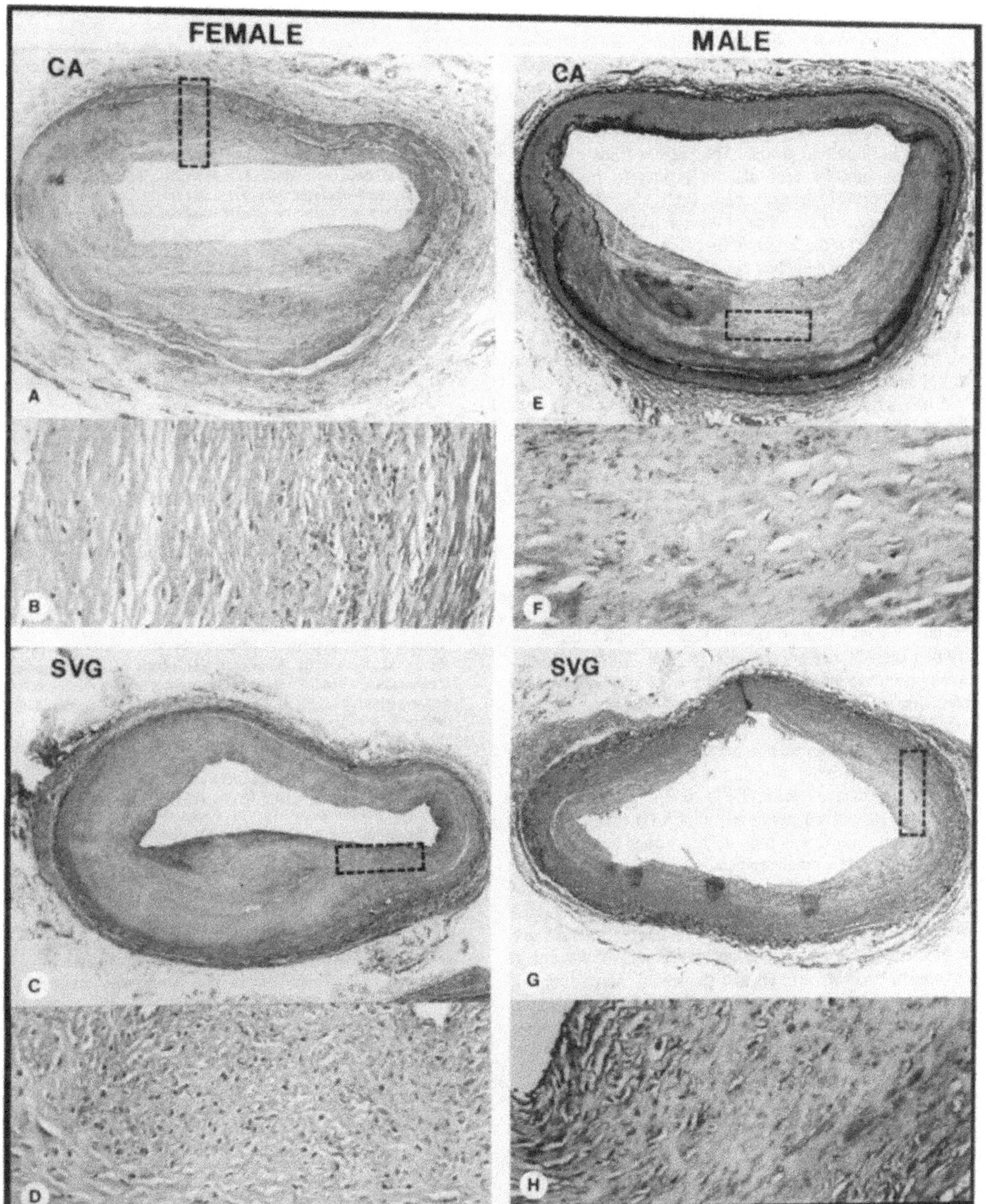
FEMALE
MALE
CA
CA
A
E
B
F
SVG
SVG
C
G
D
H

Discussion

Although several studies have compared clinical features of myocardial ischemia and results after coronary angioplasty and after bypass surgery in women versus men (16–23), no study has compared the composition of atherosclerotic plaques in the coronary arteries or in other vascular systems in those two groups. The present study compared plaque composition according to gender in both native epicardial coronary arteries and in saphenous veins used as aortocoronary conduits. The 11 women and 11 men studied were matched for the length of time that the saphenous vein aortocoronary conduits had been in place. The native coronary arteries and the saphenous vein grafts of each patient were studied by dividing their entire lengths into 5-mm segments, which then were examined histologically. In all, nearly 2,000 sections were examined by a computerized morphometric technique.

Comparison of all categories of degree of lumen narrowing of the native coronary arteries and the saphenous vein grafts revealed no difference between findings in women versus those in men.

In contrast, analysis of plaque composition disclosed that the plaques in both the native coronary arteries and saphenous vein grafts differed in women and men: in the native coronary arteries, the mean percentage of dense, acellular fibrous tissue in the plaques was much lower in women than in men (mean 50% vs. 85%), and the mean percentage of cellular fibrous tissue in the plaques was much higher in women than in men (mean 38% vs. 4%). Similar findings were present in the saphenous veins used as aortocoronary conduits: dense, acellular fibrous tissue in the plaques of the saphenous vein grafts comprised a significantly smaller percentage in women than in men (mean 25% vs. 57%) and cellular fibrous tissue constituted a higher percentage in women than in men (mean 70% vs. 36%).

It was established previously (2,4,5,13) that cellular fibrous tissue, which was present in a higher amount in the plaques of the 11 women studied, is often found at an early stage of plaque development, whereas dense fibrous tissue, the dominant component in the plaques of the 11 men studied, is seen in later stages. These differences in plaque composition, that is, the younger appearance of plaques in the native coronary arteries and saphenous venous conduit in women and the older appearance in men, might be due to differences in duration or speed of the atherosclerotic process or to different mechanisms or influences in women and men, which will require further investigation.

We thank Michael A. Proschan, PhD for statistical advice and Ricardo V. Dreyfuss and Christopher R. Dame for photographic expertise.

References

1. Roberts CS, Roberts WC. Cross-sectional area of the proximal portions of the three major epicardial coronary arteries in 98 necropsy patients with different coronary events: relationship to heart weight, age, and sex. Circulation 1980;62:953–9.
2. Dollar AL, Kragel AH, Fernicola DJ, Waclawiw MA, Roberts WC. Composition of atherosclerotic plaques in coronary arteries in women <40 years of age with fatal coronary artery disease and implication for plaque reversibility. Am J Cardiol 1991;67:1223–7.
3. Gertz SD, Malekzadeh S, Dollar AL, Kragel AH, Roberts WC. Composition of atherosclerotic plaques in the four major epicardial coronary arteries in patients ≥90 years of age. Am J Cardiol 1991;67:1228–33.
4. Kragel AH, Reddy SG, Wittes JT, Roberts WC. Morphometric analysis of the composition of atherosclerotic plaques in the four major epicardial coronary arteries in acute myocardial infarction and in sudden coronary death. Circulation 1989;80:1747–56.
5. Kragel AH, Reddy SG, Wittes JT, Roberts WC. Morphometric analysis of the composition of coronary arterial plaques in isolated unstable angina pectoris with pain at rest. Am J Cardiol 1990;66:562–7.
6. Vlodaver Z, Edwards JE. Pathologic changes in aortic coronary arterial saphenous vein grafts. Circulation 1971;64:719–28.
7. Barboriak JJ, Pintar K, Korns ME. Atherosclerosis in aortocoronary vein grafts. Lancet 1974;2:621–4.
8. Spray TL, Roberts WC. Changes in saphenous veins used as aortocoronary bypass grafts. Am Heart J 1977;94:500–16.
9. Smith SH, Geer JC. Morphology of saphenous vein-coronary artery bypass grafts. Seven to 116 months after surgery. Arch Pathol Lab Med 1983;107:13–8.
10. Atkinson JB, Forman MB, Vaughan WK, Robinowitz M, McAllister HA, Virmani R. Morphologic changes in long-term saphenous vein bypass grafts. Chest 1985;88:341–8.
11. Campeau L, Lesperance J, Corbara F, Hermann J, Grondin CM, Bourassa MG. Aortocoronary saphenous vein bypass graft changes 5 to 7 years after surgery. Circulation 1978;58(suppl I):I-170–5.
12. Kalan JM, Roberts WC. Morphologic findings in saphenous veins used as coronary arterial bypass conduits for longer than 1 year: necropsy analysis of 53 patients, 123 saphenous veins and 1865 five-millimeter segments of veins. Am Heart J 1990;119:1164–84.
13. Mautner SL, Mautner GC, Hunsberger SA, Roberts WC. Comparison of composition of atherosclerotic plaques in saphenous veins used as aortocoronary bypass conduits with plaques in native coronary arteries in the same men. Am J Cardiol 1992;70:1380–7.
14. Movat HZ. Demonstration of all connective tissue elements in a single section. Arch Pathol 1955;60:289–95.
15. Hook GR, Rasband W. Macmeasure: a low-cost, easy to operate quantitative morphometrics system for the Macintosh computer. In: Baily GW, ed: Proceedings of the 45th Annual Meeting of the Electron Microscopy Society of America. San Francisco: San Francisco Press, 1987:920–1.
16. Johansson S, Bergstrand R, Schlossman D, Selin K, Vedin A, Wilhelmsson C. Sex differences in cardioangiographic findings after myocardial infarction. Eur Heart J 1984;5:374–81.
17. Loop FD, Golding LR, MacMillan JP, Cosgrove DM, Lytle BW, Sheldon WC. Coronary artery surgery in women compared with men: analyses of risks and long-term results. J Am Coll Cardiol 1983;1:383–90.
18. Fisher LD, Kennedy JW, Davis KB, et al. Association of sex, physical size, and operative mortality after coronary artery bypass in the Coronary Artery Surgery Study (CASS). J Thorac Cardiovasc Surg 1982;84:334–41.
19. Bolooki H, Vargas A, Green R, Kaiser GA, Ghahramani A. Results of direct coronary artery surgery in women. J Thorac Cardiovasc Surg 1975;69:271–7.
20. Tyras DH, Barner HB, Kaiser GC, Codd JE, Laks H, Willman VL. Myocardial revascularization in women. Ann Thorac Surg 1978;25:449–53.
21. Golding LR, Groves LK. Results of coronary artery surgery in women. Cleve Clin Q 1976;43:113–5.
22. Killen DA, Reed WA, Arnold M, McCallister BD, Bell HH. Coronary artery bypass in women. Long-term survival. Ann Thorac Surg 1982;34:559–63.
23. Douglas JS Jr, King SB III, Jones EL, Craver JM, Bradford JM, Hatcher CR Jr. Reduced efficacy of coronary bypass surgery in women. Circulation 1981;64(suppl II):II-11–6.

Expected and unexpected changes in venous autografts used as aortocoronary conduits

WILLIAM C. ROBERTS, MD • *Baylor Cardiovascular Institute*

Since its introduction 30 years ago, numerous patients have benefited from coronary arterial bypass grafting. Despite its benefits to most patients, coronary bypass, of course, is not free of complications. Stenosis or complete occlusion of venous grafts used as aortocoronary conduits still occurs. While all venous grafts develop some morphologic changes, the degree and functional significance of the changes vary widely. This article describes structural changes observed early and late in saphenous veins that are used as aortocoronary conduits.

DEGREES OF NARROWING OF NATIVE EPICARDIAL CORONARY ARTERIES IN SYMPTOMATIC MYOCARDIAL ISCHEMIA

Before focusing on changes in saphenous veins used as aortocoronary conduits, a brief discussion on the status of native epicardial coronary arteries in patients likely to undergo aortocoronary bypass grafting appears appropriate. Examination at necropsy of coronary endarterectomy specimens or examination during life by intravascular ultrasonic imaging of the 4 major (right, left main, left anterior descending, and left circumflex) epicardial coronary arteries in patients >30 years of age with symptomatic myocardial ischemia and angiographic narrowing >50% in diameter of 1 or more major coronary arteries discloses that atherosclerotic plaques are present in virtually every 5-mm segment of the entire lengths of the arteries (1, 2) (*Figure*). In patients with angiographically so-called "single-vessel disease," approximately 40% of the lumen of each 5-mm segment of the 4 major arteries (average of 54 segments per patient) is obliterated by plaque; in patients with angiographically "double-vessel disease," approximately 50% of the total lumen is obliterated by plaque; in patients with "triple-vessel disease," approximately 60% of the total lumen is filled with plaque; and in patients with "quadruple-vessel disease," approximately 70% of the total lumen is filled with plaque. Thus, the greater the number of major coronary arteries significantly narrowed as shown by angiogram, the greater the total amount of atherosclerotic plaque in the major epicardial coronary arteries.

THE NORMAL SAPHENOUS VEIN

The normal human saphenous vein contains a thin *intima* consisting of relatively acellular fibrous tissue covered by a single layer of endothelial cells and separated from the media by a rudimentary internal elastic membrane. The *media* consists of multiple layers of smooth muscle cells separated by bundles of collagen; ground substance; and occasional short, elastic fibers. Most medial, smooth muscle layers have a circular orientation; in areas near the venous valves, however, the middle circular layers have a more longitudinal arrangement. Frequently, longitudinally oriented, smooth muscle fascicles make up the innermost layers of the media. The *adventitia* is composed of bundles of collagen with scattered fascicles of longitudinally oriented, smooth muscle cells. Broad, loose bands of elastic fibers are present in abundance. Vasa vasorum are present and may extend into the outmost portion of the media.

FINDINGS IN REMNANT SAPHENOUS VEINS EXCISED FOR AORTOCORONARY CONDUITS BUT NEVER USED

Some degree of intimal fibrous thickening commonly occurs in saphenous veins excised for aortocoronary bypass but never used. Waller and Roberts (3) examined nearly 3500 cm of unused but excised saphenous vein from 402 patients having coronary bypass surgery. The length of the unused saphenous veins ranged from 0.5 to 52 cm per patient (mean, 8.5). A histologic section was examined from each of the 6788 5-mm long segments: the lumen in 0.4% of the sections was narrowed 76% to 100% by fibrous tissue in cross-sectional area; 0.6% were narrowed 51% to 75% in cross-sectional area; 12% were narrowed 26% to 50% in cross-sectional area; and 87% were narrowed ≥25% in cross-sectional area. The percent of 5-mm segments of unused vein narrowed >75% in cross-sectional area was similar in men and women, and it was similar in each of 5 decades (31 to 40, 41 to 50, 51 to 60, 61 to 70, and 71 to 80 years). Thus, approximately 1% of saphenous veins excised for coronary bypass are narrowed >50% by fibrous tissue in cross-sectional area before they are used as aortocoronary conduits.

NUMBERS OF AORTIC ANASTOMOTIC SITES, NUMBERS OF CONDUITS, AND NUMBERS OF CORONARY ANASTOMOTIC SITES

I doubt if any 2 surgeons perform the bypass operation in quite the same manner, and these individual variations may affect patient outcome and graft outcome. The phrases "2 bypasses" or "3 bypasses" or "4 bypasses" are commonly used, but their meaning is not always precise. I suspect that most users of the phrase "3 bypasses" are referring to the number of coronary anastomoses. A patient may have 3 coronary anastomotic sites and

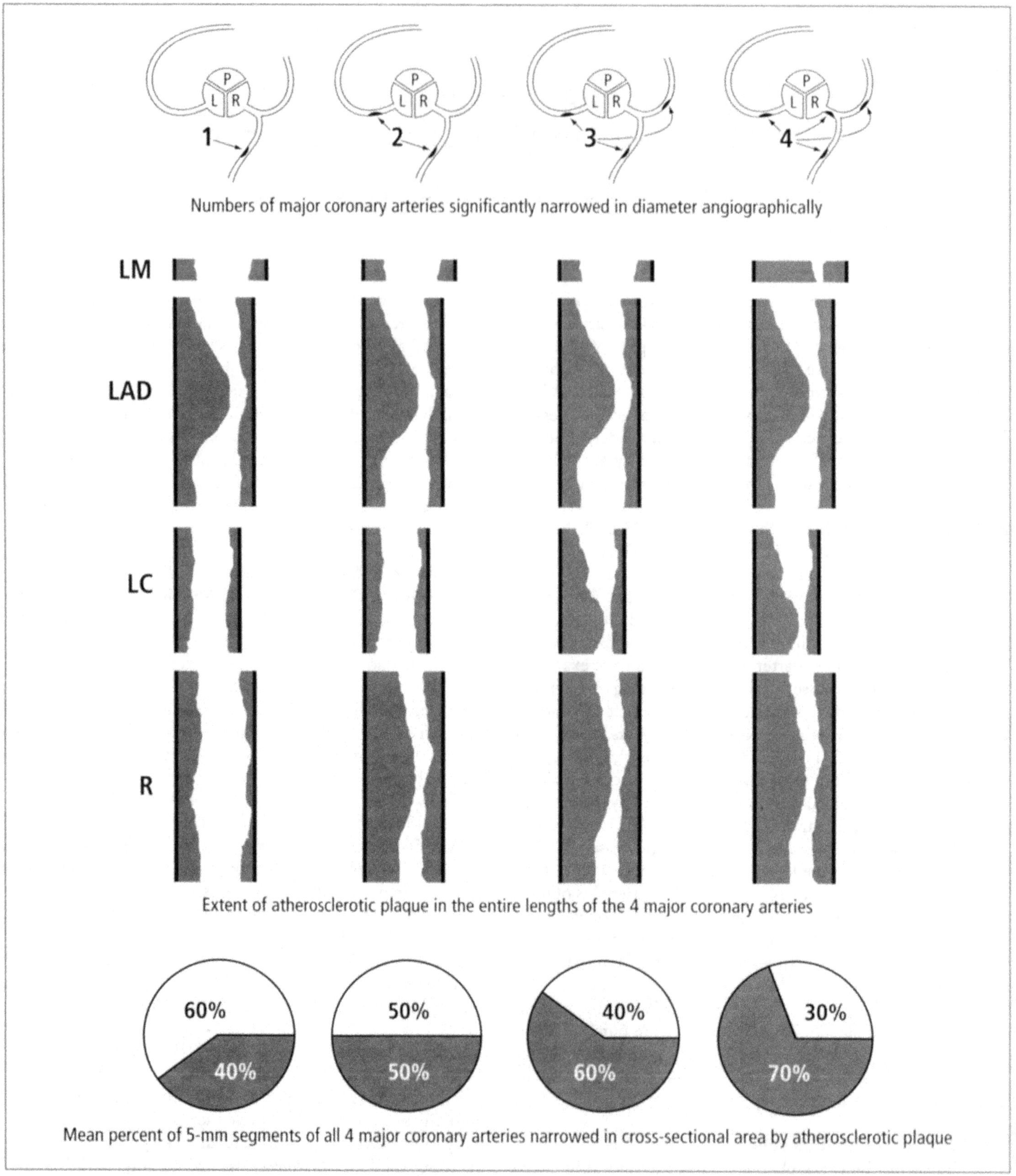

Figure. Diagram showing numbers of coronary arteries significantly narrowed by angiogram (*top*), the amounts of plaque in the entire lengths of the 4 major (left main [LM]), left anterior descending [LAD], left circumflex [LC], and right [R]) epicardial coronary arteries (*middle*), and a cross-sectional area view (*bottom*) of the average amount of plaque in each 5-mm segment of the entire lengths of the 4 major coronary arteries according to the numbers of major arteries significantly narrowed by angiogram. Reprinted by permission of the publisher from Roberts WC: Coronary lesions, coronary disease, single-vessel disease, and two-vessel disease: word and phrase misnomers providing false impressions of the extent of coronary atherosclerosis in symptomatic myocardial ischemia. *Am J Cardiol* 1990;66:121–123. Copyright 1990 by Excerpta Medica Inc.

only 1 conduit ("round-the-world" bypass) or 2 conduits or 3 conduits with similar numbers of aortic anastomotic sites. To prevent confusion, it might be best to always state the number of aortic anastomotic sites, the number of conduits, and the number of coronary anastomotic sites. To me, it seems most reasonable for each of these 3 to be the same: if a patient is to have 3 coronary anastomotic sites, it might be ideal to have 3 conduits and 3 separate aortic anastomotic sites. If only 1 conduit is used with a single aortic anastomotic site and the single conduit is anastomosed to 7 different coronary arteries, the outcome is not ideal if the single aortic anastomosis closes or the single conduit closes proximally. With similar numbers of aortic anastomotic sites, conduits, and coronary anastomotic sites, this circumstance is less likely to occur.

The location of the coronary anastomotic site appears to be relatively similar with most surgeons. The distal 1 cm of the right coronary artery probably is ideal because the most severe narrowing of this artery tends to be in its distal third rather than the proximal or middle third (4). The most common anastomotic site of the left anterior descending is probably about two thirds down its length, and this location, of course, is logical because this artery tends to be more severely narrowed in its proximal third than in either its middle or distal thirds (4). The same situation also appears reasonable for the first diagonal artery. Anastomoses in the obtuse marginal arteries usually are within 3 cm of their origin from the left circumflex.

Tension on the conduit is 1 of the various technical factors that can affect flow in aortocoronary conduits (5). Abnormal tension is indicated by grooving or indentation into the right atrial wall or right atrioventricular sulcus or by flattening of the graft passing anterior to the pulmonary trunk. If the graft is under tension, leakage at the bypass anastomosis probably is more likely than without tension. *Twisting of a conduit* may prevent successful bypass grafting (6).

EARLY CHANGES IN SAPHENOUS VEINS USED AS AORTOCORONARY CONDUITS

In 1906, Carrel and Guthrie (7) described intimal thickening of veins implanted into the arterial system in dogs and concluded that veins placed in the arterial circulation had a strong tendency to assume the character of an artery. In further vein transplantation experiments in 1908, Carrel (8) described 4 characteristic changes in veins used as arteries in the peripheral circulation: 1) intimal thickening; 2) adventitial thickening (from fibrosis); 3) loss of the inner third of the media; and 4) loss of elastic fibers, producing a fibrous tube. In addition, medial hypertrophy was observed in some grafts. These changes subsequently have been confirmed in humans in saphenous veins used for femoropopliteal and aortocoronary bypass.

Spray and Roberts (9, 10) studied a large number of saphenous vein grafts from patients dying within a year after aortocoronary bypass. Vein grafts from patients dying intraoperatively showed minimal medial edema (clear spaces between layers of smooth muscle) and disrupted adventitia (occurring during excision of the vein before grafting). By 2 weeks, mural edema was more pronounced, some medial smooth muscle cells were necrotic, and inflammatory infiltrates were present. The endothelium often was disrupted, and the intimal surface usually was covered, either partially or completely, by fibrin. By 3 weeks, cells with characteristics of smooth muscle appeared in the subendothelial portion of the intima. The cells generally were oriented such that their longest diameter was parallel to the direction of blood flow. Thereafter, the subendothelial intimal lesions became more generalized and less cellular, ground substance appeared in abundance, and short elastic fibers and vascular channels occasionally were present. The smooth muscle fibers of the media gradually diminished in number and were replaced, in part or in whole, by fibrous tissue. Fibrous tissue also increased in the adventitia, and its elastic fibers became severely disrupted or disappeared completely. Organizing fibrin on the external surface of the grafts probably contributed to the adventitial fibrosis. Capillaries were present in the adventitia and often were extended into the fibrotic media. Thus, the saphenous vein used as an artery becomes a stiff, fibrous tissue conduit.

LATE CHANGES IN SAPHENOUS VEINS USED AS AORTOCORONARY CONDUITS

Kalan and Roberts (11) described findings at necropsy in 123 saphenous vein grafts and in 1865 5-mm segments of the grafts in 53 patients who had single aortocoronary bypass operations 13 to 185 months (mean, 58) before death. Of the 53 patients, 32 (60%) died from a cardiac cause, and of their 73 saphenous vein aortocoronary conduits, 36 (49%) were narrowed at some point by atherosclerotic plaque more than 75% in cross-sectional area; the remaining 21 patients (40%) died from noncardiac causes, and of their 50 saphenous vein conduits, 10 (20%) were narrowed by plaque, at some point, more than 75% in cross-sectional area. Of the 53 patients, 31 (58%) had at least 1 bypass graft maximally narrowed at some point by fibromuscular tissue with or without lipid greater than 75% in cross-sectional area; 12 patients (23%) had maximal graft narrowing of 51% to 75%; 8 patients (15%), 26% to 50%; and 2 patients (4%), 0 % to 25%. The percent of patients with a graft narrowed over 75% at necropsy did not increase as the interval from bypass surgery to death increased.

Of the 123 saphenous vein grafts, 47 (38%) were maximally narrowed greater than 75% in cross-sectional area; 44 (36%), 51% to 75%; 22 (18%), 26% to 50%; and 10 (8%), 0% to 25%. Of the 47 grafts narrowed over 75% in cross-sectional area, 29 actually were narrowed by fibrous tissue greater than 95% in cross-sectional area. The percent of saphenous veins narrowed greater than 75% at necropsy was not affected by gender (men 38%, women 36%), presence or absence of systemic hypertension (40% vs 33%), or presence or absence of diabetes mellitus (30% vs 48%). The percent of grafts narrowed over 75% in cross-sectional area did not correlate with the interval between bypass surgery and death, or with the coronary artery to which the graft was connected.

The degree of narrowing of the saphenous vein graft was related to the degree of luminal narrowing of the native coronary artery at or within 2 cm distal to the saphenous vein-coronary artery anastomosis. Of the 49 grafts attached to a coronary artery that was narrowed greater than 75% at or distal to the anastomosis, 33 (67%) were significantly narrowed; of the 74 grafts attached to a coronary artery narrowed less than 75% distal to the anastomotic site, 14 (19%) were severely narrowed.

Analysis of the 1865 5-mm long saphenous vein segments disclosed that 209 segments (11%) were narrowed 96% to 100% in cross-sectional area; 172 (9%), 76% to 95%; 407 (22%), 51% to 75%; 685 (37%), 26% to 50%; and 392 (21%), 0% to 25%. Similar percents of segments were narrowed greater than 75% in men and women (22% vs 15%), in diabetics and nondiabetics (18% vs 26%), and in hypertensives and nonhypertensives (21% vs 20%). Further, the interval from coronary bypass to death did not correlate with the percent of segments severely narrowed.

Although the percent of saphenous vein segments narrowed greater than 75% in cross-sectional area at necropsy did not correlate with the interval from bypass grafting to death, it did relate to the mode of death. Of the 32 patients dying from a cardiac cause, 295 (27%) of 1104 saphenous vein segments were narrowed greater than 75%, whereas of the 21 patients dying from a noncardiac cause, 86 (11%) of 761 saphenous vein segments were so narrowed. The percent of segments of native coronary artery narrowed greater than 75% was similar in patients with cardiac and noncardiac modes of death, 673 of 1441 (47%) vs 333 of 895 (37%), respectively.

COMPOSITION OF TISSUE CAUSING LATE LUMINAL NARROWING IN THE SAPHENOUS VEINS USED AS AORTOCORONARY CONDUITS

Lipid was present in the wall of a graft in 39 of the 53 patients (74%). Fifteen had intracellular lipid alone (foam cells), and 24 had both foam cells and extracellular lipid. Extracellular lipid was not found in a saphenous vein graft until 26 months after bypass. Lipid was present in 69 (56%) of the 123 saphenous vein grafts from the 39 patients. Intracellular lipid was present in all 69 grafts, either alone (33 grafts) or with extracellular lipid (36 grafts). The amount of lipid present appeared to increase as the interval from coronary bypass to death increased. Foam cells were located near the luminal surfaces of the intimal fibrous tissue, and they did not appreciably narrow the lumen. Extracellular lipid deposits were located deeper in the plaque, separated from the lumen by a layer of fibrous tissue; they often contributed significantly to luminal narrowing.

Hemorrhage into plaque (into the lipid portion only) was found in 26 (21%) saphenous vein grafts from 17 (32%) patients. This condition was seen as early as 24 months after bypass and did not increase in frequency thereafter as the interval from bypass to death increased. Luminal narrowing greater than 75% in cross-sectional area was significantly more common in grafts with than without plaque hemorrhage.

Luminal thrombus was present in 16 (13%) saphenous vein grafts from 14 (26%) patients. Thrombus was not seen until 32 months after bypass, and its frequency did not increase thereafter as the interval from bypass to death increased. Thrombus within the graft lumen was present in 16 of 69 grafts that had deposits of lipid in their walls, and in none of 54 grafts devoid of lipid. In 14 of these 16 grafts, hemorrhage into plaque was found.

Calcific deposits were present in 13 (11%) of the 123 saphenous vein grafts from 11 patients, and they were first seen 34 months after coronary bypass. All of the deposits were small and were present in 18 (1%) of the 1865 5-mm saphenous vein segments.

The aforementioned data indicate that virtually all saphenous veins used as aortocoronary conduits for longer than a year develop atherosclerotic plaques in each 5-mm segment of their entire lengths. Thus, atherosclerotic plaquing late in saphenous veins used as aortocoronary conduits is diffuse, just as it is in native coronary arteries in patients with fatal myocardial ischemia (1, 2). The amounts of luminal narrowing in the saphenous veins used as aortocoronary conduits were significantly greater in those patients who died from a cardiac cause, compared with those who died from a noncardiac cause. Surprisingly, the interval from coronary bypass to death did not correlate with either the percent of vein conduits or the percent of 5-mm segments of vein conduit narrowed by plaque over 75% in cross-sectional area. Moreover, the percent of 5-mm segments of saphenous vein conduit severely narrowed was similar in the 35 patients surviving up to 5 years, compared with the 18 patients surviving over 5 years.

The composition of plaques in the saphenous venous conduits is similar to that in the native coronary arteries. Fibrous tissue or fibromuscular tissue was the dominant component of the plaques in the saphenous vein conduits, just as it is the dominant component of plaques in the native coronary arteries in patients with fatal coronary artery disease without coronary bypass (12, 13).

The frequency of the various modes of death among patients dying late after coronary bypass is a bit different from that of patients with symptomatic myocardial ischemia without coronary bypass (14). Of the 53 coronary bypass patients studied, only 32 (60%) died from a cardiac cause; therefore, 21 (40%) died from noncardiac causes. Among patients with symptomatic myocardial ischemia who do not have coronary bypass, approximately 95% die from a cardiac cause. The fact that 40% of the bypass cases studied died from noncardiac causes supports the view that the bypass operation in many patients prolongs life long enough for many to develop various fatal noncardiac conditions. Of the 53 bypass patients reported by Kalan and Roberts (11), 10 (19%) died from cancer, a percent far higher than patients with symptomatic myocardial ischemia not having coronary surgery.

The study by Kalan and Roberts (11) reemphasizes that coronary bypass is useful but that it does not deter progression of the underlying atherosclerotic process. In a slight way, the bypass operation might even cause acceleration of the atherosclerotic process, because in about 25% of persons having coronary bypass, both the serum total cholesterol and the body weight increase substantially during the first year after operation. Because lowering the serum (or plasma) total cholesterol level (and specifically the low-density lipoprotein cholesterol) decreases the chances of "heart attack" and may cause some portion of atherosclerotic plaques to regress and other portions to not progress, a strong case can be advanced for combined simultaneous initiation of both low-fat, low-cholesterol diet therapy and lipid-lowering drug therapy as soon as reasonably feasible after a coronary bypass operation (15).

In January 1997, the Post Coronary Artery Bypass Graft Trial Investigators (16) reported results of a study of 1351 patients who had undergone aortocoronary bypass grafting 1 to 11 years earlier and who had low-density lipoprotein (LDL) cholesterol levels between 130 and 175 mg/dL, triglyceride levels <300 mg/dL, and at least 1 patent vein graft on coronary angiography. The study divided the patients into those in whom an "aggressive" treatment plan was employed with the goal of lowering LDL cholesterol to 60 to 85 mg/dL and those in whom a "moderate" treatment plan was employed with the goal of lowering LDL cholesterol to 130 to 140 mg/dL. In the aggressive treatment group, a mean of 76 ± 13 mg of lovastatin was employed, and 30% also received 8 g/day of cholestyramine; in the moderate treatment group, a mean of 4 ± 1 mg of lovastatin was employed, and 5% also received 8 g/day of cholestyramine. Coronary angiography was repeated an average of 4.3 years after the baseline angiogram. The primary angiographic outcome was the mean percentage per patient of grafts with a decrease of ≥0.6 mm in lumen diameter.

As measured annually during the study, the mean LDL cholesterol level of patients who received aggressive treatment ranged from 93 to 97 mg/dL; with moderate treatment, the range was from 132 to 136 mg/dL. The mean percentage of grafts with progression of atherosclerosis was 27% for patients whose LDL cholesterol levels were lowered with aggressive treatment and 39% for those who received moderate treatment. There was no significant difference in angiographic outcome in patients receiving warfarin and those who did not receive warfarin. The rate of revascularization during the 4-year study was 29% lower in the group whose LDL cholesterol levels were lowered aggressively, compared with the group receiving moderate treatment (6.5% vs 9.2%). Thus, aggressive lowering of LDL cholesterol levels to <100 mg/dL reduced the progression of atherosclerosis in aortocoronary bypass grafts. This recent study, therefore, gives strong support to the use of lipid-lowering agents, particularly the statin drugs, after aortocoronary bypass operations to lower the LDL cholesterol to <100 mg/dL.

CAUSES OF MORPHOLOGIC CHANGES IN SAPHENOUS VEINS USED AS AORTOCORONARY CONDUITS

Although the causes of the changes in saphenous vein grafts are in many ways similar to those causing atherosclerotic plaques in native coronary arteries (17), additional mechanisms almost surely play a role when a vein is switched to an arterial location. The early changes in the saphenous veins are similar to the phlebosclerotic lesions in venous varicosities, changes presumably caused by the response of the vein to increases in hydrostatic pressure. Arteriovenous shunts of any origin (congenital, traumatic, or iatrogenic) show intimal thickening, presumably the result of increased pressure and flow. Subendothelial proliferative lesions in the pulmonary arteries of patients with pulmonary hypertension and in vena cava and portal veins in patients with chronic right-sided congestive cardiac failure or portal hypertension also are seen in the saphenous veins transferred to the aortocoronary position. Brody and colleagues (18, 19) attempted to differentiate the effects of pressure and ischemia on femoral vein grafts in dogs. Vein segments were either left intact or dissected free from their adventitia, thereby severing the vasa vasora and producing medial ischemia. Next, the vein segments were either left in the venous system or were arterialized by creation of an arteriovenous fistula. The presence of medial ischemia in the absence of elevated pressure and flow produced medial fibrosis in the vein without subendothelial, intimal proliferative lesions. Elevated intravascular pressure alone, however, without alterations in blood supply to the media by the vasa vasorum produced intimal lesions without evidence of medial fibrosis. The combination of elevated intraluminal pressure and medial ischemia resulted in medial and intimal changes similar to the changes seen in human saphenous veins used as aortocoronary conduits.

The intimal process in saphenous veins and specifically the degree of luminal narrowing in saphenous veins in the aortocoronary position are almost certainly accelerated when flow through the conduit is relatively poor. The major cause of poor flow is severe narrowing in the native coronary artery (to which the vein is attached) at or just distal to the site of anastomosis (9–11, 20). The smaller the native coronary arteries to which the graft is to be connected, the less the amount of atherosclerotic plaque necessary to cause significant luminal narrowing. Smaller hearts have smaller coronary arteries than larger hearts (21). Small patients tend to have smaller hearts than larger patients. Thus, similar amounts of plaque cause more luminal narrowing in small patients than in large patients. Women on average are smaller than men and, therefore, on average they have smaller hearts and smaller coronary arteries. Coronary bypass might be expected, therefore, to have poorer results in women than in men, because the smaller arteries might cause poor flow through the conduits by plaque in the native coronary arteries.

Kalan and Roberts (22) found the above scenario probably to be the case. Their 121 necropsy patients dying within 60 days of coronary bypass operations had significantly lower mean heart weights than did the 90 patients dying late, and this fact held true for both sexes. Most patients with normal-sized hearts were in the early death group; conversely, most patients in the late death group had hearts of increased weight. Their findings suggest that patients with normal- or near-normal–sized hearts have a higher early mortality after coronary bypass than do persons with hearts of increased weight. Furthermore, more changes leading to luminal narrowing of bypass conduits might be expected in persons with small native coronary arteries (small hearts), because the runoff through the graft may not be as good as in patients with larger native coronary arteries (larger hearts).

COMPARISON OF MORPHOLOGIC CHANGES IN SAPHENOUS VEINS WITH THOSE IN INTERNAL MAMMARY ARTERIES USED AS AORTOCORONARY CONDUITS

For practical purposes, none of the aforedescribed changes in saphenous veins used as aortocoronary conduits are found in internal mammary arteries used in the coronary position. As pointed out by others (23, 24), the patency rate early and late is splendid with the mammary artery but is much lower with the saphenous vein. Late after bypass, the internal mammary artery remains much smaller than the saphenous vein when each is used in the same patient. The internal mammary artery remains virtually devoid of intimal deposits, whereas the larger saphenous vein (in the same patient) may develop severe atherosclerotic plaque in its lumen (25, 26).

References

1. Roberts WC: Qualitative and quantitative comparison of amounts of narrowing by atherosclerotic plaques in the major epicardial coronary arteries at necropsy in sudden coronary death, transmural acute myocardial infarction, transmural healed myocardial infarction and unstable angina pectoris. *Am J Cardiol* 1989;64:324–328.
2. Roberts WC: Coronary "lesion," coronary "disease," "single-vessel disease," "two-vessel disease": word and phrase misnomers providing false impressions of the extent of coronary atherosclerosis in symptomatic myocardial ischemia. *Am J Cardiol* 1990;66:121–123.
3. Waller BF, Roberts WC: Remnant saphenous veins after aortocoronary bypass grafting: analysis of 3,394 centimeters of unused vein from 402 patients. *Am J Cardiol* 1985;55:65–71.
4. Vlodaver Z, Edwards JE: Pathology of coronary atherosclerosis. *Prog Cardiovasc Dis* 1971;14:256–274.
5. Spray TL, Roberts WC: Tension on coronary bypass conduits: a neglected cause of real or potential obstruction of saphenous vein grafts. *J Thorac Cardiovasc Surg* 1976;72:282–287.
6. Roberts WC, Lachman AS, Virmani R: Twisting of an aorto-coronary bypass conduit: a complication of coronary surgery. *J Thorac Cardiovasc Surg* 1978;75:772–776.
7. Carrel A, Guthrie CC: Results of biterminal transplantation of veins. *Am J Med Sci* 1906;132:415–422.
8. Carrel A: Results of transplantation of blood vessels, organs, and limbs. JAMA 1908;51:1662–1667.
9. Spray TL, Roberts WC: Status of the grafts and the native coronary arteries proximal and distal to coronary anastomotic sites of aortocoronary bypass grafts. *Circulation* 1977;55:741–749.
10. Spray TL, Roberts WC: Changes in saphenous veins used as aortocoronary bypass grafts. *Am Heart J* 1977;94:500–516.
11. Kalan JM, Roberts WC: Morphologic findings in saphenous veins used as coronary arterial bypass conduits for longer than 1 year: necropsy analysis of 53 patients, 123 saphenous veins, and 1865 five-millimeter segments of veins. *Am Heart J* 1990;119:1164–1184.
12. Kragel AH, Reddy SG, Wittes JT, Roberts WC: Morphometric analysis of the composition of atherosclerotic plaques in the four major epicardial coronary arteries in acute myocardial infarction and in sudden coronary death. *Circulation* 1989;80:1747–1756.
13. Kragel AH, Reddy SG, Wittes JT, Roberts WC: Morphometric analysis of the composition of coronary arterial plaques in isolated unstable angina pectoris with pain at rest. *Am J Cardiol* 1990;66:562–567.
14. Roberts WC, Potkin BN, Solus DE, Reddy SG: Mode of death, frequency of healed and acute myocardial infarction, number of major epicardial coronary arteries severely narrowed by atherosclerotic plaque, and heart weight in fatal atherosclerotic coronary artery disease: analysis of 889 patients studied at necropsy. *J Am Coll Cardiol* 1990;15:196–203.
15. Roberts WC: Lipid-lowering therapy after an atherosclerotic event. *Am J Cardiol* 1989;64:693–695.
16. The Post Coronary Artery Bypass Graft Trial Investigators: The effect of aggressive lowering of low-density lipoprotein cholesterol levels and low-dose anticoagulation on obstructive changes in saphenous-vein coronary-artery bypass grafts. *N Engl J Med* 1997;336:153–162.
17. Roberts WC: Preventing and arresting coronary atherosclerosis. *Am Heart J* 1995;130:580–600.
18. Brody WR, Kosek JC, Angell WW: Changes in vein grafts following aorto-coronary bypass induced by pressure and ischemia. *J Thorac Cardiovasc Surg* 1972;64:847–854.
19. Brody WR, Angell WW, Kosek JC: Histologic fate of the venous coronary artery bypass in dogs. *Am J Pathol* 1972;66:111–130.
20. Waller BF, Roberts WC: Amount of narrowing by atherosclerotic plaque in 44 nonbypassed and 52 bypassed major epicardial coronary arteries in 32 necropsy patients who died within 1 month of aortocoronary bypass grafting. *Am J Cardiol* 1980;46:956–962.
21. Roberts CS, Roberts WC: Cross-sectional area of the proximal portions of the three major epicardial coronary arteries in 98 necropsy patients with different coronary events: relationship to heart weight, age and sex. *Circulation* 1980;62:953–959.
22. Kalan JM, Roberts WC: Significance of cardiac weight in patients having coronary artery bypass grafting for angina pectoris. *Am J Cardiol* 1988;62:36–40.
23. Grondin CM, Campeau L, Lesperance J, Enjalbert M, Bourassa MG: Comparison of late changes in internal mammary artery and saphenous vein grafts in two consecutive series of patients 10 years after operation. *Circulation* 1984;70(Suppl I):208–212.
24. Loop FD, Lytle BW, Cosgrove DM, Stewart RW, Goormastic M, Williams GW, Golding LA, Gill CC, Taylor PC, Sheldon WC, Proudfit WL: Influence of the internal-mammary-artery graft on 10-year survival and other cardiac events. *N Engl J Med* 1986;314:1–6.
25. Barbour DJ, Roberts WC: Additional evidence for relative resistance to atherosclerosis of the internal mammary artery compared to saphenous vein when used to increase myocardial blood supply. *Am J Cardiol* 1985;56:488.
26. Kalan JM, Roberts WC: Comparison of morphologic changes and luminal sizes of saphenous vein and internal mammary artery after simultaneous implantation for coronary arterial bypass grafting. *Am J Cardiol* 1987;60:193–196.

Liver Transplantation *After* Coronary Artery Bypass Grafting

Frank Pelosi, Jr., MD, Goran B.G. Klintmalm, MD, PhD, Walter B. Simon, MD, and William C. Roberts, MD

Few patients have both coronary artery bypass grafting (CABG) and liver transplantation (LT). Indeed, only 7 patients have been reported to have had both procedures.[1–3] This article reviews findings in 12 patients who had CABG and then later had LT.

• • •

From December 1985 to July 1996, >1,150 patients have had LT at Baylor University Medical Center (BUMC) and since 1985 >8,000 patients have had CABG. The database of Baylor's LT unit was reviewed searching for patients who had had both LT and CABG. A total of 15 patients were retrieved and their clinical records were reviewed. Three patients had LT followed in 6, 36, and 72 months, respectively, by CABG. The 12 patients included in the present study had CABG followed by LT 1 to 228 months later. Pertinent data for each of these 12 patients are summarized in Table I.

Three patients (numbers 1, 2, and 3, Table I) were found to have evidence of myocardial ischemia and angiographic evidence of severe narrowing (>50% diameter reduction) of ≥3 major (right, left anterior descending, and left circumflex) epicardial coronary arteries when they were being evaluated for LT. In other words, when first seen at BUMC, each had evidence of both hepatic and cardiac dysfunction. Two of these patients underwent CABG followed within 1 month by LT; the third had LT 7 months after CABG. The cause of the hepatic dysfunction in these patients was methotrexate toxicity (treatment for psoriasis), biliary cirrhosis, and alcoholism, respectively. Patients 1 and 3 have been reported previously.[3]

From the Baylor Cardiovascular Institute; the Baylor Institute for Transplantation Sciences; and the Departments of Internal Medicine (Division of Cardiology), Pathology and Surgery, Baylor University Medical Center, Dallas, Texas. Dr. Roberts' address is: Baylor Cardiovascular Institute, 3500 Gaston Avenue, Dallas, Texas 75246. Manuscript received October 3, 1996; revised manuscript received and accepted December 24, 1996.

In the remaining 9 patients, CABG was performed before the development of serious hepatic disease. The cause of the hepatic dysfunction in these 9 patients was hepatitis C virus in 7, and habitual alcoholism in 2. These 9 patients had LT from 60 to 228 months (mean 129) after CABG. For those who had LT secondary to hepatitis C, the interval between CABG and LT ranged from 60 to 228 months (mean 134); for alcoholism, the interval was 72 and 156 months, respectively. Ten of the 12 patients had a single CABG operation, and only 2 of the 10 procedures (numbers 2 and 3, Table I) were performed at BUMC. Each of the remaining 2 patients (numbers 6 and 12, Table I) had 2 CABG procedures (1 before and 1 after LT), and none of these 4 CABG operations was performed at BUMC.

Of the 12 patients having LT after CABG, 6 are alive as of September 1996, a period ranging from 5 to 87 months (mean 59) after LT. Of the other 6, three died within 2 months of LT, and the other 3 at 42, 99, and 108 months, respectively, after LT. Patients 4 and 6 had fatal acute myocardial infarctions. The early deaths were attributed to renal failure (patient 9), gram negative sepsis (patient 8), and acute liver failure (patient 10).

• • •

This report describes 12 patients who had LT at varying intervals after CABG. Three patients were found to have coronary artery disease when they were being evaluated for LT, and in them it was elected to perform the CABG before the LT. The other 9 patients had no evidence of hepatic dysfunction at the time of CABG. In 7 of these 9 patients, hepatitis C virus was introduced via blood transfusions given at the time of CABG. The interval from CABG to LT in them is consistent with the natural course of hepatitis C infection.[4] Five of these 7 pa-

TABLE 1 Certain Findings in 12 Patients Having Liver Transplantation After Coronary Artery Bypass Grafting

Case	Age (yr) at CABG	Age (yr) at LT	Date of CABG	Date of LT	Interval CABG to LT (mo)	Etiology of Liver Disease	Liver Weight (g)	CAs Narrowed ≥50% in Diameter				TC (mg/dl)		TG (mg/dl)		Alive (interval [mo] from LT to death or last follow-up)
								LM	LAD	LC	R	Pre LT	Post LT	Pre LT	Post LT	
1*	46	46	1988 (Dec 11)	1989 (Jan 13)	1	Methotrexate	1,570	0	+	+	+	—	—	—	—	0 (0.5)
2	50	50	1995 (Apr 24)	1995 (May 30)	1	Biliary cirrhosis	2,070	0	+	+	+	85	180	72	193	+ (12)
3*	63	63	1992 (Dec 11)	1993 (Mar 3)	7	Alcoholism	1,080	0	+	+†	+†	103	154	172	273	+ (37)
4	52	57	1981	1986 (May 12)	60	Hepatitis C	—	0	+†	+†	+†	300	120	28	286	0 (99)
5	55	61	1983	1989 (Mar 28)	72	Alcoholism	1,230	0	0	+†	+†	—	237	—	213	+ (87)
6**	40, 55	50	1975, 1990	1985 (Dec 19)	120	Hepatitis C	—	0	+†	+†	+†	—	197	—	314	0 (108)
7	46	56	1979	1989 (July 8)	120	Hepatitis C	2,200	+	+†	+†	+†	—	212	—	286	+ (84)
8	49	59	1975	1985 (Aug 4)	120	Hepatitis C	900	—	—	—	—	—	—	—	—	0 (2)
9	53	63	1977	1987 (Apr 22)	120	Hepatitis C	1,050	—	+†	+	+	—	—	—	—	0 (42)
10	47	60	1983	1996 (Mar 25)	156	Alcoholism	1,475	0	+†	+†	0	129	159	115	246	0 (0.5)
11	40	54	1982	1996 (Mar 29)	168	Hepatitis C	1,090	0	+†	0	+†	163	203	214	242	+ (5)
12**	40, 62	50	1972, 1994	1991 (May 29)	228	Hepatitis C	2,250	0	+†	+†	+†	107	173	59	324	+ (63)

*Previously reported by Morris JJ et al (Reference 3).

**CABG was performed both before and after LT.

†Patent bypass conduit at the time of LT.

CAs = coronary arteries; CABG = coronary artery bypass grafting; LAD = left anterior descending; LC = left circumflex; LM = left main; LT = liver transplantation; mo = months; R = right; TC = serum total cholesterol; TG = serum triglycerides; + = positive or present; 0 = negative or absent; — = not available.

tients had undergone CABG in the 1970s and 2 in 1982. During those decades, of course, blood for transfusion was not tested for hepatitis C virus antibody, and, furthermore, far more blood transfusions were given at the time of CABG than are given today.

The estimated frequencies of hepatitis C virus infection and its consequences among the approximately 500,000 patients undergoing CABG annually in the USA before and after the introduction of hepatitis C antibody serology are summarized in Figure 1. The frequencies for blood for transfusion among the 500,000 CABG patients in the USA before and after the introduction of hepatitis C antibody serology are summarized in Figure 2.

There has been an approximate 7-fold decrease in the frequency of development of end-stage liver disease after CABG since the development of hepatitis C antibody serology.[5] Likewise, there has been an approximate 17-fold decrease in the percentage of hepatitis C virus infected blood units used in transfusions during CABG since the introduction of the hepatitis C antibody serology.[5] The risk of acquiring hepatitis C virus after CABG will, of course, diminish further as fewer units of blood are used during CABG. For example, at BUMC in 1995, an average of 2.3 units of blood were used per CABG operation, and 47% of the patients undergoing CABG at BUMC in 1995 received no transfusion at all. Therefore, the patients who did receive a blood transfusion at the time of CABG averaged 4.4 units.

Only 3 previous reports including a total of 7 patients have been published of patients having both CABG and LT.[1–3] Four of the 7 patients had LT before the CABG and 1 patient had CABG and LT at the same operation. The remaining 2 patients had LT 33 and 210 days, respectively, after CABG. Each of these 2 patients have been reported previously.[3] Each of these 2 patients are like our patients numbers 1 and 2 (Table I) in that both were found to have coronary artery disease during their work-up for hepatic dysfunction and it was elected to do the CABG before the LT. None of the previously reported patients had LT late after CABG and normal hepatic function at the time of CABG, the situation in 9 of our 12 patients.

In summary, 12 patients are described who had LT after CABG. Nine of them had normal hepatic function at the time of LT and cirrhosis was precipitated by hepatitis C virus in 7 of the 9 patients. Because of the present policy of testing blood for hepatitis C before transfusion and because of the small numbers of blood transfusions now given at the time of CABG, it is predicted that LT after CABG will be much less of a problem in the future. Liver transplantation can be a life-saving procedure for serious hepatic dysfunction developing late after CABG.

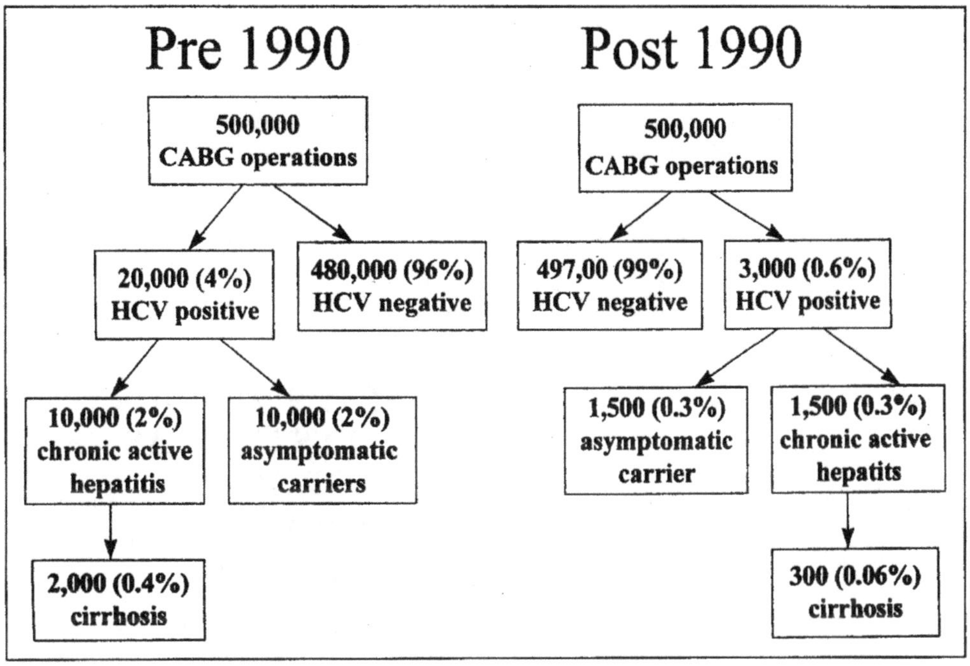

FIGURE 1. Estimated annual frequencies of sequelae of hepatitis C virus (HCV) infection from transfused blood products at the time of coronary artery bypass grafting (CABG) before and after the availability of hepatitis C antibody for donor screening.

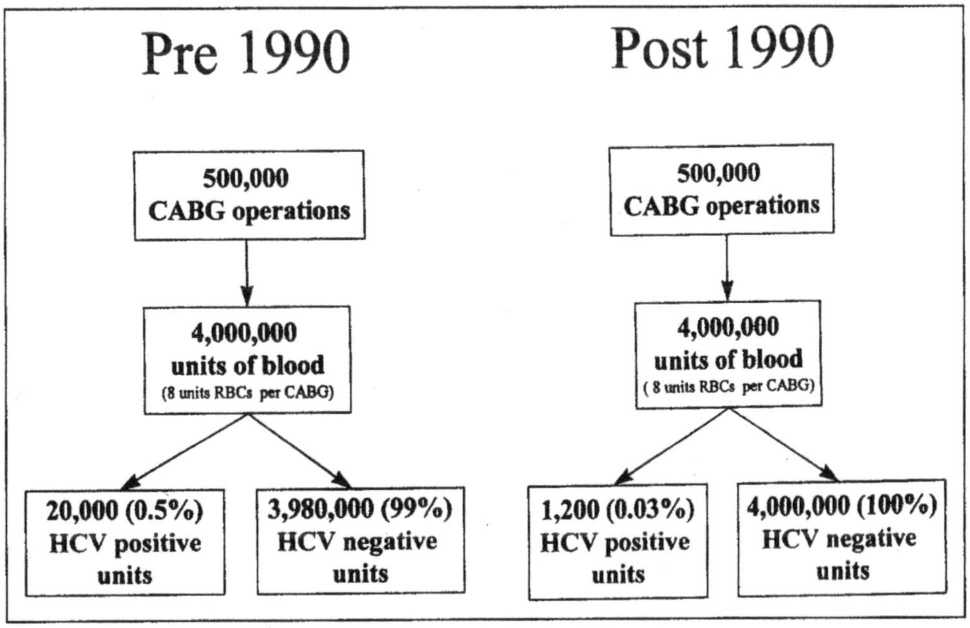

FIGURE 2. Estimated annual frequency of hepatitis C virus (HCV) seropositivity in transfused units of red blood cells (RBCs) at the time of coronary artery bypass grafting (CABG) before and after the availability of hepatitis C antibody for donor screening.

1. Dillow JR, Larrieu AJ, Fine RH. Emergency coronary revascularization in liver transplant recipient. *Chest* 1995;108:1763–1764.

2. Dunton RF, Karlson KJ, Leonardi HK, Jenkins RL, Berger RL. Coronary artery bypass grafting in patients with transplanted livers. *Ann Thorac Surg* 1994;58:1054–1058.

3. Morris JJ, Hellman CL, Gawey BJ, Ramsey MAE, Valek TR, Gunning TC, Swygert TH, Shore-Lesserson L, Lalehzarian F, Brayman KL, Brennan TA. Three patients requiring both coronary artery bypass grafting and orthotopic liver transplantation. *J Cardiothorac Vasc Anesth* 1995;9:322–332.

4. Alter HJ. The hepatitis C virus and its relationship to the clinical spectrum of NANB hepatitis. *J Gastroenterol Hepatol* 1990;5(suppl 1):78–94.

5. Donahue JG, Munoz A, Ness PM, Brown DE, Yawn DH, McAllister HA, Reitz BA, Nelson KE. The declining risk of post-transfusion hepatitis C virus infection. *N Engl J Med* 1992;327:369–373.

6. CHANGES IN VENOUS AUTOGRAFTS USED AS AORTOCORONARY CONDUITS

William C. Roberts, M.D.

The most important contribution to therapy for patients with symptomatic myocardial ischema has been the coronary bypass operation. Since its introduction over 2 decades ago, numerous patients have benefited from this procedure. Despite its benefits to most patients, coronary bypass is not free of complications. Stenosis or complete occlusion of venous grafts used as aortocoronary conduits still occurs too frequently. Whereas all venous grafts develop some morphologic changes, the degree and functional significance of the changes vary widely. The structural changes observed early and late in saphenous veins used as aortocoronary conduits are presented in this section.

Degrees of Narrowing of the Native Epicardial Coronary Arteries in Symptomatic Myocardial Ischemia

Before the changes in saphenous veins used as aortocoronary conduits are focused on, a brief discussion on the status of the native epicardial coronary arteries in patients likely to undergo aortocoronary bypass grafting appears appropriate. As summarized in Figure 1, examination at necropsy (or during life by intravascular ultrasonic imaging) of the four major (right, left main, left anterior descending, and left circumflex) epicardial coronary arteries in patients over 30 years of age with symptomatic myocardial ischemia and angiographic narrowing greater than 50 per cent in diameter of one or more major coronary arteries discloses that atherosclerotic plaques are present in nearly every 5-mm. segment of the entire length of the arteries.[17,18] In patients with angiographically "single-vessel disease," approximately 40 per cent of the lumen of each 5-mm. segment of the four major arteries (average of 54 segments per patient) is obliterated by plaque; in patients with angiographically "double-vessel disease," approximately 50 per cent of the total lumen is obliterated by plaque; in patients with "triple-vessel disease," approximately 60 per cent of the total lumen is filled with plaque; and in patients with "quadruple-vessel disease," approximately 70 per cent of the total lumen is filled with plaque. Thus, the greater the number of major coronary arteries significantly narrowed, the greater the total amount of atherosclerotic plaque in the major epicardial coronary arteries.

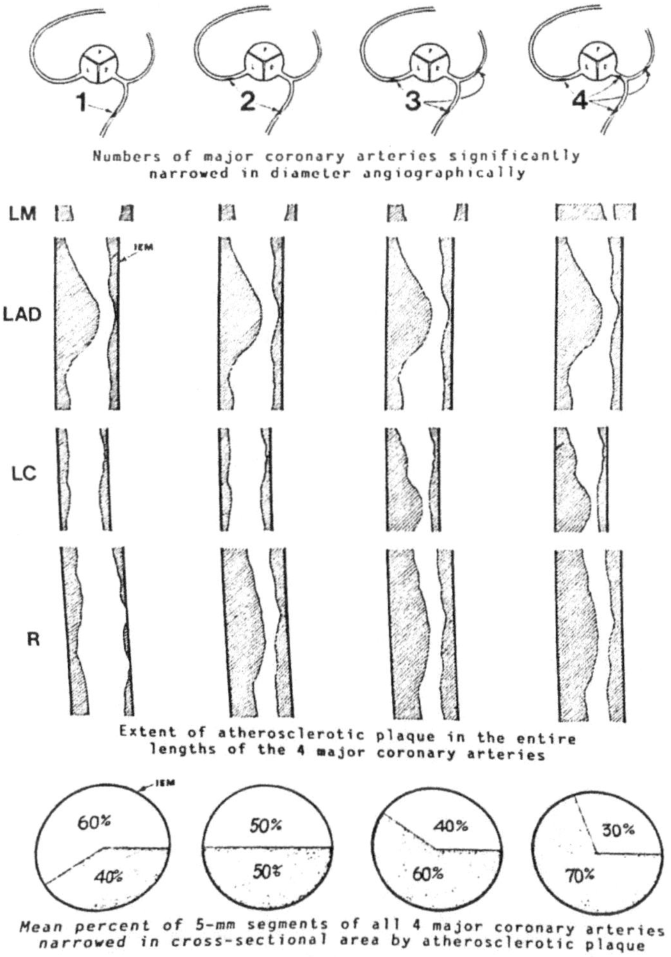

Figure 1. Diagram showing the number of major coronary arteries severely narrowed in diameter by angiogram (upper); the average amount of atherosclerotic plaque in the left main (LM), left anterior descending (LAD), left circumflex (LC), and ight (R) coronary arteries in full length according to the number of coronary arteries ignificantly narrowed by angiogram (middle); and the average amount of cross-ctional area narrowing by atherosclerotic plaque in each 5-mm. segment of the ır major epicardial coronary arteries (lower). (From Roberts, W. C.: Coronary sion," coronary "disease," "single-vessel disease," "two-vessel disease": rd and phrase misnomers providing false impressions of the extent of coronary ·rosclerosis in symptomatic myocardial ischemia. Am. J. Cardiol., 66:121,).)

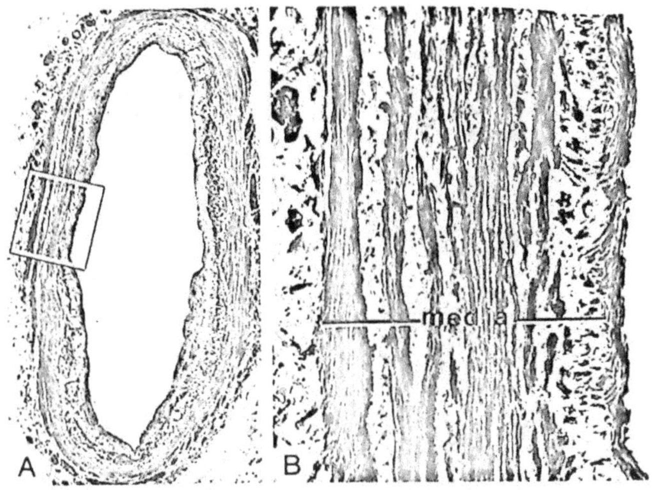

Figure 2. Normal saphenous vein. *A*, Low-power view showing medial circular and longitudinal smooth muscle layers (Movat stain, ×20). *B*, High-power view of area enclosed in box in *A* (Movat stain, ×130). Multiple layers of circular smooth muscle separated by layers of fibrous tissue form the media. Occasional longitudinal smooth muscle fascicles are present near the lumen. (From Spray, T. L., and Roberts, W. C.: Changes in saphenous veins used as aortocoronary bypass grafts. Am. Heart J., 94:500, 1977.)

The Normal Saphenous Vein

The normal human saphenous vein contains a thin *intima* consisting of relatively acellular fibrous tissue covered by a single layer of endothelial cells and separated from the media by a rudimentary internal elastic membrane (Fig. 2). The *media* consists of multiple layers of smooth muscle cells, separated by bundles of collagen, ground substance, and occasional short elastic fibers. Most medial smooth muscle layers have a circular orientation; in areas near the venous valves, however, the middle circular layers have a more longitudinal arrangement. Frequently, longitudinally oriented smooth muscle fascicles form the innermost layers of the media. The *adventitia* is composed of bundles of collagen with scattered fascicles of longitudinally oriented smooth muscle cells. Broad loose bands of elastic fibers are present in abundance. Vasa vasorum are present and may extend into the outermost portion of the media.

Findings in Remnant Saphenous Veins Excised for Aortocoronary Conduits but Unused

Some degree of intimal fibrous thickening occurs commonly in saphenous veins excised but unused for aortocoronary bypass. Waller and Roberts[26] examined nearly 3500 cm. of unused but excised saphenous veins from 402 patients undergoing coronary bypass surgery. The length of the unused saphenous veins ranged from 0.5 to 52 cm. per patient (mean 8.5 cm.). A histologic section was examined from each of the 6788 5-mm. long segments: the lumen in 0.4 per cent of the sections was narrowed 76 to 100 per cent in cross-sectional areas by fibrous tissue; 0.6 per cent were narrowed 51 to 75 per cent in cross-sectional areas; 12 per cent were narrowed 26 to 50 per cent; and 87 per cent were narrowed 25 per cent or less in cross-sectional

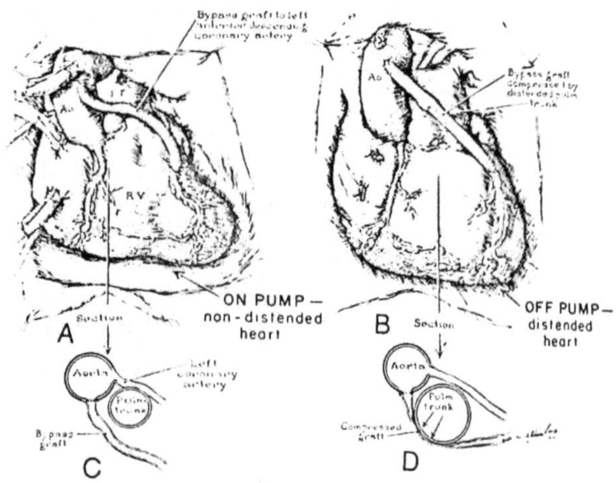

Figure 3. Schematic showing how a graft to the left anterior descending coronary artery can be placed under tension. (From Spray, T. L., and Roberts, W. C.: Tension on coronary bypass conduits. A neglected cause of real or potential obstruction of saphenous vein grafts. J. Thorac. Cardiovasc. Surg., 72:282, 1976.)

areas. The percentage of 5-mm. segments of unused vein narrowed more than 75 per cent in cross-sectional areas was similar in males and females, and it was similar in each of 5 decades (31 to 40, 41 to 50, 51 to 60, 61 to 70, and 71 to 80 years). Thus, approximately 1 per cent of saphenous veins excised for coronary bypass are narrowed more than 50 per cent in cross-sectional area by fibrous tissue before they are used as aortocoronary conduits.

Numbers of Aortic Anastomotic Sites, Conduits, and Coronary Anastomotic Sites

It is doubtful that any two surgeons perform the bypass operation in quite the same manner, and these individual variations may affect patient and graft outcome. The phrases "two bypasses" or "three bypasses" or "four bypasses" are commonly used, but their meaning is not always precise. It is suspected that most users of the phrase "three bypasses" are referring to the number of coronary anastomoses. A patient may have three coronary anastomotic sites and only one conduit ("round-the-world" bypass) or two or three conduits with similar numbers of aortic anastomotic sites. To prevent confusion, it might be best to always state the number of aortic anastomotic sites, the number of conduits, and the number of coronary anastomotic sites. To the author, it appears most reasonable for each of these three to be the same: if a patient is to have three coronary anastomotic sites, it might be ideal to have three conduits and three separate aortic anastomotic sites. If only one conduit is used with a single aortic anastomotic site and the single conduit is anastomosed to seven different coronary arteries, the outcome is not ideal if the single aortic anastomosis closes or the single conduit closes proximally. With similar numbers of aortic anastomotic sites, conduits, and coronary anastomotic sites, this circumstance is less likely to occur.

The location of the coronary anastomotic site appears to be relatively similar with most surgeons. The distal 1 cm. of the right coronary artery is probably ideal because the most severe narrowing of this artery tends to be its distal third rather than the proximal or middle third.[24] The most common anastomotic site of the left anterior descending is probably about two thirds down its length, and this location, of course, is logical because this artery tends to be more severely narrowed in its proximal third than in either its middle or distal thirds.[24] The same situation also appears reasonable for the first diagonal artery. Anastomoses in the obtuse marginal arteries are usually within 3 cm. of their origin from the left circumflex.

Of the various technical factors that can affect flow in aortocoronary conduits, *tension on the conduit* is one.[21] Abnormal tension is indicated by grooving or indentation into the right atrial wall or right atrioventricular sulcus or by flattening of the graft passing anterior to the pulmonary trunk. Several explanations for the occurrence of this tension are probable and summarized in Figure 3. If the graft is under tension, leakage at the bypass anastomosis is probably more likely than it is without tension (Fig. 4). *Twisting of a conduit*, as illustrated in Figures 5 and 6, may prevent successful bypass grafting.[19]

Early Changes in Saphenous Veins Used as Aortocoronary Conduits

In 1906, Carrel and Guthrie[5] described intimal thickening of veins implanted into the arterial system in dogs and concluded that veins placed in the arterial circulation had a strong tendency to assume the character of an artery. In further vein transplantation experiments in 1908, Carrel[4] described four characteristic changes in veins used as arteries in the peripheral circulation: (1) intimal thickening, (2) adventitial thickening (from fibrosis), (3) loss of the inner third of the media, and (4) loss of elastic fibers producing a fibrous tube. In addition, medial hypertrophy was observed in some grafts. These changes have subsequently been confirmed in humans in saphenous veins used for femoropopliteal and aortocoronary bypass.

Spray and Roberts[22,23] studied a large number of saphenous vein grafts from patients dying within a year after aortocoronary bypass (Fig. 7). Vein grafts from patients dying intraoperatively showed minimal medial edema (clear spaces between layers of smooth muscle) and disrupted adventitia (occurring during excision of the vein before grafting). By 2 weeks, mural edema was more pronounced, some medial smooth muscle cells were necrotic, and inflammatory infiltrates were present. The endothelium often was disrupted, and the intimal surface usually was covered, either partially or completely, by fibrin. By 3 weeks, cells with characteristics of smooth muscle appeared in the subendothelial portion of the intima. The cells generally were oriented such that their longest diameter was parallel to the direction of blood flow. Thereafter, the subendothelial intimal lesions became more generalized and less cellular, ground substance appeared in abundance, and short elastic fibers and vascular channels occasionally were present. The smooth muscle fibers of the media gradually diminished in number and were replaced, in part or in whole, by fibrous tissue. Fibrous tissue also increased in the adventitia, and its elastic fibers became severely disrupted or disappeared completely. Organizing

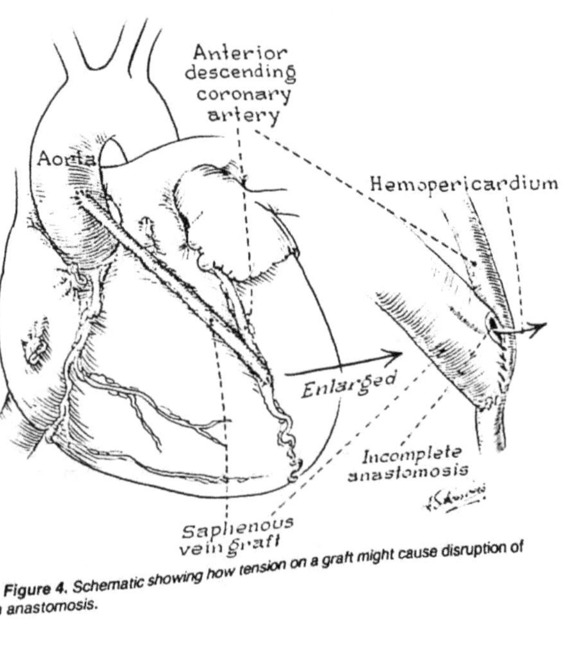

Figure 4. Schematic showing how tension on a graft might cause disruption of an anastomosis.

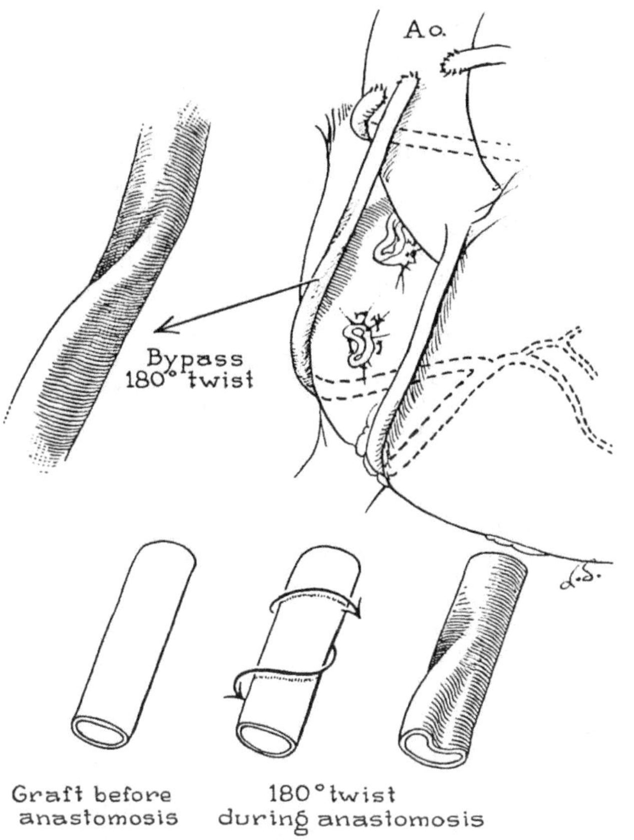

Figure 5. Schematic showing mild twisting of a graft to the right coronary artery. (From Roberts, W. C., Lachman A. S., and Virmani, R.: Twisting of an aorta-coronary bypass conduit. A complication of coronary surgery. J. Thorac. Cardiovasc. Surg., *75*:772, 1978.)

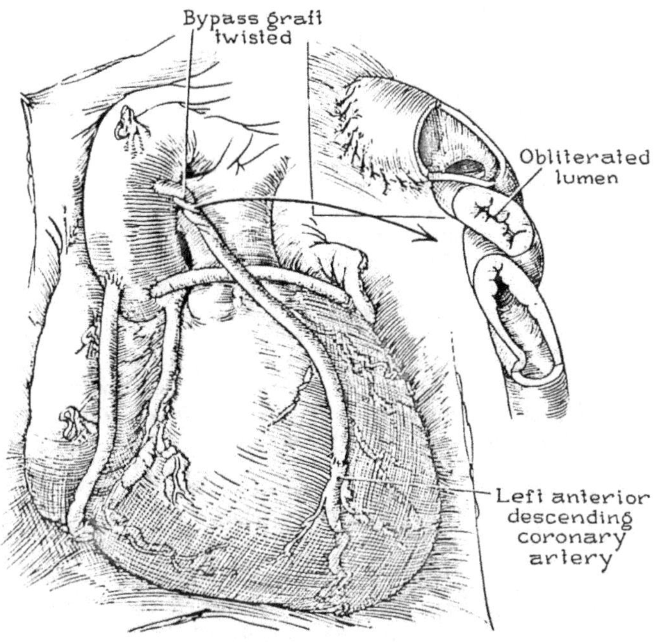

***Figure 6.** Schematic showing severe twisting of a graft to the left anterior scending coronary artery. (From Roberts, W. C., Lachman, A. S., and Virmani, Twisting of an aorta-coronary bypass conduit. A complication of coronary gery. J. Thorac. Cardiovasc. Surg., 75:772, 1978.)*

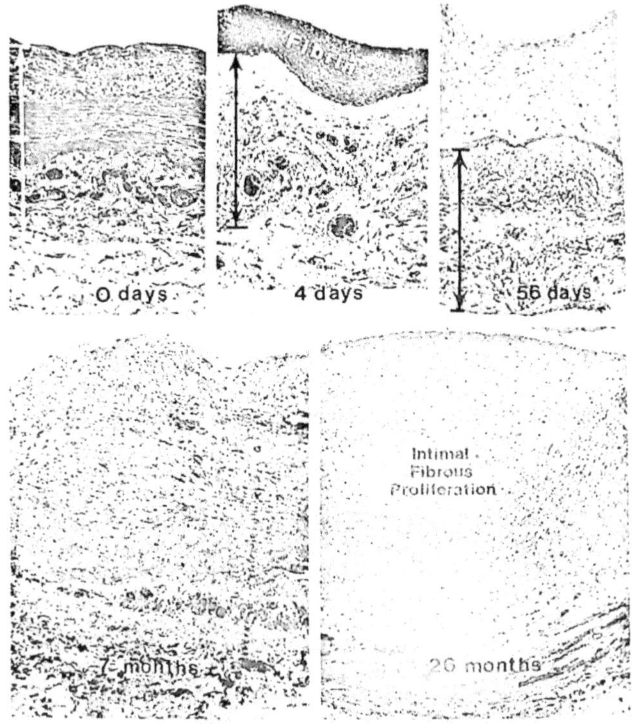

Figure 7. Composite of changes seen in saphenous vein aortocoronary grafts from 0 days (normal vein) to 26 months after implantation at the same magnification (×54). Arrows indicate normal wall thickness (media plus adventitia): 0 days, intima thin, marked medial smooth muscle layers in both circular and longitudinal directions, loose adventitial tissue; 4 days, large deposit of fibrin over slightly thickened intima, marked loss of medial smooth muscle with cellular infiltration; 56 days, thickened vein wall with marked intimal fibrous proliferation, medial smooth muscle cells depleted and replaced by fibrous tissue; 7 months, severe intimal fibrous proliferation is present containing some neovascular channels, and marked loss of medial smooth muscle and replacement fibrosis is present; 26 months, the vein wall has become almost completely replaced by fibrous tissue creating a fibrous tube, and only small areas of medial smooth muscle cells remain. (All Movat stains. From Spray, T. L., and Roberts, W. C.: Changes in saphenous veins used as aortocoronary bypass grafts. Am. Heart J., *94*:500, 1977.)

fibrin on the external surface of the grafts probably contributed to the adventitial fibrosis. Capillaries were present in the adventitia, and they often extended into the fibrotic media. Thus, the saphenous vein used as an artery becomes a stiff, fibrous tissue conduit.

Late Changes in Saphenous Veins Used as Aortocoronary Conduits

Kalan and Roberts[9] described at necropsy findings in 123 saphenous vein grafts and in 1865 5-mm. segments of the grafts in 53 patients who had had a single aortocoronary bypass operation 13 to 185 months (mean 58 months) before death. Of the 53 patients, 32 (60 per cent) died from a cardiac cause, and of their 73 saphenous vein aortocoronary conduits, 36 (49 per cent) were narrowed at some point more than 75 per cent in cross-sectional area by atherosclerotic plaque; the remaining 21 patients (40 per cent) died of noncardiac causes, and of their 50 saphenous vein conduits, 10 (20 per cent) were narrowed at some point more than 75 per cent in cross-sectional area by plaque. Of the 53 patients, 31 (58 per cent) had at least one bypass graft maximally narrowed greater than 75 per cent in cross-sectional area at some point by fibromuscular tissue with or without lipid; 12 patients (23 per cent) had maximal graft narrowing of 51 to 75 per cent; 8 patients (15 per cent), 26 to 50 per cent; and 2 patients (4 per cent), 0 to 25 per cent. The percentage of patients with a graft narrowed over 75 per cent at necropsy did not increase as the interval from bypass surgery to death increased.

Of the 123 saphenous vein grafts, 47 (38 per cent) were maximally narrowed greater than 75 per cent in cross-sectional area; 44 (36 per cent), 51 to 75 per cent; 22 (18 per cent), 26 to 50 per cent; and 10 (8 per cent), 0 to 25 per cent. Of the 47 grafts narrowed over 75 per cent in cross-sectional area, 29 actually were narrowed greater than 95 per cent in cross-sectional area by fibrous tissue. The percentage of saphenous veins narrowed greater than 75 per cent at necropsy was not affected by sex (males 38 per cent, females 36 per cent), presence or absence of systemic hypertension (40 per cent versus 33 per cent), or presence or absence of diabetes mellitus (30 per cent versus 48 per cent). The percentage of grafts narrowed over 75 per cent in cross-sectional area did not correlate with the interval between bypass surgery and death or with the coronary artery to which the graft was connected.

The degree of narrowing of the saphenous vein graft was related to the degree of luminal narrowing of the native coronary artery at, or within 2 cm. distal to, the saphenous vein–coronary artery anastomosis. Of the 49 grafts attached to a coronary artery that was narrowed greater than 75 per cent at or distal to the anastomosis, 33 (67 per cent) were significantly narrowed. Of the 74 grafts attached to a coronary artery narrowed less than 75 per cent distal to the anastomotic site, 14 (19 per cent) were severely narrowed.

Analysis of the 1865 5-mm. long saphenous vein segments disclosed that 209 segments (11 per cent) were narrowed 96 to 100 per cent in cross-sectional area; 172 (9 per cent), 76 to 95 per cent; 407 (22 per cent), 51 to 75 per cent; 685 (37 per cent), 26 to 50 per cent; and 392 (21 per cent), 0 to 25 per cent. Similar percentages of segments were narrowed greater than 75 per cent in males and females (22 per cent versus 15 per cent); in diabetic and nondiabetic patients (18 per cent versus 26 per cent); and in hypertensive and nonhypertensive patients (21 per cent versus 20 per cent). Moreover, the interval from coronary bypass to death did not correlate with the percentage of segments severely narrowed.

Although the percentage of saphenous vein segments narrowed greater than 75 per cent in cross-sectional area at necropsy did not correlate with the interval from bypass grafting to death, it did relate to the mode of death. Of the 32 patients dying from a cardiac cause, 295 (27 per cent) of 1104 saphenous vein segments were narrowed greater than 75 per cent, whereas of the 21 patients dying from a noncardiac cause, 86 (11 per cent) of 761 saphenous vein segments were so narrowed. The percentage of segments of native coronary artery narrowed greater than 75 per cent was similar in patients with cardiac and noncardiac modes of death (673 of 1441 [47 per cent] versus 333 of 895 [37 per cent]).

Composition of Tissue Causing Luminal Narrowing Late in the Saphenous Veins Used as Aortocoronary Conduits

Lipid was present in the wall of a graft in 39 of the 53 patients (74 per cent). Fifteen had intracellular lipid alone (foam cells), and 24 had both foam cells and extracellular lipid. Extracellular lipid was not found in a saphenous vein graft until 26 months after bypass. Lipid was present in 69 (56 per cent) of the 123 saphenous vein grafts from the 39 patients. Intracellular lipid was present in all 69 grafts either alone (33 grafts) or along with extracellular lipid (36 grafts). The amount of lipid present appeared to increase as the interval from coronary bypass to death increased. Foam cells were located near the luminal surfaces of the intimal fibrous tissue, and they did not appreciably narrow the lumen. Extracellular lipid deposits were located deeper in the plaque separated from the lumen by a layer of fibrous tissue, and they often contributed significantly to luminal narrowing.

Hemorrhage into plaque (into the lipid portion only) was found in 26 (21 per cent) saphenous vein grafts from 17 (32 per cent) patients. It was observed as early as 24 months after bypass, and it did not increase in frequency thereafter as the interval from bypass to death increased. Luminal narrowing greater than 75 per cent in cross-sectional area was significantly more common in grafts with than in those without plaque hemorrhage.

Luminal thrombus was present in 16 (13 per cent) saphenous vein grafts from 14 (26 per cent) patients. Thrombus was not seen until 32 months after bypass, and its frequency did not increase thereafter as the interval from bypass to death increased. Thrombus within the graft lumen was present in 16 of 69 grafts that had deposits of lipid in the walls and in none of 54 grafts devoid of lipid. In 14 of these 16 grafts, hemorrhage into plaque also was found.

Calcific deposits were present in 13 (11 per cent) of the 123 saphenous vein grafts from 11 patients, and they were first seen 34 months after coronary bypass. All the deposits were small. They were present in 18 (1 per cent) of the 1865 5-mm. saphenous vein segments.

The aforementioned data indicate that nearly all saphenous veins used as aortocoronary conduits for longer than a year develop atherosclerotic plaques in each 5-mm. segment of the entire length. Thus, the atherosclerotic plaquing late in saphenous veins used as aortocoronary conduits is diffuse, just as it is in native coronary arteries in patients with fatal myocardial ischemia.[17,18] The amount of luminal narrowing in the saphenous veins used as aortocoronary conduits was significantly greater in those patients who died from a cardiac cause, compared with those who died from a noncardiac cause. Surprisingly, the interval from coronary bypass to death did not correlate with either the percentage of vein conduits or the percentage of 5-mm. segments of vein conduit narrowed over 75 per cent in cross-sectional area by plaque. Moreover, the percentage of 5-mm. segments of saphenous vein conduit severely narrowed was similar in the 35 patients surviving up to 5 years, compared with the 18 patients surviving more than 5 years.

The composition of the plaques in the saphenous venous conduits is similar to that in the native coronary arteries. Fibrous tissue or fibromuscular tissue was the dominant component of the plaques in the saphenous vein conduits, just as it is the dominant component of plaques in the native coronary arteries in patients with fatal coronary artery disease without coronary bypass.[10,11]

The frequency of the various modes of death among the patients dying late after coronary bypass is different from that of patients with symptomatic myocardial ischemia without coronary bypass.[20] Of the 53 coronary bypass patients studied, only 32 (60 per cent) died from a cardiac cause, and 21 (40 per cent) died from a noncardiac cause. Among patients with symptomatic myocardial ischemia who do not have coronary bypass, approximately 95 per cent die from a cardiac cause. The fact that 40 per cent of the bypass patients studied died from a noncardiac cause supports the view that the bypass operation in many patients prolongs life, long enough in many to develop various fatal noncardiac conditions. Of the 53 bypass patients reported by Kalan and Roberts,[9] 10 (19 per cent) died from cancer, a percentage far higher than in patients with symptomatic myocardial ischemia not undergoing coronary surgery.

The study by Kalan and Roberts[9] re-emphasizes that coronary bypass is useful but that it does not deter progression of the underlying atherosclerotic process. In a minor way, the bypass operation might even cause acceleration of the atherosclerotic process because in about 25 per cent of individuals who undergo coronary bypass, the serum total cholesterol increases and the body weight increases substantially during the first year after operation. Because lowering of the serum (or plasma) total cholesterol level (and specifically the low-density lipoprotein cholesterol) decreases the likelihood of heart attack and may cause some portion of atherosclerotic plaques to regress and other portions to at least not progress, a strong case can be advanced for combined simultaneous initiation of both low-fat, low-cholesterol diet therapy and lipid-lowering drug therapy as soon as is reasonably feasible after a coronary bypass operation.[15]

Causes of Morphologic Changes in Saphenous Veins Used as Aortocoronary Conduits

Although the causes of the changes in saphenous vein grafts are in many ways similar to those of atherosclerotic plaques in native coronary arteries,[14,16] additional mechanisms almost surely have a role when a vein is switched to an arterial location. The changes in the saphenous veins are similar early to the phlebosclerotic lesions in venous varicosities, changes presumably caused by the response of the vein to increases in hydrostatic pressure. Arteriovenous shunts of any origin (congenital, traumatic, or iatrogenic) show intimal thickening, presumably the result of increased pressure and flow. Subendothelial proliferative lesions in the pulmonary arteries of patients with pulmonary hypertension and in the vena cava and portal veins in patients with chronic right-sided congestive cardiac failure or portal hypertension are also seen in the saphenous veins transferred to the aortocoronary position. Brody and colleagues[2,3] attempted to differentiate the effects of pressure and ischemia on femoral vein grafts in dogs. Vein segments were either left intact or dissected free from their adventitia, thereby severing the vasa vasorum and producing medial ischemia. The vein segments were then either left in the venous system or were arterialized by creation of an arteriovenous fistula. The presence of medial ischemia in the absence of elevated pressure and flow produced medial fibrosis in the vein without subendothelial intimal proliferative lesions. Elevated intravascular pressure alone, however, without alterations in blood supply to the media by the vasa vasorum, produced intimal lesions without evidence of medial fibrosis. The combination of both elevated intraluminal pressure and medial ischemia caused medial and intimal changes similar to the changes seen in human saphenous veins used as aortocoronary conduits (Table 1).

The intimal process in saphenous veins and specifically the degree of luminal narrowing in saphenous veins in the aortocoronary position is almost certainly accelerated when flow through the conduit is relatively poor. The major cause of poor flow is severe narrowing in the native coronary artery (to which the vein is attached) at or just distal to the site of anastomosis.[9,22,23,25] The smaller the native coronary arteries to which the graft is to be connected, the less the amount of atherosclerotic plaque necessary to cause significant luminal narrowing. Smaller sized hearts have smaller coronary arteries than do larger sized hearts.[13] Small patients tend to have smaller hearts than larger patients have. Thus, similar amounts of plaque cause more luminal narrowing in small patients than in large patients. Females, on average, are smaller than males and, therefore, generally have smaller hearts and smaller coronary arteries. Coronary bypass might be expected therefore to have poorer results in females than in males because the smaller arteries might cause poorer flow through the conduits by plaque in the native coronary arteries. Kalan and Roberts[8] found this scenario to probably be the case. Their 121 necropsy patients dying within 60 days of a coronary bypass operation had significantly lower mean heart weights than did the 90 patients dying late, and this fact held true for both sexes. Most patients with normal sized hearts were in the early death group; conversely, most patients in the late death group had hearts of increased weight. Their findings suggest that patients with normal or near-normal sized hearts have a higher early mortality after coronary bypass than do those with hearts of increased weight. Moreover, more changes causing luminal narrowing of bypass conduits might be expected in individuals with small native coronary arteries (small hearts) because the run-off through the graft may not be as good as in patients with larger native coronary arteries (larger hearts).

TABLE 1. Effects of Pressure and Ischemia on Venous Conduits

Vasa Vasorum Intact	
Low pressure (venous)	High pressure (arterial)
↓	↓
Normal histology	Intimal proliferation and fibrosis
Intact myocytes	Intact myocytes
Vasa Vasorum Interrupted	
Low pressure (venous)	High pressure (arterial)
↓	↓
Medical fibrosis	Intimal Proliferation and fibrosis
Loss of myocytes	Medial fibrosis
	Loss of myocytes

fter Brody, W. R., Kosek, J. C., and Angell, W. W.: Changes in vein 's following aortocoronary bypass induced by pressure and ische- J. Thorac. Cardiovasc. Surg., 64:847, 1972.

Comparison of Morphologic Changes in Saphenous Veins to Those in Internal Mammary Arteries Used as Aortocoronary Conduits

For practical purposes, none of the aforedescribed changes in saphenous veins used as aortocoronary conduits are found in internal mammary arteries used in the coronary position. As emphasized by others, clinically[6,12] the patency rate both early and late is excellent with the mammary artery and much less with the saphenous vein. Although the internal mammary artery late after bypass remains much smaller than does the saphenous vein when each is utilized in the same patient, the internal mammary artery remains nearly devoid of intimal deposits, whereas the saphenous vein, although much larger, may develop severe atherosclerotic plaque in the lumen.[1,7]

REFERENCES

1. Barbour, D. J., and Roberts, W. C.: Additional evidence for relative resistance to atherosclerosis of the internal mammary artery compared to saphenous vein when used to increase myocardial blood flow. Am. J. Cardiol., *56*:488, 1985.
2. Brody, W. R., Angell, W. W., and Kosek, J. C.: Histologic fate of the venous coronary artery bypass in dogs. Am. J. Pathol., *66*:111, 1972.
3. Brody, W. R., Kosek, J. C., and Angell, W. W.: Changes in vein grafts following aortocoronary bypass induced by pressure and ischemia. J. Thorac. Cardiovasc. Surg., *64*:847, 1972.
4. Carrel, A.: Results of transplantation of blood vessels, organs, and limbs. J.A.M.A., *51*:1662, 1908.
5. Carrel, A., and Guthrie, C. C.: Results of biterminal transplantation of veins. Am. J. Med. Sci., *132*:415, 1906.
6. Grondin, C. M., Campeau, L., Lesperance, J., Enjalbert, M., and Bourassa, M. G.: Comparison of late changes in internal mammary artery and saphenous vein grafts in two consecutive series of patients 10 years after operation. Circulation, *70*(Suppl. I): I-208, 1984.
7. Kalan, J. M., and Roberts, W. C.: Comparison of morphologic changes and luminal sizes of saphenous vein and internal mammary artery after simultaneous implantation for coronary arterial bypass grafting. Am. J. Cardiol., *60*:193, 1987.
8. Kalan, J. M., and Roberts, W. C.: Significance of cardiac weight in patients having coronary artery bypass grafting for angina pectoris. Am. J. Cardiol., *62*:36, 1988.
9. Kalan, J. M., and Roberts, W. C.: Morphologic findings in saphenous veins used as coronary arterial bypass conduits for longer than 1 year: Necropsy analysis of 53 patients, 123 saphenous veins, and 1,865 five-millimeter segments of veins. Am. Heart J., *119*:1164, 1990.
10. Kragel, A. H., Reddy, S. G., Wittes, J. T., and Roberts, W. C.: Morphometric analysis of the composition of atherosclerotic plaques in the four major epicardial coronary arteries in acute myocardial infarction and in sudden coronary death. Circulation, *80*:1747, 1989.
11. Kragel, A. H., Reddy, S. G., Wittes, J. T., and Roberts, W. C.: Morphometric analysis of the composition of coronary arterial plaques in isolated unstable angina pectoris with pain at rest. Am. J. Cardiol., *66*:562, 1990.
12. Loop, F. D., Lytle, B. W., Cosgrove, D. M., Stewart, R. W., Goormastic, M.,

Williams, G. W., Golding, L. A. R., Gill, C. C., Taylor, P. C., Sheldon, W. C., and Proudfit, W. L.: Influence of the internal-mammary-artery graft on 10-year survival and other cardiac events. N. Engl. J. Med., *314*:1, 1986.

13. Roberts, C. S., and Roberts, W. C.: Cross-sectional area of the proximal portions of the three major epicardial coronary arteries in 98 necropsy patients with different coronary events. Relationship to heart weight, age, and sex. Circulation, *62*:953, 1980.
14. Roberts, W. C.: Factors linking cholesterol to atherosclerotic plaques. Am. J. Cardiol., *62*:495, 1988.
15. Roberts, W. C.: Lipid-lowering after an atherosclerotic event. Am. J. Cardiol., *64*:693, 1989.
16. Roberts, W. C.: Atherosclerotic risk factors—are there ten or is there only one? Am. J. Cardiol., *64*:552, 1989.
17. Roberts, W. C.: Qualitative and quantitative comparison of amounts of narrowing by atherosclerotic plaques in the major epicardial coronary arteries at necropsy in sudden coronary death, transmural acute myocardial infarction, transmural healed myocardial infarction and unstable angina pectoris. Am. J. Cardiol., *64*:324, 1989.
18. Roberts, W. C.: Coronary "lesion," coronary "disease," "single-vessel disease," "two-vessel disease": Word and phrase misnomers providing false impressions of the extent of coronary atherosclerosis in symptomatic myocardial ischemia. Am. J. Cardiol., *66*:121, 1990.
19. Roberts, W. C., Lachman, A. S., and Virmani, R.: Twisting of an aorta-coronary bypass conduit. A complication of coronary surgery. J. Thorac. Cardiovasc. Surg., *75*:772, 1978.
20. Roberts, W. C., Potkin, B. N., Solus, D. E., and Reddy, S. G.: Mode of death, frequency of healed and acute myocardial infarction, number of major epicardial coronary arteries severely narrowed by atherosclerotic plaque, and heart weight in fatal atherosclerotic coronary artery disease: Analysis of 889 patients studied at necropsy. J. Am. Coll. Cardiol., *15*:196, 1990.
21. Spray, T. L., and Roberts, W. C.: Tension on coronary bypass conduits. A neglected cause of real or potential obstruction of saphenous vein grafts. J. Thorac. Cardiovasc. Surg., *72*:282, 1976.
22. Spray, T. L., and Roberts, W. C.: Status of the grafts and the native coronary arteries proximal and distal to coronary anastomotic sites of aortocoronary bypass grafts. Circulation, *55*:741, 1977.
23. Spray, T. L., and Roberts, W. C.: Changes in saphenous veins used as aortocoronary bypass grafts. Am. Heart J., *94*:500, 1977.
24. Vlodaver, Z., and Edwards, J. E.: Pathology of coronary atherosclerosis. Prog. Cardiovasc. Dis., *14*:256, 1971.
25. Waller, B. F., and Roberts, W. C.: Amount of narrowing by atherosclerotic plaque in 44 nonbypassed and 52 bypassed major epicardial coronary arteries in 32 necropsy patients who died within 1 month of aortocoronary bypass grafting. Am. J. Cardiol., *46*:956, 1980.
26. Waller, B. F., and Roberts, W. C.: Remnant saphenous veins after aortocoronary bypass grafting: Analysis of 3,394 centimeters of unused vein from 402 patients. Am. J. Cardiol., *55*:65, 1985.

Cardiac Observations Late After Operative Transmyocardial Laser "Revascularization"

John H. Summers, MD, A. Carl Henry III, MD, and William C. Roberts, MD

Transmyocardial laser "revascularization" (TLR) is a relatively new surgical technique developed with the intent of producing channels within the left ventricular wall so that the intracavitary blood will perfuse the myocardium. The procedure initially was applied to patients deemed unsuitable for conventional revascularization procedures and with symptoms refractory to maximal medical therapy. Few patients having this procedure have been studied at necropsy. This report describes a patient who underwent TLR, became asymptomatic, and was later killed in a motor vehicle accident.

• • •

B.H., a 60-year-old man, had an acute myocardial infarction at age 39 years (1977) and underwent coronary artery bypass grafting at that time. He apparently did well thereafter until age 52 (1990) when angina pectoris appeared. A second coronary bypass was performed at that time and he became asymptomatic until age 59 (1997; 13 months before death) when angina reappeared. The angina rapidly worsened to Canadian Cardiovascular Society class IV despite antianginal drug therapy. Cardiac catheterization showed total occlusions of the aortocoronary saphenous venous conduits to the left obtuse marginal and right coronary arteries and a patent left internal mammary artery to a diffusely and severely narrowed native left anterior descending coronary artery. Small fixed anterior wall and moderate-sized reversible inferolateral wall perfusion defects were seen by dual-isotope, single-photon emission computed tomography perfusion scanning. The left ventricular cavity was mildly dilated, the lateral and anterior walls were hypokinetic, and ejection fraction was 44%.

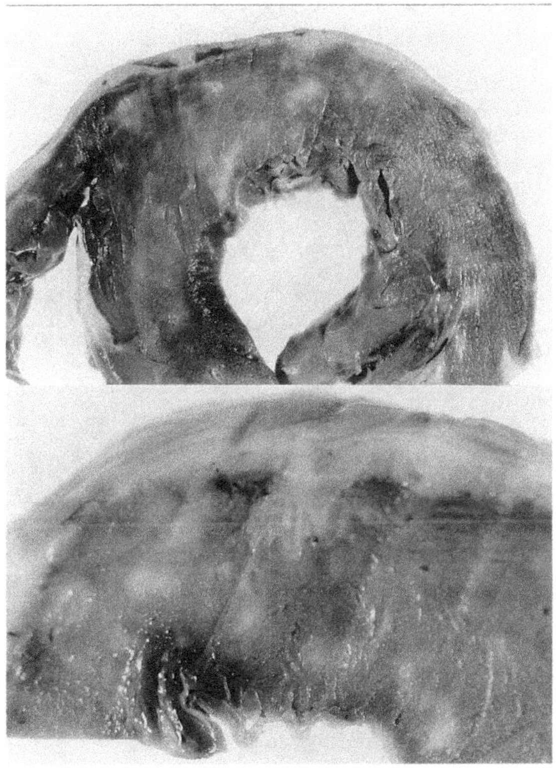

FIGURE 1. Gross photographs of portions of left ventricular wall in the patient described showing numerous focal scars.

Laser transmyocardial revascularization via thoracotomy was performed in 19 November 1997 using a carbon dioxide laser: 31 transmyocardial left ventricular channels were created using an average energy of 50 J per application. Myocardial penetration was confirmed by transesophageal echo through visualization of spontaneous echo contrast within the left ventricular cavity with each application of laser energy. The hospital course was uncomplicated and when seen 3 and 6 months after TLR he was asymptomatic. He

TABLE I Previously Reported Cardiac Patients Having Left Ventricular Laser Therapy >30 Days Before Necropsy

Author (reference number)	Year of Report	Days After Therapy	Age (yr) & Sex	Symptoms Lessened After TLR	Patent Channels in LV Wall		LV Scar	
					Macro	Micro	Macro	Micro
Mirhoseini[1]	1990	1,460	–	+	0	+	0	0
Cooley[2]	1994	90	56M	+	0	+	+	+
Burkhoff[3]	1996	31	71M	0	0	0	+	+
Gassler[4]	1997	150	48F	0	0	0	0	+
Frazier[5]	1998	55	54M	0	0	+	–	+

LV = left ventricular; + = present; 0 = absent; – = no information.

From the Departments of Medicine (Cardiology), Thoracic and Cardiovascular Surgery, and Pathology, and the Baylor Cardiovascular Institute, Baylor University Medical Center, Dallas, Texas. Dr. Roberts' address is: Baylor Cardiovascular Institute, Baylor University Medical Center, 3500 Gaston Avenue, Dallas, Texas 75246. Manuscript received April 8, 1999, and accepted April 13.

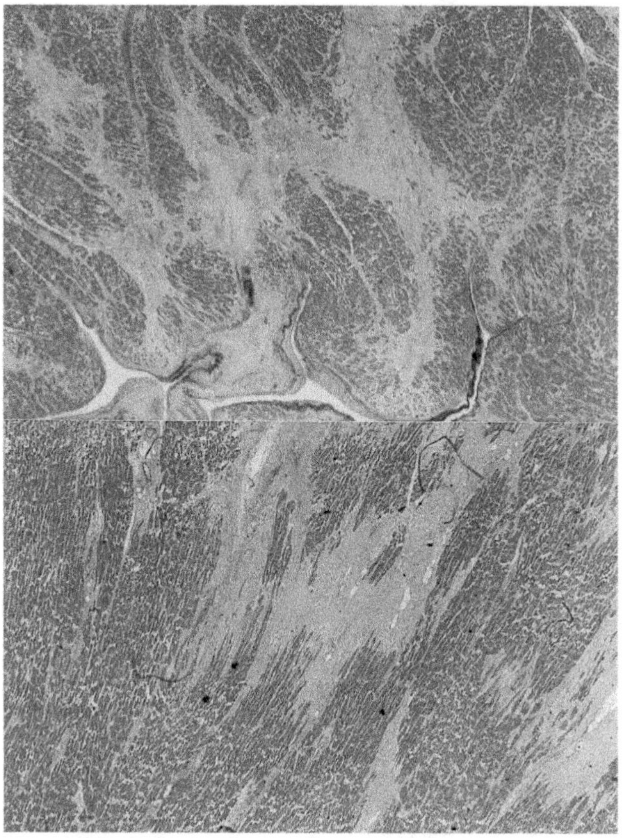

FIGURE 2. Photomicrographs of scars in the left ventricular free wall in the patient described. *Upper view* also shows endocardium; *lower view* is in the more midportion of the left ventricular wall. Each magnified × 12.5; Movat stains.

died in a motor vehicle accident on 7 August 1998 (261 days after TLR).

At autopsy, the heart weighed 570 g. The left ventricular wall at the apex was transmurally scarred. The left ventricular free wall in its basal half contained numerous focal scars, usually larger in the epicardial half than in the endocardial half (Figure 1). Many of these scars were roughly perpendicular to the epicardial surface. No vascular channels were visible grossly within the scars or in the adjacent normal-appearing myocardium. The ventricular septum contained few scars, and those present were small. Other than a few small blood vessels, no vascular channels were observed histologically in the focal scars or in adjacent scars (Figure 2).

• • •

The hitherto described findings at necropsy in an asymptomatic patient who died from a noncardiac condition nearly 9 months after TLR suggest that the left ventricular vascular channels created at operation completely close and are replaced by dense scar tissue containing few blood vessels. In the patient described, no vascular channels were seen in the left ventricular wall connecting it to the left ventricular cavity.

At least 5 patients having TLR >30 days before autopsy have been reported[1–5] (Table I). Vascular channels were reported in the first patient having TLR,[1] but more recent reports have shown few or no left ventricular myocardial channels. The earlier reports showed vascular channels by relatively high-power photomicrographs but without supporting gross photographs of the left ventricular wall.

Despite the lack of left ventricular myocardial channels in our patient, he was asymptomatic after recovering from the TLR operation. Preoperatively, he had had severe angina pectoris. Thus, the procedure either decreases myocardial ischemia by a mechanism other than by producing left ventricular myocardial wall channels or there is a major placebo effect of TLR.

1. Mirhoseini M, Shelgikar S, Cayton M. Clinical and histologic evaluation of laser myocardial revascularization. *J Clin Laser Med Surg* 1990;8:73–77.
2. Cooley DA, Frazier OH, Kadipasaoglu KA, Pahlivanoglu S, Shannon RL, Angelini P. Transmyocardial laser revascularization anatomic evidence of long-term channel patency. *Tex Heart Inst J* 1994; 21:220–224.
3. Burkhoff D, Fisher PE, Apfelbaum M, Kohmoto T, DeRosa CM, Smith CR. Histologic appearance of transmyocardial laser channels after 4½ weeks. *Ann Thorac Surg* 1996;61:1532–1535.
4. Gassler N, Wintzer HO, Stubbe HM, Wullbrand A, Helmchen U. Transmyocardial laser revascularization Histologic features in human nonresponder myocardium. *Circulation* 1997;95:371–375.
5. Frazier OH, Kadipasaoglu KA, Radovancevic B, Cihan HB, March RJ, Mirhoseini M, Cooley DA. Transmyocardial laser revascularization in allograft coronary artery disease. *Ann Thorac Surg* 1998;65: 1138–1141.

Thrombotic occlusion of the aortic ostia of saphenous venous grafts early after coronary artery bypass grafting by using the Symmetry aortic connector system

Alan S. Donsky, MD,[a,d] Jeffrey M. Schussler, MD,[a,d] Michael S. Donsky, MD,[a,d] William C. Roberts, MD,[b,d] and Baron L. Hamman, MD,[c,d] Dallas, Tex

St Jude Medical (St Paul, Minn) received Food and Drug Administration approval in May 2001 for a device to aid in the anastomosis of vein grafts to the aorta during coronary artery bypass grafting. This device, known as the Symmetry aortic connector system, allows the surgeon to connect a vein graft to the aorta without the use of sutures or an aortic clamp. To our knowledge, no reports have appeared describing complications from the use of this device. In this report we describe 2 patients who had complete thrombotic occlusions of the aortic ostia of saphenous venous grafts early postoperatively after the use of this device.

Clinical Summaries

PATIENT 1. A 66-year-old obese (body mass index, 45 kg/m^2) woman with type 2 diabetes mellitus, systemic hypertension, abdominal aortic aneurysm resection 4 years earlier, and heparin-induced thrombocytopenia was admitted for unstable angina pectoris. Coronary angiography disclosed that the left circumflex artery arose from the right sinus of Valsava and coursed in a retroaortic position to the left atrioventricular sulcus and distally was small and diffusely narrowed. The left anterior descending coronary artery was totally occluded in its midportion, and the right coronary artery was narrowed up to 75% in diameter. Left ventricular angiography disclosed normal systolic function with an estimated ejection fraction of 70%.

Off-pump coronary artery bypass grafting was performed through a left thoracotomy. Two saphenous venous grafts were attached to the ascending aorta by using the Symmetry system. One graft was anastomosed to the posterior descending branch of the right coronary artery, and the other graft was anastomosed to an obtuse marginal branch of the left circumflex coronary artery. The left internal thoracic artery (LITA) was anastomosed to the left anterior descending artery, but poor blood flow was noted through it, and a proximal obstruction of the LITA was assumed to be present. As a consequence, the LITA was severed, and the remaining 3-cm end was anastomosed to the vein graft supplying the obtuse marginal coronary artery, creating a Y-type composite graft. Lepirudin, instead of heparin, was used during the procedure because circulating heparin-associated antibodies were present.

The patient was extubated on the first postoperative day and transferred to the telemetry floor on aspirin and furosemide. Her recovery was complicated by persistent hypoxemia and increasing oxygen requirements despite rigorous diuresis. On postoperative day 7, severe hypoxemia and bradycardia occurred, followed by asystole; appropriate resuscitation efforts were unsuccessful.

Necropsy disclosed thrombi completely filling the ostia of both vein grafts at their anastomosis with the ascending aorta (Figure 1). The lumen of the vein graft to the posterior descending artery was otherwise widely patent. The LITA and the vein graft to the obtuse marginal artery were completely filled with thrombus. The left ventricular cavity was of normal size, and the heart weighed 515 g. A small area of necrosis (acute myocardial infarction) was seen in the myocardium adjacent to the anastomotic site of the vein graft to the obtuse marginal coronary artery.

From the Departments of Internal Medicine (Division of Cardiology),[a] Pathology,[b] and Cardiothoracic Surgery[c] and the Heart and Vascular Institute,[d] Baylor University Medical Center, Dallas, Tex.

Received for publication Jan 22, 2002; accepted for publication Feb 16, 2002.

Address for reprints: Baron L. Hamman, MD, Baylor University Medical Center, Division of Cardiothoracic Surgery, 3500 Gaston Ave, Dallas, TX 75246 (E-mail: Bhamman@CDM.net).

J Thorac Cardiovasc Surg 2002;124:397-9

0022-5223/2002 $35.00+0 **12/54/124236**

doi:10.1067/mtc.2002.124236

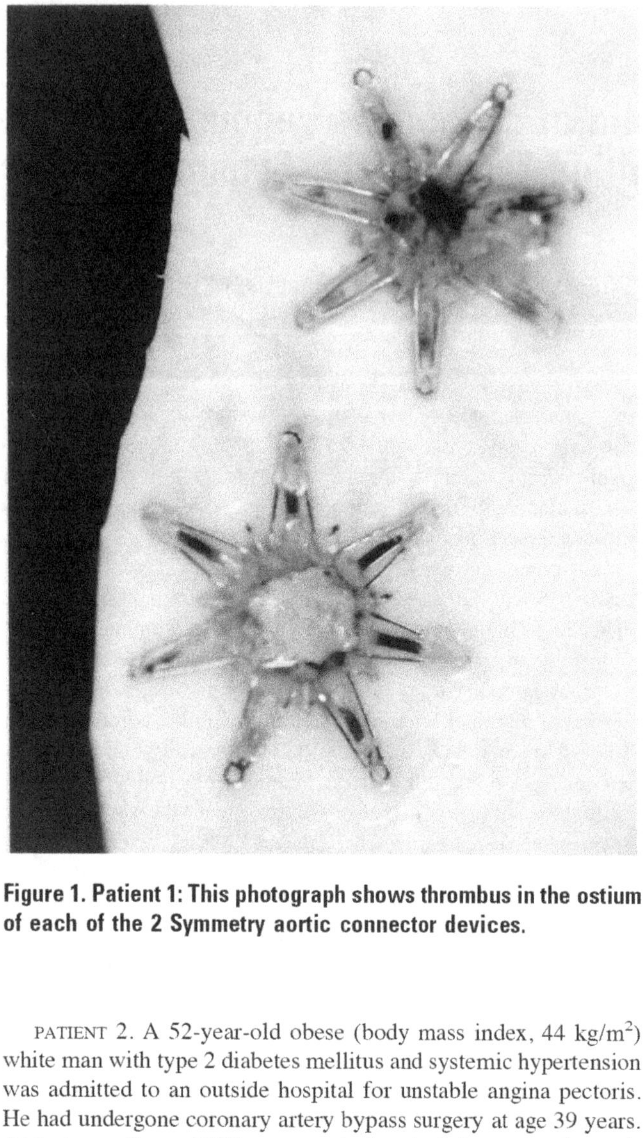

Figure 1. Patient 1: This photograph shows thrombus in the ostium of each of the 2 Symmetry aortic connector devices.

PATIENT 2. A 52-year-old obese (body mass index, 44 kg/m^2) white man with type 2 diabetes mellitus and systemic hypertension was admitted to an outside hospital for unstable angina pectoris. He had undergone coronary artery bypass surgery at age 39 years. At that operation, a LITA was attached to the left anterior descending coronary artery, and 2 saphenous venous grafts were attached to the obtuse marginal and right coronary arteries, respectively. He was transferred to Baylor University Medical Center on clopidogrel and enoxaparin. Coronary angiography showed complete occlusion of the vein graft to the obtuse marginal. The other 2 conduits were widely patent. The left main coronary artery was narrowed to 70% in diameter, and the proximal portion of the left circumflex was narrowed up to 95% in diameter. The ejection fraction by left ventricular angiography was estimated to be 30%.

Off-pump coronary artery bypass surgery through a left thoracotomy was performed. The Symmetry system was used in the anastomosis of a saphenous venous graft to the descending aorta, and it was then anastomosed to the obtuse marginal coronary artery. He was transferred to the telemetry floor on aspirin, metoprolol, and furosemide. On postoperative day 4, he had recurrent chest pain that was unresponsive to nitrates. An electrocardiogram now showed new T-wave inversions in the lateral precordial leads, and the troponin level was increased (1.9 ng/mL). Coronary angiography showed that contrast material injected into the left main coronary artery filled the distal end of the vein graft through the obtuse marginal coronary artery. However, contrast material injected into the descending aorta demonstrated total occlusion of the new vein graft at its ostium (Figure 2). Balloon angioplasty and stent placement was performed to the left main artery and the proximal portion of the circumflex artery with excellent angiographic results. The patient had no recurrence of chest pain and was discharged 2 days later.

Discussion

The Symmetry aortic connector system is a nitinol metallic device that functions somewhat like a grommet to attach a saphenous vein to a punched out portion of the aorta. This anastomosis is performed without sutures or an aortic clamp. This system has several potential advantages over the traditional suturing method. First, the time required to perform the anastomosis is reduced, and that might shorten recovery time. Second, minimizing aortic manipulation might reduce the risk of embolic events and thus reduce the incidence of neurologic complications. Finally, the size of the incision might be reduced because only limited exposure is needed to safely and consistently deploy the connector. Eckstein and associates[1] reported on their initial experience with this device in 20 patients undergoing off-pump coronary artery bypass surgery. They had excellent results, with no patient having any cardiac-related event within 3 months.

Each of the 2 patients described herein had thrombotic occlusion of the aortic ostia of saphenous venous grafts early after bypass surgery with the Symmetry aortic connector system. Such an occurrence in the early postoperative period with standard suture techniques is exceedingly uncommon. One of us (B.L.H.) has used this device in many patients, and the 2 described herein were the first encountered with known thrombotic complications at the aortic anastomotic sites.

Before concluding that the thrombotic complications were the direct result of one or more defects in the Symmetry system, several factors must be considered. Patient 1 had a history of heparin-induced thrombocytopenia with circulating antibodies, a circumstance recognized to be associated with a prothrombotic state. The saphenous venous graft attached to the left obtuse marginal coronary artery in the patient was totally occluded by thrombus, as was the LITA attached to it. The saphenous venous graft to the posterior descending artery, in contrast, was widely patent, except at its ostium. Patient 2 had the aortic anastomosis performed in the descending thoracic aorta. Both patients were extremely obese (grade 3/3) and had diabetes mellitus and systemic hypertension, features characteristic of the metabolic syndrome (insulin resistance syndrome), a condition recognized to be a prothrombotic state.[2,3] Whether these complicating factors played a role in the thrombotic occlusions of the aortic ostia in these 2 patients is, of course, unclear.

It is possible that the acute thrombosis seen in these 2 patients is similar in pathophysiology to that seen in acute stent thrombosis. The early experience with coronary artery stenting showed that acute thrombosis was a significant limiting factor. Improvements in stent design, deployment techniques, and the use of antiplatelet agents (ticlopidine and clopidogrel) dramatically reduced the incidence of acute stent thrombosis to less than 1%.[4] Although the use of clopidogrel is standard therapy after coronary artery stent-

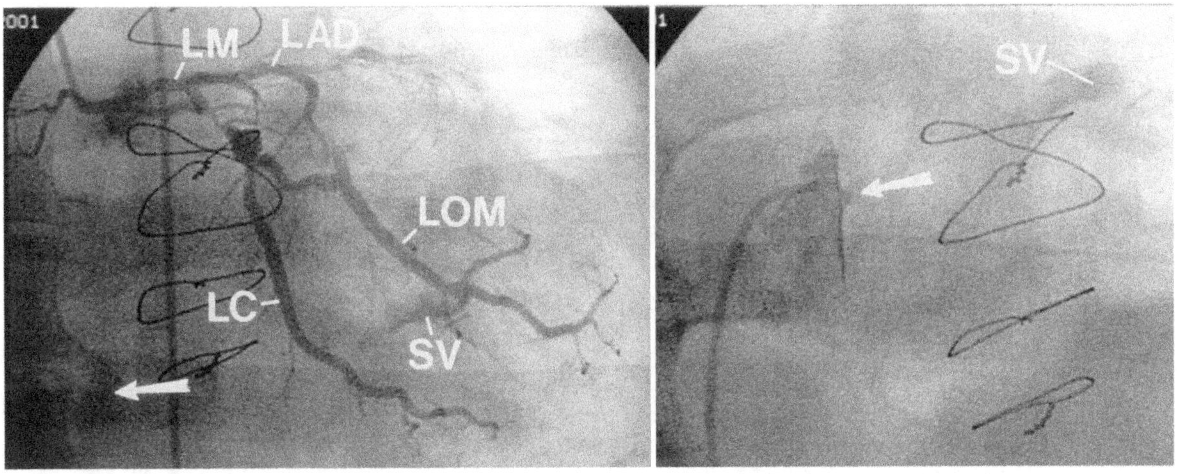

Figure 2. Patient 2: Coronary angiogram. *Left,* This photograph was taken after injection of contrast material into the left main *(LM)* coronary artery. The distal end of the saphenous venous graft *(SV)* fills through the left obtuse marginal *(LOM)*. *LAD,* Left anterior descending artery; *LC,* left circumflex. *Right,* This photograph was taken after injection of contrast material into the descending aorta at the sight of the saphenous venous conduit *(arrow)*. The ostium of the conduit is occluded. The upper right portion shows residual contrast material in the saphenous venous graft, which remained after the injection into the left main coronary artery.

ing, its use after placement of the Symmetry device has not been carefully studied.

In summary, 2 patients are described who underwent off-pump coronary artery bypass grafting with the Symmetry aortic connector system for the aortic anastomosis. Necropsy in one patient showed that the ostia of both aortic anastomotic sites were occluded by thrombus. In the second patient the aortic anastomotic site (in descending thoracic aorta) was demonstrated by angiography to be occluded. Although both patients had conditions predisposing to thrombus, such thrombotic occlusion of the aortic anastomotic sites are exceedingly rare in patients with an aortic anastomosis inserted by means of suture.

References

1. Eckstein FS, Bonilla LF, Strauffer E, Berg TA, Schmidli J, Carrel TP. Minimizing aortic manipulation during OPCAB using the Symmetry aortic connector system for proximal vein graft anastomosis. *Ann Thorac Surg*. 2001;72:S995-8.
2. Grundy SM. Hypertriglyceridemia, atherogenic dyslipidemia, and the metabolic syndrome. *Am J Cardiol*. 1998;81:18B-25B.
3. Juhan-Vague I, Alessi MC, Vague P. Increased plasma plasminogen activator inhibitor 1 levels: a possible link between insulin resistance and atherothrombosis. *Diabetologia*. 1991;34:457-62.
4. Schog A, Neumann FJ, Kastrati A, Schuhlen H, Blasini R, Hadamitzky M, et al. A randomized comparison of antiplatelet and anticoagulant therapy after the placement of coronary-artery stents. *N Engl J Med*. 1996;334:1084-9.

www.ingramcontent.com/pod-product-compliance
Lightning Source LLC
LaVergne TN
LVHW062148200926
848484LV00007B/1882
9798886800784